The Complete Nutrition and Diet Guide for POTS, EDS and MCAS

Evidence-Based Meal Plans, Recipes & Dietary Strategies for Dysautonomia, Ehlers-Danlos Syndrome & Mast Cell Activation Syndrome

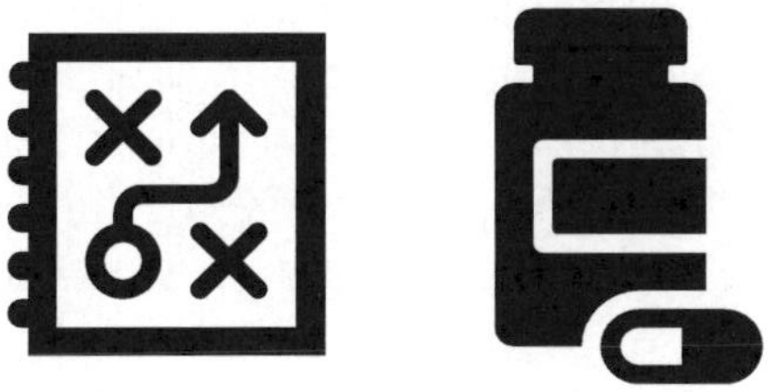

Sabia Roberta Sutton

This book is intended for educational and informational purposes only and does not constitute medical advice, diagnosis, or treatment. The dietary strategies, recipes, food lists, supplement discussions, and clinical information presented in this book are drawn from published research and established nutritional science and are not intended to replace the guidance of qualified healthcare professionals. Readers should consult their physicians, registered dietitians, and other members of their medical team before making any changes to their diet, supplement regimen, or medication schedule, particularly those managing postural orthostatic tachycardia syndrome, Ehlers-Danlos syndrome, mast cell activation syndrome, or any other medical condition.

The author and publisher disclaim any liability, loss, or risk incurred as a consequence, directly or indirectly, of the use or application of any content in this book. Individual results will vary based on medical history, condition subtype, medication interactions, food sensitivities, and other clinical factors that no book can fully account for. All sodium targets, elimination protocols, and supplement considerations should be verified with a prescribing provider before implementation.

All case studies, clinical scenarios, and patient examples presented in this book are composites created for educational illustration. They do not represent any specific individual, living or deceased, and any resemblance to actual persons is entirely coincidental. Names, ages, locations, and identifying details used in case studies and scenarios are fictional. No endorsement of any product, brand, supplement manufacturer, or pharmaceutical company is intended or implied. Mention of specific products or brands is for informational context only. The author has no financial relationship with any company or product referenced in this text.

First Edition:2026

ISBN: 978-1-7645291-1-2

Table of Contents

Preface

The idea for this book began with a spreadsheet, not a manuscript.

A woman I will call Diane had been diagnosed with postural orthostatic tachycardia syndrome by her cardiologist, hypermobile Ehlers-Danlos syndrome by her geneticist, and probable mast cell activation syndrome by her allergist. Each specialist had given her dietary instructions. The cardiologist prescribed 8 to 10 grams of sodium daily and told her to drink three liters of fluid. The allergist handed her a low-histamine food list and told her to eliminate aged cheeses, fermented foods, cured meats, and anything that had been sitting in the refrigerator for more than twenty-four hours. The geneticist suggested she increase her intake of vitamin C, zinc, and foods that support collagen production.

Diane went home and tried to follow all three instructions at once. Within a week she realized she had a problem. Several of the high-sodium foods she relied on, such as sauerkraut, soy sauce, and cured deli meats, were on the allergist's list of high-histamine foods to avoid. Some of the collagen-supporting foods the geneticist recommended were also histamine liberators. The low-histamine recipes she found online were uniformly bland and contained almost no sodium, which left her lightheaded and tachycardic by mid-afternoon. She could follow one set of instructions or another, but following all three at the same time felt impossible.

So she built a spreadsheet. She cross-referenced every food across all three dietary sheets, color-coding items that were safe for all three conditions versus those that conflicted. She tracked her sodium intake alongside her histamine reactions. She modified recipes one ingredient at a time, testing substitutions and recording what triggered symptoms and what did not. Over several months, she developed a personal food system that addressed POTS, EDS, and MCAS simultaneously.

That spreadsheet, multiplied by the published clinical evidence, is the foundation of the book you are holding.

The medical literature on nutrition for each of these three conditions has grown substantially over the past decade. Researchers have documented the role of sodium and fluid loading in POTS management. Studies have mapped the histamine content of foods, the behavior of the diamine oxidase enzyme, and the dietary triggers of mast cell degranulation. Nutritional science has identified the specific micronutrients required for collagen synthesis and the gastrointestinal manifestations of connective tissue disorders that shape how and what EDS patients can eat. What the literature has not produced, until now, is a single resource that integrates all three bodies of evidence into one unified dietary framework.

That gap has real consequences. Patients managing the trifecta, the clinical cluster of POTS, EDS, and MCAS, receive fragmented dietary advice from multiple providers who are each expert in their own domain but rarely in communication with each other. The cardiologist does not check with the allergist before recommending sodium-rich foods. The allergist does not ask the geneticist which nutrients the patient needs for connective tissue support. The patient is left to reconcile these competing instructions alone, usually through trial and error, often at the cost of symptom flares that could have been prevented.

This book was written to close that gap.

Every chapter in this book approaches nutrition from all three conditions simultaneously. The recipes were developed to be low-histamine, high-sodium, anti-inflammatory, collagen-supportive, and gastroparesis-accommodating by default, not as modifications or afterthoughts but as baseline design criteria. The elimination and reintroduction protocol accounts for mast cell reactivity while preserving the sodium and fluid intake that POTS management requires. The supplement chapter evaluates each supplement through the lens of all three conditions, flagging interactions and evidence quality for each.

The clinical science in this book is drawn from peer-reviewed research, and every recommendation includes the physiological reasoning behind it. Understanding the why behind a dietary recommendation matters. When you know that histamine accumulates in food as a function of bacterial activity over time, you can make informed decisions about freshness and storage that no food list can fully capture. When you understand how sodium affects plasma volume and venous return in POTS, you can adapt your intake to the demands of a particular day rather than following a rigid number. When you know which micronutrients feed the collagen synthesis pathway and which ones compete for absorption, you can time your meals and supplements for maximum effect.

But clinical science alone does not feed a person. The second half of this book is relentlessly practical. Recipes include sodium content per serving, histamine risk classification, and modification options. Meal plans adapt to flare days, stable days, and the energy constraints that come with managing chronic illness. The appendices are designed to be photocopied, posted on the refrigerator, and brought to medical appointments. The food and symptom journal template turns subjective experience into data that your healthcare team can act on.

This book does not replace your doctors. It does not diagnose, prescribe, or treat. What it does is give you and your medical team a shared framework, an evidence-based starting point that saves everyone the weeks or months of trial and error that most trifecta patients currently endure. The dietary strategies in these pages should be discussed with your treating physicians and adapted to your individual clinical picture. The most effective use of this book is collaborative: you bring the lived experience, your providers bring the clinical judgment, and this book brings the nutritional evidence that connects the two.

The pages that follow were written with one guiding principle. A person managing POTS, EDS, and MCAS should not have to choose between their conditions at every meal. They should be able to open one book, find one framework, and eat one dinner that serves all three.

That is what this book delivers.

PART ONE: THE SCIENCE OF THE TRIFECTA

Introduction

What This Book Is

A 38-year-old woman sits in her fourth specialist's office in six months. She has a POTS diagnosis from her cardiologist, an hEDS diagnosis from her geneticist, and a probable MCAS diagnosis from her allergist. Each specialist handed her a dietary sheet. The cardiologist's sheet says to increase sodium. The allergist's sheet says to eliminate histamine. The geneticist mentioned something about collagen-supporting nutrients. None of the three sheets reference each other. Two of them contradict each other on specific foods. She is holding all three, staring at them, trying to figure out what she's actually supposed to eat for dinner tonight.

That scenario plays out in waiting rooms and kitchens every day, and it is the reason this book was written. It is a practical companion for people managing one, two, or all three of the conditions that frequently travel together: **postural orthostatic tachycardia syndrome (POTS)**, **Ehlers-Danlos syndrome (EDS)**, and **mast cell activation syndrome (MCAS)**. These three conditions, increasingly recognized as a clinical cluster (Cheung & Vadas, 2015; Seneviratne et al., 2017), create dietary demands that overlap, compete, and sometimes conflict. Managing them through food requires a framework that accounts for all three simultaneously, not three separate handouts taped to the refrigerator.

This book provides that framework. It translates the clinical evidence on nutrition for each condition into a unified dietary strategy, complete with recipes, meal plans, food lists, tracking templates, and the physiological reasoning behind every recommendation. It explains not just *what* to eat but *why* specific foods affect specific symptoms through specific mechanisms.

What This Book Is Not

This book does not replace your medical team. It does not diagnose conditions, prescribe treatments, or recommend medication changes. The dietary strategies presented here are drawn from published research, clinical guidelines, and established nutritional science, but they are educational tools, not medical prescriptions. Every recommendation in this book should be discussed with your treating physicians, particularly your prescribing provider, your gastroenterologist if you have one, and ideally a registered dietitian familiar with these conditions.

The reason for this boundary is simple. POTS, EDS, and MCAS each present differently across individuals. Your specific subtype, your medication regimen, your comorbidities, your food sensitivities, and your nutritional status create a clinical picture that no book can fully account for. What this book can do is give you and your healthcare team a shared language, a structured approach, and evidence-based starting points that save everyone time and frustration.

If you are currently under the care of a physician for any of these conditions, bring this book to your next appointment. Show them the dietary framework. Ask if the sodium targets, the elimination protocol, and the supplement considerations apply to your specific situation. The most effective use of this book is as a bridge between the clinical guidance your doctors provide and the practical reality of what goes on your plate.

Working with Your Healthcare Team

The dietary framework in this book was built to complement standard medical treatment for each trifecta condition. The chapters on sodium and fluid loading (Chapter 5.0) support the pharmacological management of POTS. The histamine elimination and reintroduction protocol (Chapters 6.0 and 7.0) works alongside mast cell stabilizers and antihistamines. The connective tissue nutrition strategies (Chapter 4.0) supplement the physical therapy and joint protection strategies used in EDS management.

To get the most from this book alongside your medical care:

- Share the daily sodium targets from Chapter 5.0 with your cardiologist or POTS specialist, particularly if you are on fludrocortisone or midodrine, since dietary sodium interacts with these medications (as discussed in section 23.3).
- Discuss the elimination diet protocol from Chapter 6.0 with your allergist or immunologist before starting, especially if you are already on cromolyn sodium or ketotifen. The medication timing guidance in Chapter 23.0 explains why this coordination matters.
- If you take a proton pump inhibitor, review section 23.5 with your gastroenterologist. Long-term PPI use affects the absorption of several nutrients that are already at risk in trifecta patients.
- Bring your food and symptom journal (Chapter 12.0, template in Appendix B) to specialist appointments. Tracked data communicates more useful information than verbal recall, and gives your provider concrete patterns to evaluate.
- If you are considering any supplement from Chapter 22.0, discuss it with your prescribing physician before starting. Some supplements interact with medications commonly used in trifecta management.

How to Read This Book

Not every reader needs every chapter in order. The book is structured so that foundational science comes first (Chapters 1.0 through 5.0), followed by the dietary framework (Chapters 6.0 through 12.0), then recipes and practical application (Chapters 13.0 through 21.0), and finally supplementary guidance (Chapters 22.0 through 24.0). But depending on which condition is your primary concern, different chapters will carry different weight.

If POTS is your primary condition, start with Chapter 5.0 (Sodium and Fluid Strategies). This chapter establishes the foundation that every other dietary recommendation builds on for POTS management. From there, read Chapter 3.0 (Digestive Dysfunction) for the gastroparesis and motility considerations that affect how POTS patients can practically consume the volumes of sodium and fluid they need. Then move to Chapter 13.0 (Meal Planning Foundations) and Chapter 20.0 (Beverages and Electrolytes) for the practical application. The exercise and nutrition timing guidance in section 24.1 is particularly relevant if you are following a reconditioning protocol like the Dallas or CHOP Protocol.

If MCAS is your primary condition, start with Chapter 6.0 (The Elimination Framework) and Chapter 7.0 (Strategic Reintroduction). These two chapters form the core dietary intervention for mast cell activation. Read Chapter 4.0 (Histamine and Food Chemistry) first if you want to understand the science behind the elimination protocol, specifically how histamine accumulates in food, which foods are histamine liberators versus high-histamine content, and how the diamine oxidase enzyme works. Chapter 22.0 (Supplements and Evidence) covers quercetin, vitamin C, and DAO supplements with the research behind each. The hormonal effects on mast cell reactivity in section 24.3 are essential reading for menstruating patients.

If EDS is your primary condition, start with Chapter 4.0 (Nutrition and the Trifecta) for the collagen synthesis pathway and the specific micronutrients required to support connective tissue. Chapter 3.0 covers the GI manifestations of EDS (gastroparesis, visceroptosis, and motility disorders) that shape how and what you can eat. Chapter 22.0 addresses the collagen supplement question directly, including what the evidence actually shows for EDS versus the general population.

If you have all three conditions (the full trifecta), read the book in order. The chapters are sequenced to build understanding progressively, and the dietary framework in Chapters 6.0 through 12.0 integrates all three conditions simultaneously. The recipes in Chapters 13.0 through 21.0 were developed to be trifecta-compatible by default (low-histamine, high-sodium, anti-inflammatory, gastroparesis-accommodating), so they apply to the full clinical picture without requiring modification for individual conditions.

If you are a healthcare provider (physician, dietitian, nurse practitioner, physical therapist), Chapters 1.0 through 5.0 provide the clinical and scientific rationale for the dietary framework. Chapter 23.0 (Diet and Medication Interactions) and Chapter 22.0 (Supplements and Evidence) contain the pharmacological and evidence-based information most relevant to clinical decision-making. The appendices provide reproducible tools you can share with patients.

A Note on the Structure

Each chapter in this book follows a consistent format designed for both sequential reading and quick reference. Chapters open with a real scenario drawn from the clinical patterns common to trifecta patients, followed by the relevant science, practical applications, case studies showing the concepts in action, and a reference list documenting the evidence base. Subheadings are numbered (for example, section 5.3 or section 12.4) so that cross-references between chapters point you to specific locations rather than vague "as discussed earlier" directions.

The recipes in Chapters 13.0 through 21.0 include sodium content per serving, histamine risk classification, prep time, FODMAP notes where relevant, and modification options for gastroparesis. The appendices consolidate the food lists, tracking templates, and resource directories into photocopiable reference pages that can be posted on the refrigerator, kept in a purse, or brought to a medical appointment.

This book was written to be used. The pages should get stained. The appendices should get photocopied until they're dog-eared. The food journal template should be filled in, reviewed, brought to your doctor, and then filled in again. The recipes should be tried, modified, annotated with notes about what worked and what didn't, and shared with the people who cook for you. The best outcome this book can produce is not that you read it, but that you eat differently because of it, and that eating differently changes how you feel.

Chapter 1.0: The Trifecta Explained

Imagine waking up one morning and the simple act of standing to brush your teeth sends your heart racing to 140 beats per minute. Your vision grays at the edges. Your skin erupts in hives from seemingly nothing. Your joints ache, your stomach rebels against breakfast, and the brain fog is so thick you cannot remember if you took your morning medications. Now imagine explaining all of this to a doctor who looks at you with skepticism because each symptom, taken in isolation, seems unremarkable. For millions of people living with the intersection of Postural Orthostatic Tachycardia Syndrome, Ehlers-Danlos Syndrome, and Mast Cell Activation Syndrome, this is not a hypothetical scenario. This is Tuesday.

This chapter lays the groundwork for understanding each of these three conditions individually, the biological mechanisms connecting them, the post-COVID surge that has expanded this patient population dramatically, and the reasons why nutrition stands as the recommended first line of management before medications are even considered.

1.1 Understanding POTS

Postural Orthostatic Tachycardia Syndrome, commonly abbreviated as **POTS**, is a form of **dysautonomia**, a dysfunction of the autonomic nervous system that controls involuntary body processes such as heart rate, blood pressure, digestion, and temperature regulation (Sheldon et al., 2015). The hallmark diagnostic criterion is an increase in heart rate of 30 or more beats per minute in adults (or 40 or more in adolescents) within 10 minutes of standing, without a corresponding drop in blood pressure that would indicate classic orthostatic hypotension (Vernino et al., 2021). Between one and three million Americans are estimated to live with POTS, and that number has grown substantially since the COVID-19 pandemic (Bryarly et al., 2019).

But POTS is not a single, uniform condition. Understanding the subtypes is critical because each responds differently to dietary and lifestyle interventions.

Neuropathic POTS is the most common subtype and results from damage to small nerve fibers, particularly in the legs and feet. These damaged nerves fail to signal blood vessels to constrict when a person stands, allowing blood to pool in the lower body. The result is reduced blood return to the heart, prompting a compensatory spike in heart rate (Raj, 2013). Dietary intervention for neuropathic POTS centers on increasing blood volume through high sodium and fluid intake, because more circulating volume partially compensates for the pooling problem.

Hypovolemic POTS involves abnormally low blood volume, sometimes up to 13% below normal levels. Patients with this subtype may have dysregulated renin-angiotensin-aldosterone system activity, meaning their kidneys excrete too much sodium and water (Raj, 2013). For these patients, aggressive sodium and fluid loading is particularly effective because the intervention directly addresses the root cause of their symptoms.

Hyperadrenergic POTS is characterized by elevated levels of norepinephrine upon standing, often exceeding 600 pg/mL. These patients frequently experience tremor, anxiety, and significant blood pressure fluctuations in addition to tachycardia (Grubb, 2008). And here is where dietary management becomes nuanced. While most POTS patients benefit from high sodium intake, hyperadrenergic patients may actually worsen with excessive salt because their systems are already in a state of sympathetic overdrive. Dietary strategies for this subtype emphasize stable blood sugar, avoidance of stimulants, and careful, individualized sodium dosing rather than the blanket recommendation of 10 grams per day.

The distinction between subtypes matters enormously for nutrition planning. A strategy that stabilizes one patient may destabilize another. This is precisely why the standard advice of "just eat more salt" falls short.

1.2 Understanding EDS

Ehlers-Danlos Syndrome refers to a group of 13 heritable connective tissue disorders affecting the skin, joints, blood vessels, and gastrointestinal tract (Malfait et al., 2017). The type most frequently associated with the trifecta is **hypermobile EDS (hEDS)** and the related **Hypermobility Spectrum Disorder (HSD)**, both characterized by generalized joint hypermobility, chronic pain, skin hyperextensibility, and a broad range of systemic complications.

Connective tissue is the structural scaffolding of the body. It forms the walls of blood vessels, the lining of the gastrointestinal tract, the ligaments stabilizing joints, and the matrix supporting organs. When the genetic instructions for building this tissue contain errors, the consequences ripple through virtually every system (Tinkle et al., 2017).

For nutritional purposes, the gastrointestinal impact of EDS demands the most attention. Research demonstrates that approximately 85 to 90 percent of people with hEDS experience gastrointestinal symptoms (Fikree et al., 2017). These are not minor inconveniences. A large case-control study found that patients with EDS had 12.26 times higher odds of a concurrent gastroparesis diagnosis compared to patients without EDS (Tai et al., 2020). Gastroesophageal reflux disease, irritable bowel syndrome, functional constipation, and dysmotility are all reported at elevated rates (Thwaites et al., 2022). The structural changes in collagen within the smooth muscle of the GI tract create anatomical vulnerabilities including diverticulosis, prolapse, and rectal abnormalities (Steiner et al., 2023).

These GI complications create a cascade of nutritional problems. When eating causes pain, nausea, or bloating, patients eat less. When the gut moves food too slowly or too quickly, nutrient absorption suffers. When restricted diets eliminate entire food groups in an attempt to control symptoms, micronutrient deficiencies develop. A 2024 cross-sectional study published in The American Journal of Gastroenterology found that 62.1% of hEDS/HSD patients had altered their diet in the previous year, 62.3% regularly skipped meals, and 25.3% required some form of nutritional support (Topan et al., 2024).

Understanding EDS as a connective tissue disorder rather than "just" a joint condition reframes the entire approach to nutrition. The goal is not simply to avoid foods that cause discomfort. The goal is to provide adequate building blocks for compromised tissue while navigating a digestive system that often works against you.

1.3 Understanding MCAS

Mast Cell Activation Syndrome is a condition in which mast cells, a type of immune cell found throughout the body, become inappropriately activated and release excessive amounts of chemical mediators (Afrin et al., 2017). Most people associate mast cells primarily with **histamine**, and histamine is indeed one of the most well-known mediators responsible for symptoms like flushing, itching, hives, and GI distress. But mast cells release over 1,000 different mediators, including **tryptase**, **prostaglandins**, **leukotrienes**, and **cytokines**, each capable of triggering distinct sets of symptoms across multiple body systems (Theoharides et al., 2019).

This distinction matters for dietary management. A person with MCAS might not react to dietary histamine at all if their symptoms are driven primarily by prostaglandin or leukotriene release. Conversely, a person whose mast cells are dumping large amounts of histamine may find dietary histamine reduction enormously helpful. The Mast Cell Action organization emphasizes that MCAS involves the abnormal release of various mediators, not just histamine, and that someone with MCAS may not necessarily react to dietary histamine depending on which mediators dominate their symptom picture (Mast Cell Action, 2024).

MCAS can produce symptoms in virtually any organ system. Skin reactions (flushing, hives, itching), GI symptoms (abdominal pain, diarrhea, nausea), cardiovascular symptoms (tachycardia, hypotension), respiratory symptoms (wheezing, nasal congestion), and neurological symptoms (brain fog, headache) are all common (Molderings et al., 2011). The triggers are equally varied and can include foods, temperature changes, stress, fragrances, chemicals, medications, and physical exertion.

A study examining food hypersensitivities among patients with mast cell disorders found that 20.6% of patients self-reported food reactions. However, only 3.4% of these reactions were confirmed by relevant IgE sensitization testing (Vlieg-Boerstra et al., 2005). This finding illustrates a point that separates MCAS-related food reactions from true food allergies. The reaction pathways are different, which means standard allergy testing often comes back negative even in patients who clearly react to certain foods.

For practical dietary management, the **low-histamine diet** is the most commonly recommended starting point for MCAS patients. This involves reducing intake of aged, fermented, and processed foods where histamine accumulates, prioritizing fresh foods prepared and consumed quickly, and being attentive to food storage and preparation methods (The Mast Cell Disease Society, 2022). But the low-histamine diet is a general guideline requiring individual experimentation, not a rigid prescription that should be followed identically by every patient.

1.4 Biological Connections

The trifecta is not three conditions randomly coexisting in the same body. There are plausible biological mechanisms linking them.

The connection between EDS and POTS begins with blood vessels. Blood vessel walls are made of connective tissue. In hEDS, these walls may be excessively compliant, stretching more easily than they should. When a person stands, gravity pulls blood downward. Normally, blood vessels constrict to push blood back toward the heart. In hEDS, the overly elastic vessels are less effective at this constriction, allowing blood to pool in the lower extremities. The heart compensates by beating faster. This is POTS (Gazit et al., 2003; Rowe et al., 1999).

The connection between EDS and MCAS involves the physical relationship between mast cells and connective tissue. Mast cells are embedded throughout connective tissue, residing in skin, gut lining, respiratory mucosa, and around blood vessels. When the connective tissue matrix is structurally abnormal, the mechanical environment around mast cells changes. A 2022 review documented higher rates of immune-mediated and allergic conditions in hEDS/HSD populations, suggesting that structural connective tissue abnormalities may contribute to immune dysregulation (Seneviratne et al., 2017).

The data support these connections quantitatively. A study by Chopra and colleagues found that the percentage of MCAS within a group of patients who had both POTS and EDS was 31%, compared to approximately 2% in patients without POTS and EDS. The odds ratio between the two groups was 32.46, a statistically striking result (Cheung & Vadas, 2015; as referenced in clinical literature by Chopra et al.).

1.5 Case Study: Recognizing the Trifecta

Background

Dorothea, a 28-year-old graphic designer, had been experiencing dizziness upon standing, chronic fatigue, and unexplained skin flushing since her early twenties. She was initially told she had anxiety and was prescribed an SSRI. Her symptoms worsened after a bout of influenza at age 26, and she began experiencing episodes of rapid heart rate, abdominal pain after meals, and hives that appeared and disappeared without obvious cause. Her joints had always been "flexible," and she frequently rolled her ankles during walks.

Presentation

During evaluation at a dysautonomia clinic, Dorothea's heart rate increased from 72 beats per minute supine to 118 beats per minute after eight minutes of standing. Her Beighton score was 7 out of 9, indicating generalized joint hypermobility. She reported avoiding multiple foods after noticing skin reactions and GI distress, and she had lost 12 pounds over six months without intending to. Blood work revealed low vitamin D and borderline low B12.

Analysis

Dorothea's presentation illustrates the classic trifecta pattern. The orthostatic tachycardia (POTS) likely relates to the vascular laxity associated with her joint hypermobility (hEDS). Her skin flushing, unexplained hives, and food-associated GI symptoms are consistent with mast cell activation. The dietary restriction driven by fear of reactions had created nutritional deficiencies, compounding her fatigue and orthostatic intolerance. Each condition was amplifying the others.

Intervention

Dorothea's care team, including a cardiologist familiar with POTS and a registered dietitian, initiated a structured approach. Fluid intake was increased to 2.5 liters daily with added electrolytes providing 5 grams of sodium. A guided low-histamine dietary framework was introduced while ensuring adequate caloric and protein intake. Vitamin D3 supplementation at 5,000 IU daily and B12 supplementation were started. Food reintroduction was planned after a four-week stabilization period.

Outcome

After eight weeks, Dorothea's standing heart rate increase had reduced to 24 beats per minute. Her skin flushing episodes decreased in frequency. She regained four of the 12 lost pounds. She reported that the structured dietary approach reduced her anxiety about eating because she had a framework for making safe choices rather than avoiding food out of fear.

Teaching Points

- The trifecta often presents as overlapping symptoms that are initially misattributed to anxiety or stress, delaying appropriate diagnosis and treatment
- Nutritional deficiencies caused by fear-driven dietary restriction can worsen the very symptoms the restriction was intended to manage
- Addressing hydration and sodium intake first can produce measurable improvement in POTS symptoms relatively quickly

1.6 The Long COVID Acceleration

The COVID-19 pandemic fundamentally altered the landscape of POTS and, by extension, the trifecta. A 2025 study analyzing electronic medical records from over 65 million U.S. patients found that the incidence rate of POTS increased from 1.42 per million person-years before COVID to 20.3 per million person-years after the pandemic began, representing a greater than fivefold increase (Dulal et al., 2025). Monthly new case diagnoses jumped from an estimated 4.21 per month to 22.66 per month.

Among patients with long COVID specifically, POTS is strikingly common. A 2025 prospective analysis of 467 highly symptomatic long COVID patients found that 31% met diagnostic criteria for POTS (Björnson et al., 2025). The LISTEN study at Yale reported that 28.9% of long COVID participants had new-onset POTS (Mouslmani et al., 2025). These patients were younger, predominantly female, and reported higher rates of mast cell disorders alongside their autonomic dysfunction.

What this means for nutrition is straightforward. Millions of people who had no prior experience with dysautonomia are now managing conditions that require specific dietary interventions. They are searching for guidance. And most standard nutritional advice, designed for the general population, not only fails to address their needs but may actively worsen their symptoms.

1.7 Nutrition as First Line Treatment

The 2015 Heart Rhythm Society Expert Consensus Statement on the Diagnosis and Treatment of Postural Tachycardia Syndrome explicitly recommends non-pharmacological interventions, including dietary modifications and fluid management, as the first line of treatment before medication is considered (Sheldon et al., 2015). The British Dietetic Association similarly states that a nutritional assessment should be offered to all patients with POTS, and that dietary changes and fluid adjustments should be trialed before pharmacological treatment (BDA, 2023). The Canadian Cardiovascular Society Position Statement recommends 10 grams of salt via high-salt foods, salt sticks, and tablets, along with at least 3 liters of oral fluids daily (Raj et al., 2020).

This consensus exists because dietary interventions address the physiological mechanisms underlying symptoms. Increased sodium and fluid intake expands blood volume, directly countering the hypovolemia that worsens orthostatic intolerance. Smaller, more frequent meals reduce postprandial blood pooling. Low-histamine dietary approaches can lower the total mediator burden on an overactive immune system. Adequate protein supports connective tissue integrity. Micronutrient repletion corrects deficiencies that impair autonomic function.

Nutrition is not a complementary therapy or an afterthought. For the trifecta population, it is the foundation upon which all other management strategies are built.

1.8 Case Study: Post COVID Onset

Background

Marius, a 35-year-old high school teacher and former recreational runner, contracted COVID-19 in early 2023. His acute illness was moderate, requiring no hospitalization. However, six weeks after his initial recovery, he began experiencing persistent tachycardia upon standing, crushing fatigue, brain fog that made lesson planning impossible, and episodes of abdominal cramping with diarrhea after eating.

Presentation

Marius's primary care physician initially attributed his symptoms to deconditioning and anxiety. After four months of worsening symptoms, he was referred to a cardiologist who performed a tilt table test revealing a heart rate increase of 42 beats per minute within seven minutes of upright positioning. He had no prior history of joint hypermobility or allergic symptoms. He reported that his diet had become increasingly restricted as he eliminated foods that seemed to trigger GI episodes, and that he was now eating primarily plain rice, chicken, and water.

Analysis

Marius represents the rapidly growing population of post-viral POTS patients. His case demonstrates how COVID-19 can trigger autonomic dysfunction in individuals with no predisposing connective tissue disorder. His self-directed dietary restriction, while understandable, had reduced his sodium intake to approximately 1.5 grams per day (well below the 3 to 10 grams recommended for POTS) and his caloric intake to roughly 1,200 calories, insufficient for a man of his size and activity level. The inadequate sodium was worsening his orthostatic symptoms, while the caloric deficit was compounding his fatigue.

Intervention

A registered dietitian specializing in dysautonomia restructured Marius's diet. Sodium intake was increased to 6 grams daily through salted foods, electrolyte drinks, and salt tablets. Fluid intake was raised to 3 liters. Meals were divided into five smaller eating occasions throughout the day. Foods were reintroduced systematically, one at a time, with a food and symptom diary to identify genuine triggers versus coincidental reactions.

Outcome

Within six weeks, Marius's resting-to-standing heart rate differential dropped to 26 beats per minute. He reported a 40% reduction in brain fog severity and was able to return to work part-time. His GI symptoms decreased substantially once he stopped eating primarily refined carbohydrates (which were actually worsening his POTS through postprandial blood pooling) and increased his protein, fat, and sodium intake.

Teaching Points

- Post-viral POTS can emerge in individuals with no prior history of the trifecta conditions, meaning new patients often have no established knowledge of dysautonomia-specific dietary needs

- Self-directed dietary restriction without guidance frequently leads to inadequate sodium and caloric intake, paradoxically worsening the very symptoms patients are trying to manage
- Simple nutritional interventions, particularly sodium loading and meal restructuring, can produce measurable autonomic improvement within weeks

1.9 Summary

POTS, EDS, and MCAS are distinct conditions with their own diagnostic criteria, pathophysiology, and symptom profiles. But they share biological connections rooted in connective tissue structure, autonomic nervous system regulation, and immune system activity. Understanding each condition individually provides the foundation for understanding why they co-occur and, more importantly, why dietary management must account for all three simultaneously.

The three POTS subtypes (neuropathic, hypovolemic, and hyperadrenergic) respond differently to sodium and fluid loading, making subtype identification relevant to nutritional planning. The GI dysfunction inherent to hEDS creates obstacles to nutrient intake and absorption that must be addressed proactively rather than ignored. MCAS introduces variable food sensitivities driven by mast cell mediator release that goes far beyond simple histamine, requiring individualized dietary assessment rather than a one-size-fits-all elimination diet.

The post-COVID expansion of the POTS population has made nutritional guidance for dysautonomia more urgently needed than at any point in the history of these conditions. And the expert consensus across multiple medical societies is unambiguous: dietary and lifestyle modifications come first. The chapters that follow will build on this foundation, moving from understanding toward practical application.

Chapter 2.0: The Dietary Paradox

Picture three specialists standing in front of a whiteboard, each writing dietary instructions for the same patient. The cardiologist writes: "Increase sodium to 10 grams per day. Drink 3 liters of fluid. Add electrolytes." The immunologist writes: "Avoid fermented foods. Eliminate aged cheeses, cured meats, and anything with vinegar. Keep all foods as fresh as possible." The gastroenterologist writes: "Eat small meals. Reduce fiber if gastroparesis is present. Consider low-FODMAP. Ensure adequate protein for bone density." Now step back and look at the whiteboard. Some of those instructions complement each other. Some directly contradict each other. And the patient standing in front of that whiteboard has to figure out what to eat for lunch.

This chapter examines the central nutritional conflict inherent to managing POTS, EDS, and MCAS simultaneously, explores why standard dietary advice fails this population, introduces the concept of the histamine bucket, and presents the Trifecta-Compatible dietary framework that guides the remainder of this book.

2.1 The Core Tension

Each condition in the trifecta makes specific nutritional demands, and those demands sometimes push in opposing directions.

POTS requires increased sodium intake, typically 3 to 10 grams per day according to expert consensus guidelines (Sheldon et al., 2015; Raj et al., 2020). This is two to four times the sodium recommended for the general population by the American Heart Association (AHA, 2024). POTS also demands 2 to 3 liters of fluid daily and benefits from blood volume expansion through both dietary sodium and adequate caloric intake. Many commonly recommended high-sodium foods, however, are processed items like canned soups, deli meats, and pickled vegetables, which happen to be among the highest histamine foods available.

MCAS management frequently involves a low-histamine dietary approach that restricts aged, fermented, cured, and long-stored foods (The Mast Cell Disease Society, 2022). Histamine accumulates in food through bacterial action over time, meaning that the very foods promoted for gut health in the general population (yogurt, kefir, sauerkraut, kombucha, aged cheeses) can be the worst triggers for someone with mast cell overactivation (Maintz & Novak, 2007). Additionally, MCAS patients may react to food additives, preservatives, and certain naturally occurring compounds like salicylates and oxalates, further narrowing the dietary window.

EDS creates GI dysfunction that limits what and how much a patient can physically tolerate eating. Gastroparesis (delayed stomach emptying) makes large meals painful and may require reduced fiber and fat. GERD demands avoiding acidic and spicy foods. IBS symptoms may necessitate a low-FODMAP approach. And underlying all of this is the need for adequate protein to support compromised connective tissue and sufficient micronutrients (particularly vitamin C, vitamin D, and B vitamins) to address common deficiencies (Steiner et al., 2023; Tseng et al., 2021).

The tension becomes concrete in everyday food decisions. Bone broth, for instance, is frequently recommended for POTS patients because it provides sodium, fluid, and minerals in a single serving. But traditional bone broth simmered for 12 to 24 hours is one of the highest histamine foods a person can consume, because prolonged cooking at warm temperatures creates ideal conditions for histamine-producing bacteria. A POTS patient with concurrent MCAS who follows the standard "drink more bone broth" advice may trigger a full mast cell flare.

2.2 Why Standard Advice Fails

Generic "healthy eating" recommendations from mainstream nutrition guidance can actively harm trifecta patients, and understanding why is essential before attempting any dietary changes.

The Dietary Guidelines for Americans recommend limiting sodium intake to 2,300 milligrams per day (USDA, 2020). For a POTS patient who needs 3,000 to 10,000 milligrams, following this advice could worsen orthostatic symptoms, increase fainting episodes, and reduce quality of life. The standard advice is based on cardiovascular risk reduction in the general population, which is entirely reasonable for that population. But POTS patients are not the general population. Their cardiovascular physiology operates under different rules, and applying general guidelines to a specialized condition produces poor outcomes.

Similarly, mainstream nutrition promotes fermented foods as beneficial for gut health based on evidence about the microbiome (Marco et al., 2017). Yogurt, kimchi, sauerkraut, and kombucha are staples of "gut-friendly" dietary advice. For a patient with MCAS or histamine intolerance, these foods can trigger flushing, tachycardia, GI distress, hives, and headaches. The patient who follows popular gut health advice and loads up on fermented foods may experience a dramatic symptom flare and conclude, incorrectly, that their body simply cannot tolerate any dietary intervention.

High-fiber diets are recommended for general digestive health. For a patient with EDS-related gastroparesis, high fiber can worsen gastric retention, increase bloating and pain, and slow an already sluggish digestive system to a halt. The advice that helps the general population harms this specific population because the underlying physiology is different.

Recognizing this disconnect is not about dismissing standard nutritional science. The science is sound for the populations studied. The problem is applying population-level guidance to a clinical subpopulation with distinct pathophysiology.

2.3 The Histamine Bucket

One of the most useful conceptual models for understanding MCAS-related food reactions is the **histamine bucket** (also called the histamine load or histamine threshold model). This concept helps explain why a person might tolerate a food on Monday and react to the identical food on Wednesday.

Every person has a threshold for total histamine and mast cell mediator load before symptoms appear. Imagine a bucket that can hold a certain volume before overflowing. Multiple sources contribute to filling that bucket throughout any given day: histamine from food, histamine released by mast cells in response to environmental triggers (heat, stress, fragrances), histamine produced by gut bacteria, and any other inflammatory inputs the body is processing (Comas-Basté et al., 2020).

When the bucket is relatively empty, a moderate-histamine food might be tolerated without difficulty. The body's histamine-degrading enzymes, primarily **diamine oxidase (DAO)** and **histamine N-methyltransferase (HNMT)**, can handle the additional load (Maintz & Novak, 2007). But when the bucket is already near full, perhaps because of poor sleep the night before (which increases mast cell reactivity), exposure to perfume at the office (a common MCAS trigger), menstrual cycle hormonal fluctuations (estrogen stimulates mast cells), and cumulative stress, that same moderate-histamine food pushes the total load over the threshold. The bucket overflows. Symptoms appear.

This model has profound practical implications. It means that identifying food triggers is far more complex than simple cause-and-effect. A food diary that only tracks what was eaten will miss the picture. An effective diary must also capture sleep quality, stress level, environmental exposures, hormonal timing, and symptom severity to reveal patterns.

2.4 Case Study: Conflicting Dietary Advice

Background

Jessamine, a 32-year-old veterinary technician, was diagnosed with hEDS at age 24, POTS at age 27, and MCAS at age 30. She saw three specialists in three different health systems. Her cardiologist recommended increasing salt intake to 8 grams per day and drinking 3 liters of fluid with electrolytes. Her allergist recommended a strict low-histamine elimination diet. Her gastroenterologist, noting her GERD and IBS symptoms, recommended a low-FODMAP diet.

Presentation

Jessamine attempted to follow all three sets of dietary instructions simultaneously. The low-histamine diet eliminated most high-sodium convenience foods she had been relying on. The low-FODMAP diet eliminated onions, garlic, and many fruits she enjoyed. The overlap between the two restriction lists left her eating essentially plain rice, fresh chicken, cucumber, and salt tablets. Her caloric intake dropped to 900 calories per day. She developed worsening fatigue, her hair began thinning, and her POTS symptoms deteriorated because she could not consume enough food volume to support her sodium and fluid goals.

Analysis

Jessamine's experience illustrates what happens when condition-specific dietary advice is given in isolation without considering the full clinical picture. Each recommendation was individually reasonable. But when layered together without coordination, they created a restriction so severe that it became medically harmful. The ARFID (Avoidant/Restrictive Food Intake Disorder) risk in this population is real. Topan et al. (2024) found that a positive ARFID screening was associated with a 7.55 odds ratio with dietary alterations in hEDS patients, and that those with ARFID had a four-fold increased risk of requiring nutritional support.

Intervention

A registered dietitian with experience in dysautonomia conducted a comprehensive nutritional assessment and developed a coordinated plan. Rather than following three separate restrictive diets, the dietitian identified a core group of foods that satisfied all three sets of requirements simultaneously: fresh, low-histamine, low-FODMAP, and preparable in high-sodium versions. Meals were restructured into five daily eating occasions. Sodium was incorporated through sea salt added during cooking, electrolyte drinks, and salt tablets, rather than relying on processed foods. Caloric intake was gradually increased to 1,800 calories.

Outcome

Over 10 weeks, Jessamine's caloric intake stabilized, her weight loss reversed, and her hair thinning slowed. Her POTS symptoms improved with adequate sodium delivery. Her MCAS flares became less frequent as her stress level decreased (stress from not knowing what to eat had been a significant mast cell trigger). She described the experience as "finally having permission to eat again."

Teaching Points

- Specialist dietary advice given in isolation can create combined restriction severe enough to cause malnutrition, particularly when multiple conditions each require their own dietary modifications
- A coordinated dietary approach that identifies foods meeting all condition-specific criteria simultaneously is more sustainable and effective than layering separate restrictive diets
- Psychological stress from dietary confusion and food fear functions as a mast cell trigger, meaning that reducing food anxiety is itself a therapeutic intervention

2.5 Carbohydrates and Blood Pooling

A specific dietary concern for POTS patients involves the relationship between carbohydrate intake and postprandial symptoms. After eating, blood flow increases to the gastrointestinal tract to support digestion. This is normal physiology. But in POTS, where the autonomic nervous system already struggles to maintain adequate blood distribution, the additional diversion of blood to the gut can produce a significant drop in blood available to the brain and heart. The result is worsened tachycardia, dizziness, brain fog, and fatigue after meals (Mehr et al., 2018).

High-glycemic carbohydrates produce larger and faster insulin responses, which in turn cause greater postprandial blood shifts. Research has demonstrated that high-carbohydrate meals exacerbate POTS symptoms more than meals with equivalent calories from protein and fat (Mehr et al., 2018). Additionally, blood sugar spikes may independently trigger mast cell degranulation. For patients with concurrent MCAS, this creates a double problem: the meal worsens both autonomic and immune symptoms simultaneously.

A related and encouraging finding involves gluten. Penny et al. (2016) discovered that POTS patients had a higher prevalence of celiac disease (4% compared to 1% in the background population) and gluten intolerance (42% compared to 19%). A survey by Zha et al. (2022) found that 20 POTS patients who had self-selected a gluten-free diet for more than four weeks reported an average 45% self-reported reduction in POTS symptoms. While this was a small, uncontrolled study based on self-report, the magnitude of the finding warrants attention.

The practical takeaway is not that all trifecta patients should eliminate gluten. Rather, the data suggest that reducing high-glycemic carbohydrate loads and considering a trial gluten elimination may benefit a substantial subgroup of POTS patients.

2.6 The Trifecta Compatible Framework

Given the competing demands of these three conditions, this book introduces the **Trifecta-Compatible** dietary framework. This is not a rigid diet plan. It is a set of guiding principles that allow patients and their healthcare providers to make food choices that address all three conditions simultaneously rather than sacrificing one condition's management for another's.

The core principles are:

Freshness first. Because histamine accumulates in food over time, the framework prioritizes the freshest possible ingredients. Meat purchased fresh and cooked immediately or frozen immediately after purchase. Vegetables bought in small quantities and consumed within days. Leftovers cooled rapidly and frozen within one to two hours rather than stored in the refrigerator for days. This single principle addresses MCAS dietary concerns without requiring the memorization of extensive food lists.

Sodium through whole food preparation. Rather than relying on processed high-sodium foods (which tend to be histamine-rich), sodium is added through sea salt during cooking, electrolyte beverages, and salt tablets. This allows POTS patients to meet their sodium targets without introducing the processed foods that MCAS patients need to avoid.

Protein at every eating occasion. Adequate protein supports connective tissue integrity (relevant for EDS), stabilizes blood sugar (relevant for POTS), and helps prevent the muscle wasting that can accompany restricted diets. The framework targets 1.2 to 1.6 grams of protein per kilogram of body weight daily, distributed across multiple meals.

Small, frequent meals. Eating four to six times per day rather than three large meals reduces postprandial blood pooling (helping POTS), decreases gastric distension (helping EDS-related gastroparesis and GERD), and spreads dietary histamine intake across the day rather than concentrating it in large loads (helping MCAS).

Individualization over elimination. The framework avoids blanket elimination of entire food groups. Instead, it begins with a core group of well-tolerated foods, stabilizes symptoms, and then systematically reintroduces foods one at a time to identify genuine individual triggers rather than applying generic avoidance lists.

2.7 Case Study: The Fermentation Trap

Background

Faramond, a 41-year-old software engineer diagnosed with POTS and suspected MCAS, read extensively about gut health and decided to add fermented foods to his diet. He began consuming kefir daily, started making his own sauerkraut, added miso soup as a regular lunch, and supplemented with a probiotic containing multiple Lactobacillus strains.

Presentation

Within two weeks, Faramond's POTS symptoms worsened. His standing heart rate, which had been managed at a 25 beat-per-minute differential, increased to a 38 beat-per-minute differential. He developed facial flushing after meals, intermittent hives on his chest and arms, and worsening GI symptoms including cramping and diarrhea. He attributed these changes to stress at work and continued the fermented food regimen for another month before his symptoms became severe enough to seek urgent care.

Analysis

Faramond had inadvertently created a massive histamine load through his dietary changes. Kefir, sauerkraut, and miso are among the highest dietary sources of histamine due to the fermentation process that generates them. Additionally, certain Lactobacillus strains used in probiotic supplements are histamine-producing bacteria (Lactic acid bacteria vary in their histamine production; L. reuteri and L. casei are notable producers) (Patel et al., 2020). His well-intentioned gut health protocol had dramatically increased both exogenous histamine intake and endogenous histamine production, overwhelming his already compromised mast cell stability.

Intervention

All fermented foods were removed. Faramond was transitioned to a low-histamine dietary framework with fresh foods prepared and consumed within 24 hours. If probiotic use was desired, strains with evidence of histamine-lowering properties (such as Bifidobacterium infantis and Lactobacillus rhamnosus GG) were discussed as potential alternatives after symptom stabilization (Dev et al., 2008).

Outcome

Within three weeks of removing fermented foods, Faramond's heart rate differential returned to 24 beats per minute. Flushing and hives resolved. GI symptoms improved substantially. He described the experience as "shocking, because everything I read said fermented foods were supposed to help."

Teaching Points

- Fermented foods, while beneficial for the general population's gut microbiome, can be among the most potent histamine triggers for MCAS patients, creating a direct conflict between mainstream gut health advice and mast cell management
- Not all probiotic strains are equivalent in their relationship to histamine; some strains produce histamine while others help degrade it, making strain selection critical for this population
- Worsening of POTS symptoms can sometimes be driven by increased histamine load rather than cardiovascular deconditioning, and identifying the dietary cause can lead to rapid resolution

2.8 Essential Points to Remember

The dietary paradox at the heart of trifecta management is not a problem to be solved by choosing one condition's needs over another's. It is a challenge to be navigated through informed, coordinated decision-making. POTS demands sodium and fluid. MCAS demands freshness and histamine awareness. EDS demands GI-gentle eating with nutritional adequacy. These demands can be met simultaneously, but only through a framework that understands all three conditions and their interactions.

Standard nutritional advice designed for the general population fails trifecta patients because their physiology operates under different rules. What improves cardiovascular risk in a healthy person (low sodium) can worsen autonomic function in POTS. What supports gut health in most people (fermented foods) can trigger immune flares in MCAS. What promotes general digestive health (high fiber) can worsen gastroparesis in EDS.

The histamine bucket model provides a practical lens for understanding why food reactions are variable and context-dependent. The Trifecta-Compatible framework provides a set of guiding principles (freshness, sodium through whole food preparation, protein prioritization, small frequent meals, individualization over blanket elimination) that address all three conditions without creating the dangerous levels of dietary restriction that lead to malnutrition and ARFID.

Chapter 3.0: Digestive System Under Siege

Imagine sitting down to a simple dinner of grilled chicken, steamed rice, and roasted vegetables. For most people, this is an unremarkable meal. But for you, each bite triggers a cascade of uncertainty. Will the chicken cause flushing and hives because your mast cells have decided it is a threat today? Will the rice sit in your stomach for hours because your gastroparesis has slowed digestion to a crawl? Will the vegetables trigger bloating and cramping because your irritable bowel syndrome has flared again? You are not imagining this. The gastrointestinal system is one of the most commonly affected organ systems in patients living with the trifecta, and understanding why is the first step toward reclaiming some control over what you eat.

This chapter will cover the following:

- Why the autonomic nervous system directly controls digestion and how POTS disrupts that control
- How connective tissue abnormalities in EDS affect the physical structure and motility of the GI tract
- The overlapping roles of IBS, GERD, gastroparesis, dysmotility, and MCAS in creating GI chaos
- The psychological impact of chronic GI symptoms, including the risk of avoidant restrictive food intake disorder (ARFID)
- How to build a "safe foods foundation" before attempting any elimination protocol

3.1 The Autonomic Gut Connection

The autonomic nervous system (ANS) manages every aspect of digestion that happens without conscious effort. It controls the contractions that move food through the esophagus, the secretion of stomach acid, the rhythmic churning of the stomach, the wave-like movements (called **peristalsis**) that push food through the intestines, and even the release of digestive enzymes from the pancreas. When the ANS malfunctions, as it does in dysautonomia, every stage of this process can go wrong.

Research from the British Dietetic Association indicates that up to 90% of patients with POTS experience gastrointestinal symptoms (Fikree et al., 2017). This is not a coincidence. The **vagus nerve**, the longest cranial nerve in the body, serves as the primary communication highway between the brain and the gut. It carries signals that regulate stomach acid production, intestinal motility, and the coordination of digestive muscle contractions. In many POTS patients, vagal tone is impaired

(Vernino et al., 2021). The result is a digestive system that cannot properly coordinate its own functions.

The practical consequences are wide-ranging. Reduced gastric motility means food sits in the stomach longer than it should, causing nausea, early fullness, and bloating. Altered intestinal motility can swing between sluggish movement (causing constipation) and overactive movement (causing diarrhea). Blood flow redistribution after eating, known as **postprandial hypotension**, can worsen orthostatic symptoms because the body diverts blood to the digestive organs and away from the brain and heart (Mehr et al., 2018). This explains why many POTS patients feel their worst after meals, particularly large ones or those high in carbohydrates.

For patients with EDS, the problem compounds. The connective tissue that provides structural support to the gastrointestinal tract is inherently weaker in EDS patients. The smooth muscle walls of the stomach and intestines rely on collagen and elastin for their tone and shape (Thwaites et al., 2022). When these structural proteins are defective, the GI tract becomes floppy, distensible, and less efficient at moving food along. This creates a biological double hit: the nervous system cannot properly direct digestion, and the physical structure of the digestive organs cannot properly execute those directions even if they arrive correctly.

3.2 Gastroparesis and EDS

Gastroparesis is a condition in which the stomach empties its contents into the small intestine too slowly, in the absence of any mechanical obstruction. Symptoms include nausea, vomiting, early satiety (feeling full after eating very little), bloating, upper abdominal pain, and poor appetite. For many trifecta patients, gastroparesis is one of the most functionally limiting GI conditions they face.

The relationship between EDS and gastroparesis is striking. A large case-control study comparing hospitalized patients with and without EDS found that EDS patients exhibited a 12.26 times higher odds ratio of having a concurrent gastroparesis diagnosis (Beckers et al., 2017, as cited in Practical Gastroenterology; see also Thwaites et al., 2022). Another study found that 52% of patients with GI symptoms and joint hypermobility syndrome were diagnosed with gastroparesis through formal gastric emptying studies (Fikree et al., 2013). These numbers are extraordinary. They tell us that gastroparesis is not a rare complication for EDS patients. It is a common one.

So what does a 12.26 times higher odds ratio actually mean for meal planning? It means that any nutritional strategy for EDS patients must account for the strong probability that food will not leave the stomach at a normal rate. Practical implications include the following:

- **Meal size matters enormously.** Smaller, more frequent meals (four to six eating occasions per day rather than three large meals) reduce the volume the stomach must process at any given time. A stomach that struggles to empty 500 milliliters will often manage 200 milliliters without significant distress (Ganesh et al., 2020).
- **Food texture affects emptying speed.** Liquids and pureed foods generally empty faster than solid foods. On days when gastroparesis is severe, shifting toward smoothies, soups, and softer foods can maintain caloric and nutritional intake while reducing the mechanical burden on the stomach (Steiner et al., 2023).
- **Fat slows gastric emptying further.** While healthy fats are a necessary part of nutrition, very high-fat meals can worsen gastroparesis symptoms. Distributing fat intake across multiple small meals rather than concentrating it in one or two meals is a practical adjustment.
- **Fiber is a double-edged sword.** In a normally functioning GI tract, fiber supports healthy motility and feeds beneficial gut bacteria. But in a gastroparetic stomach, insoluble fiber (found in raw vegetables, whole grains, and fruit skins) can form bezoars, which are compacted masses of undigested fiber that can obstruct the stomach outlet. For patients with confirmed gastroparesis, fiber modification under dietitian guidance is often necessary (Thwaites et al., 2022).

3.3 IBS and Functional Disorders

Irritable bowel syndrome (IBS) is a functional gastrointestinal disorder characterized by recurrent abdominal pain associated with changes in stool frequency or form. It is classified into subtypes: IBS-C (constipation predominant), IBS-D (diarrhea predominant), IBS-M (mixed), and IBS-U (unsubtyped). Research suggests that up to 62% of patients with hypermobile EDS (hEDS) meet diagnostic criteria for IBS (Choudhary et al., 2021). One study using the Rome IV diagnostic criteria found that nearly 98% of subjects with hypermobility spectrum disorder met criteria for at least one adult functional gastrointestinal disorder (Lam et al., 2021).

These are not just statistical curiosities. They represent lived experiences of daily uncertainty about bowel function. The challenge for trifecta patients is that IBS in the context of EDS and POTS may have different underlying mechanisms than IBS in the general population. In the general population, IBS is often driven primarily by gut-brain axis dysfunction, visceral hypersensitivity, and psychological factors. In hEDS patients, structural changes to connective tissue in the bowel wall, impaired motility from autonomic dysfunction, and mast cell activation within the intestinal mucosa may all contribute simultaneously (Choudhary et al., 2021).

This distinction matters for treatment. Standard IBS dietary interventions, such as the **low-FODMAP diet** (which restricts fermentable oligosaccharides, disaccharides, monosaccharides, and polyols), may help some trifecta patients but not others. When the primary driver is motility dysfunction rather than fermentation-related gas production, restricting FODMAPs may not address the root cause. A 2024 cross-sectional study of 680 hEDS patients found that 62.1% had altered their diet in the past year, often without clear benefit, and 62.3% regularly skipped meals entirely (Topan et al., 2024). The study authors emphasized the need for a multidisciplinary approach rather than patients self-directing multiple restrictive diets simultaneously.

3.4 Upper GI Dysfunction Patterns

Beyond gastroparesis and IBS, trifecta patients commonly experience **gastroesophageal reflux disease (GERD)** and **functional dyspepsia (FD)**. These conditions are so prevalent in this population that they form part of the baseline experience of eating, making every meal feel like a potential minefield.

GERD occurs when stomach acid flows back into the esophagus, causing heartburn, chest pain, regurgitation, and sometimes difficulty swallowing. In EDS patients, the lower esophageal sphincter (the muscular valve between the esophagus and stomach) may be laxer due to connective tissue weakness, allowing acid to reflux more easily (Thwaites et al., 2022). Additionally, gastroparesis increases GERD risk because food sitting in the stomach for extended periods increases pressure against that weakened sphincter.

Functional dyspepsia involves chronic or recurring pain and discomfort centered in the upper abdomen. Patients describe a gnawing or burning sensation, uncomfortable fullness after eating, and early satiety. In the Topan et al. (2024) study, functional dyspepsia was independently associated with dietary alterations (OR 1.73, $p < 0.008$), meaning patients with FD were significantly more likely to restrict their diets. Lower adherence to the Mediterranean dietary pattern has been associated with worsening FD symptoms, suggesting that dietary quality, not just restriction, influences outcomes (Duncanson et al., 2021).

Dysmotility, the broader term for abnormal movement of the GI tract, ties these conditions together. When peristalsis is uncoordinated, food does not move through the system in an orderly fashion. The stomach empties too slowly (gastroparesis), the small intestine contracts irregularly (potentially contributing to bacterial overgrowth), and the colon alternates between inactivity and spasm (IBS). POTS amplifies these problems by creating hemodynamic instability during digestion. And MCAS, as we will see next, adds an inflammatory layer that makes everything more reactive.

3.5 Mast Cells Beyond Allergies

A critical misconception about MCAS-related GI symptoms is that they function like food allergies. They do not. A retrospective study examining 204 patients with mastocytosis or monoclonal mast cell activation syndrome found that while 20.6% self-reported food hypersensitivities, only 3.4% of these were confirmed by relevant IgE sensitization and allergy testing (Vlieg-Boerstra et al., 2005). The majority of reactions consisted of localized skin reactions (86%) and gastrointestinal symptoms (45%), and they were primarily mild and very seldom immunologically mediated.

This finding has profound implications for dietary management. In classic food allergy, the immune system produces specific IgE antibodies against a particular protein in a food. The reaction is reproducible: if you are allergic to peanuts, you will react to peanuts consistently. In MCAS, the mechanism is entirely different. **Mast cells** in the intestinal lining release histamine, tryptase, prostaglandins, leukotrienes, and over 1,000 other chemical mediators in response to triggers that are often unpredictable and inconsistent (Afrin et al., 2016). A food that was tolerated yesterday may cause cramping, diarrhea, or nausea today, because the threshold for mast cell activation fluctuates with stress, hormonal changes, temperature, sleep quality, and the cumulative load of other triggers.

This inconsistency is one of the most frustrating aspects of MCAS. It can lead patients to eliminate more and more foods in a desperate attempt to identify reliable patterns, when the pattern may not be about the food itself but about the total **mast cell mediator burden** at that moment. As discussed in Chapter 2.0, the concept of the "histamine bucket" helps explain why the same food can be tolerated one day and trigger symptoms another. The bucket overflows not from any single food but from the combined load of dietary histamine, environmental triggers, stress hormones, and internal mast cell activity.

3.6 SIBO and Motility Issues

Small intestinal bacterial overgrowth (SIBO) occurs when bacteria that normally reside in the large intestine migrate into the small intestine, where they ferment carbohydrates and produce gas. Symptoms include bloating, distension, abdominal pain, diarrhea, and in some cases, nutrient malabsorption. The connection to the trifecta is mechanical: the migrating motor complex (MMC), a pattern of electrical activity that sweeps residual food and bacteria out of the small intestine between meals, depends on normal autonomic nervous system function and adequate intestinal motility (Pimentel et al., 2020).

In patients with EDS-related dysmotility and POTS-related autonomic dysfunction, the MMC may not fire properly or with sufficient force. This allows bacteria to accumulate in the small intestine, creating a self-perpetuating cycle. The bacterial overgrowth itself produces toxins that can further impair motility, and the resulting inflammation can activate mast cells, worsening MCAS symptoms (Weinstock et al., 2021).

SIBO also contributes to nutrient deficiencies. Bacteria in the small intestine can consume B12 before the host absorbs it, interfere with fat absorption (causing fat-soluble vitamin deficiencies), and damage the intestinal lining, reducing the absorptive surface area. As we will explore in Chapter 5.0, these malabsorption issues compound the nutritional challenges that trifecta patients already face from restricted diets and poor appetite.

3.7 Ivo's Complex GI Presentation

Background

Ivo, a 29-year-old graduate student, was diagnosed with hEDS at age 24 following years of joint subluxations and chronic pain. Over the subsequent five years, he developed progressively worsening GI symptoms including daily nausea, bloating after every meal, alternating constipation and diarrhea, and episodes of flushing and abdominal cramping that seemed unrelated to any specific food. He had been diagnosed with IBS-M at age 26 and POTS at age 27. Despite following a strict low-FODMAP diet for eight months, his symptoms had not improved.

Presentation

Ivo reported eating only five foods consistently: white rice, boiled chicken, steamed sweet potatoes, peeled cucumbers, and pears. He described intense anxiety before meals, stating that "every time I eat, I'm bracing for what's going to happen." He had lost 14 pounds over the previous year and reported increasing fatigue, brain fog, and difficulty concentrating on his academic work. Gastric emptying testing revealed moderately delayed emptying consistent with gastroparesis. Breath testing was positive for hydrogen-dominant SIBO.

Analysis

Ivo's case illustrates the layered nature of GI dysfunction in the trifecta. His gastroparesis (related to EDS-associated connective tissue changes and POTS-related autonomic dysfunction) slowed stomach emptying, creating an environment favorable for SIBO development. The SIBO produced gas and bloating that he attributed to food intolerances, leading him to restrict his diet further. His low-FODMAP restriction, while theoretically sensible for IBS-M, removed prebiotic fibers that support healthy gut bacteria, potentially worsening the dysbiosis. Meanwhile, his increasing malnutrition from a five-food diet was contributing to fatigue and cognitive difficulties that compounded his autonomic symptoms.

Intervention

Ivo's gastroenterologist treated the SIBO with a targeted antibiotic protocol. Simultaneously, a registered dietitian specializing in EDS began gradually reintroducing foods one at a time, starting with low-histamine, easily digestible options. Small, frequent meals (six per day) replaced his pattern of two large meals. A prokinetic medication was added to support gastric motility. Food and symptom journals tracked reactions to reintroduced foods.

Outcome

After three months, Ivo had expanded his diet to include 22 foods. His weight stabilized and he regained four pounds. Nausea decreased from daily to two to three times weekly. Most importantly, his meal-related anxiety diminished as he developed a structured framework for food introduction rather than an all-or-nothing approach.

Teaching Points

- Multiple GI conditions frequently coexist in trifecta patients, and treating one (such as IBS) without addressing others (such as gastroparesis and SIBO) often produces incomplete results
- Progressive dietary restriction without professional guidance can create nutritional deficiencies that worsen the underlying conditions
- A systematic reintroduction protocol guided by a dietitian is safer and more effective than self-directed elimination

3.8 ARFID and Dietary Fear

Avoidant restrictive food intake disorder (ARFID) is a feeding and eating disorder characterized by avoiding or restricting food intake based on the sensory characteristics of food, fear of aversive consequences of eating (such as choking, vomiting, or GI pain), or apparent lack of interest in eating. Unlike anorexia nervosa, ARFID is not driven by body image concerns. It is driven by genuine, often well-founded fear that eating will cause physical suffering.

The Topan et al. (2024) study found that a positive screening for ARFID was independently associated with dietary alteration in hEDS patients (OR 7.55, 95% CI 3.27-17.40, $p < 0.001$). Patients who screened positive for ARFID, specifically the "fear of eating" and "low interest" subtypes, had a fourfold increased risk of requiring nutritional support such as oral nutritional supplements, enteral feeding, or intravenous nutrition. This is a clinical red flag. It indicates that the psychological impact of chronic GI distress is itself a medical problem requiring intervention, not just a predictable response to be expected and tolerated.

The cycle operates as follows: a patient eats a food and experiences pain, nausea, or another adverse symptom. The brain encodes this food as dangerous. The patient avoids that food. The next time a similar symptom occurs with a different food, that food is also eliminated. Over months and years, the diet narrows. But because the underlying GI dysfunction (gastroparesis, dysmotility, mast cell activation) can cause symptoms with almost any food, the elimination never reaches a point of symptom freedom. The patient continues to restrict, losing both nutritional adequacy and the enjoyment of eating.

3.9 Dorothea's Restriction Pattern

Background

Dorothea, a 35-year-old elementary school teacher, was diagnosed with MCAS at age 31 after two years of unexplained hives, flushing, and episodic abdominal cramping. She had subsequently been diagnosed with POTS and suspected hEDS. After reading extensively online about low-histamine diets, she had progressively eliminated aged cheeses, fermented foods, tomatoes, strawberries, spinach, avocados, citrus fruits, canned foods, chocolate, and most leftovers from her diet. She then eliminated gluten, dairy, and soy. Over the following year, she removed nightshade vegetables, high-oxalate foods, and most nuts.

Presentation

Dorothea was eating approximately 800 calories daily, primarily from fresh chicken breast, white rice, peeled zucchini, and blueberries. She had lost 22 pounds and her BMI had dropped to 17.2. She experienced severe fatigue, hair loss, easy bruising, frequent muscle cramps, and worsening POTS symptoms including near-syncope episodes multiple times daily. Her menstrual cycle had stopped. Despite these alarming signs, Dorothea believed she needed to eliminate more foods because she was "still reacting to everything."

Analysis

Dorothea's case demonstrates the dangerous trajectory of unsupported dietary restriction. Her caloric intake was severely inadequate. Her protein intake was insufficient to support connective tissue maintenance, which is especially critical in EDS. Her micronutrient intake was profoundly deficient: no calcium, minimal iron, almost no vitamin D, and inadequate B vitamins. Her worsening POTS symptoms were at least partially attributable to malnutrition-related hypovolemia and electrolyte imbalances. Her hair loss reflected protein and zinc deficiency. Her amenorrhea indicated that her body had entered an energy conservation state due to starvation.

The core issue was that Dorothea had conflated multiple dietary frameworks (low-histamine, low-FODMAP, low-oxalate, gluten-free, dairy-free) into a single impossibly restrictive protocol, without any professional guidance about which restrictions were appropriate for her individual situation and without monitoring for nutritional adequacy.

Intervention

A multidisciplinary team including a gastroenterologist, allergist, and registered dietitian evaluated Dorothea's actual triggers through structured challenge testing rather than self-reported avoidance. The dietitian prioritized caloric and protein adequacy before any elimination protocol. An oral nutritional supplement was added between meals. Mast cell-stabilizing medication (cromolyn sodium) was started to reduce baseline mast cell reactivity, making food reintroduction safer.

Outcome

Over six months, Dorothea regained 15 pounds and restored her menstrual cycle. Formal testing revealed that she tolerated the majority of the foods she had eliminated. Her actual confirmed triggers were limited to aged cheeses, red wine, and canned tuna. Her POTS symptoms improved as her nutritional status and blood volume recovered. She described the experience as "learning that my body was reacting to starvation, not to food."

Teaching Points

- Layering multiple restrictive diets without professional supervision creates a high risk of severe malnutrition that worsens all three trifecta conditions
- Worsening POTS symptoms during dietary restriction should trigger evaluation for nutritional deficiency as a contributing cause
- Structured food challenge testing under medical supervision provides more reliable information about true triggers than self-directed elimination

3.10 Building Safe Food Foundations

Before attempting any elimination protocol, trifecta patients need what we call a **safe foods foundation**. This is a core group of at least 15 to 20 foods from multiple categories (proteins, carbohydrates, fats, fruits, and vegetables) that are consistently tolerated, nutritionally adequate, and practically accessible. This foundation serves as the dietary floor below which you do not go, regardless of if new symptoms emerge or if you are eliminating potential triggers.

Building this foundation requires patience, a food and symptom journal, and ideally the guidance of a registered dietitian who understands the trifecta. The process works as follows:

First, identify foods you already tolerate reasonably well most of the time. The key phrase is "most of the time," not "always." In MCAS, no food will be tolerated 100% of the time because mast cell reactivity fluctuates. A food you tolerate 80% of the time is a safe food.

Second, ensure your safe foods list includes at least two to three options from each macronutrient category. You need protein sources (such as chicken, turkey, or fresh fish), complex carbohydrate sources (such as rice, sweet potatoes, or quinoa), fat sources (such as olive oil, coconut oil, or ghee), vegetables (such as zucchini, carrots, or broccoli), and fruits (such as blueberries, pears, or apples).

Third, protect your safe foods fiercely. When you begin any elimination or reintroduction protocol (which will be discussed in Chapter 6.0), your safe foods remain constant. You add and remove only the foods you are testing, never your foundation.

This approach accomplishes several goals. It prevents the dangerous spiral of progressive restriction illustrated in Dorothea's case. It ensures minimum caloric and macronutrient adequacy throughout any dietary experimentation. And it provides psychological safety, because you always have foods you can fall back on during flare days.

3.11 Bringing It All Together

The gastrointestinal system in trifecta patients operates under triple jeopardy. Autonomic dysfunction from POTS impairs the nervous system's ability to coordinate digestion. Connective tissue abnormalities from EDS compromise the physical structure and motility of the GI tract. Mast cell overactivation from MCAS creates an inflammatory environment that makes the entire system hypersensitive and unpredictable. These three mechanisms interact and amplify each other, explaining why up to 90% of POTS patients experience gut symptoms and why GI complaints are among the most debilitating features of the trifecta.

Gastroparesis, IBS, GERD, functional dyspepsia, dysmotility, and SIBO are not separate problems requiring separate diets. They are interconnected manifestations of the same underlying pathophysiology, and they require a coordinated nutritional strategy. The risk of ARFID and disordered eating in this population is real and documented, with a fourfold increase in the likelihood of needing nutritional support when ARFID is present. Restrictive diets pursued without professional guidance can cause malnutrition that worsens every condition in the trifecta.

The path forward begins with building a safe foods foundation, establishing a relationship with a registered dietitian who understands these conditions, and approaching dietary change as a structured, monitored process rather than a desperate series of eliminations. In Chapter 4.0, we will turn to the most universally recommended dietary intervention for POTS: optimizing hydration, sodium, and electrolyte intake.

Chapter 4.0: The Hydration Imperative

A 26-year-old woman with POTS collapses in the shower on a Tuesday morning. She drank two cups of coffee and nothing else before stepping into the hot water. The combination of heat-induced vasodilation, overnight dehydration, and caffeine-related diuresis dropped her already low blood volume below the threshold her body could compensate for. She wakes up on the bathroom floor with a bruised elbow and a racing heart. This scenario, or something close to it, plays out daily for POTS patients who have not yet learned that hydration is not a suggestion for their condition. It is a medical intervention as important as any prescription medication.

This chapter will cover the following:

- The evidence base for fluid and sodium recommendations in POTS, including expert consensus guidelines
- Why the sodium requirements for POTS patients differ drastically from general population guidelines
- How the sodium-glucose co-transport system affects hydration efficiency
- Practical strategies for meeting fluid and electrolyte targets, including cost comparisons of commercial versus homemade options
- Timing strategies for fluid intake around meals, mornings, and exercise

4.1 Fluid Needs in POTS

The 2021 POTS Expert Consensus Review, authored by Vernino and colleagues following a National Institutes of Health Expert Consensus Meeting, endorses patients consuming at least 2 to 3 liters of water per day along with significant sodium supplementation (Vernino et al., 2021). The 2015 Heart Rhythm Society Expert Consensus Statement recommended up to 2 to 3 liters of water and 10 to 12 grams of salt (sodium chloride) daily (Sheldon et al., 2015). The Canadian Cardiovascular Society Position Statement on POTS recommended 10 grams of salt via high-salt foods, salt sticks, and tablets, and at least 3 liters of oral fluids (Raj et al., 2020).

These are not aspirational targets. They are clinical recommendations from the highest-level consensus bodies in cardiovascular and autonomic medicine. To put them in perspective, 2 liters of fluid is approximately 8.5 cups of water. Three liters is 12.7 cups. The average American drinks approximately 5.5 cups of plain water daily (USDA Agricultural Research Service, 2016). A POTS patient needs to roughly double or triple that baseline.

The reason is straightforward. Many POTS patients have **hypovolemia**, a medical condition in which total blood volume is lower than normal (Raj, 2013). When blood volume is already reduced, the cardiovascular system has less fluid to work with. Upon standing, gravity pulls blood into the lower extremities. In a healthy person with adequate blood volume, compensatory mechanisms constrict blood vessels and maintain blood flow to the brain. In a POTS patient with reduced blood volume, these mechanisms are overwhelmed, and the heart compensates by beating faster, producing the characteristic tachycardia.

Increasing fluid intake directly increases blood volume. A study by Mehdirad et al. (2019) found that acute water ingestion of 473 milliliters (approximately two cups) produced measurable improvements in hemodynamic parameters in POTS patients within minutes. The effect was temporary, which is why sustained hydration throughout the day, not just a single large drink, is necessary.

4.2 Sodium Targets and Evidence

The general population is advised to consume no more than 2,300 milligrams (2.3 grams) of sodium daily, according to the Dietary Guidelines for Americans. Many POTS patients need 3,000 to 10,000 milligrams (3 to 10 grams) daily. This represents a two- to fourfold increase above the standard recommendation, and it can feel deeply counterintuitive. Patients raised on messages about the dangers of salt must recalibrate their understanding entirely.

The rationale is physiological. Sodium is the primary electrolyte responsible for retaining water in the bloodstream. When sodium intake increases, the kidneys retain more water, expanding **plasma volume** (the liquid portion of blood). This expansion directly counteracts the hypovolemia that drives many POTS symptoms (Garland et al., 2021). In a 2021 study examining the effects of high dietary sodium in POTS patients, increased sodium intake was associated with improved orthostatic tolerance, meaning patients could stand longer and with fewer symptoms.

Ten grams of salt translates to roughly two teaspoons of table salt daily (Harris, 2022). One teaspoon of table salt contains approximately 2,300 milligrams of sodium. To reach 10 grams of salt (approximately 4,000 milligrams of sodium from salt alone, with additional sodium from food), patients can use a combination of:

- **Salting food liberally during cooking and at the table.** This is the simplest and most palatable approach for many patients.
- **High-sodium foods.** Broth and soups, olives, pickles (if tolerated from a histamine perspective), salted nuts, and certain cheeses can contribute substantial sodium. As discussed in Chapter 2.0, histamine-compatible

high-sodium options must be selected carefully for patients with concurrent MCAS.

- **Salt tablets.** Products like Vitassium (a medical food formulated for POTS) and sodium chloride tablets provide measured doses of sodium that can be taken throughout the day.
- **Electrolyte drinks and powders.** These combine sodium with fluid, addressing both needs simultaneously.

4.3 The Hyperadrenergic Exception

Not all POTS is the same, and not all POTS subtypes respond identically to high sodium intake. The **hyperadrenergic subtype** of POTS is characterized by elevated levels of norepinephrine, a stress hormone, particularly upon standing. Patients with this subtype often have high blood pressure spikes rather than the low blood pressure seen in hypovolemic POTS. They may experience tremor, anxiety, headaches, and excessive sweating (Vernino et al., 2021).

For hyperadrenergic POTS patients, aggressive sodium loading may not be appropriate and could worsen hypertensive episodes. The Dysautonomia International guidelines note that except for the hyperadrenergic subtype, increased fluid and salt intake is typically recommended. This distinction is critical. It means that knowing your POTS subtype, as determined through formal autonomic testing and clinical evaluation, directly affects your nutritional strategy.

If you have been diagnosed with hyperadrenergic POTS, work closely with your cardiologist or autonomic specialist to determine your individual sodium targets. The general recommendation of 3 to 10 grams may not apply to you, and blindly following it could cause harm. This is one of several reasons why the advice in this book, while evidence-based, is not a substitute for individualized medical guidance.

4.4 Sodium Glucose Transport Science

You may have noticed that some electrolyte products contain sugar, while others are sugar-free. This is not just a taste preference. There is a specific physiological reason why combining sodium with a small amount of glucose improves hydration efficiency.

In the small intestine, a protein called the **sodium-glucose co-transporter 1 (SGLT1)** moves sodium and glucose across the intestinal wall and into the bloodstream simultaneously. The two molecules must be present together for this transporter to function. When sodium and glucose arrive at the intestinal lining at the same time, water follows them through osmosis, creating a rapid and efficient absorption pathway (Rao, 2004). This is the same principle behind the World

Health Organization's **oral rehydration solution (ORS)**, which has saved millions of lives in developing countries by treating cholera-related dehydration.

For POTS patients, this means that an electrolyte drink containing both sodium and a small amount of sugar will hydrate more effectively than plain salted water. The optimal ratio, based on ORS formulations, involves approximately 2.6 grams of glucose per liter of solution along with 2.6 grams of sodium chloride (WHO, 2006). Commercial products like NormaLyte are formulated based on this WHO-recommended concentration.

The catch is that too much sugar defeats the purpose. Highly sugary sports drinks like standard Gatorade contain far more sugar than is needed for co-transport, and the excess glucose can cause blood sugar spikes. For POTS patients, high-glycemic loads are already problematic because they worsen postprandial symptoms (Mehr et al., 2018). Sugar-free electrolyte options work well for patients who are eating regular meals (and thus getting glucose from food) and primarily need supplemental sodium. But for patients who are fasting, vomiting, or unable to eat, the glucose component of an ORS-style product can make the difference between adequate and inadequate rehydration.

4.5 Faustina's Electrolyte Strategy

Background

Faustina, a 32-year-old graphic designer diagnosed with POTS and hEDS at age 28, had been told by her cardiologist to "drink more water and eat more salt." She interpreted this as drinking an additional glass of water daily and occasionally eating pretzels. Her symptoms of lightheadedness upon standing, brain fog, and afternoon fatigue had not improved.

Presentation

A dietary recall revealed that Faustina consumed approximately 1.2 liters of fluid daily, including coffee, and estimated her sodium intake at 2,500 milligrams per day, which was within the general population recommendation but far below POTS targets. She disliked the taste of very salty food and found commercial electrolyte drinks too expensive at $1.50 per serving, given that she would need three to four servings daily.

Analysis

Faustina's case illustrates a common gap between medical advice and practical implementation. The instruction to "drink more water and eat more salt" is technically correct but insufficiently specific. It does not communicate the magnitude of increase required, offer practical strategies for achieving it, or address the cost barrier. Her 2,500 milligrams of daily sodium was appropriate for a healthy adult but left her approximately 1,500 to 7,500 milligrams short of POTS recommendations. Her 1.2 liters of fluid was less than half the minimum recommendation.

Intervention

Faustina worked with a dietitian to develop a structured hydration plan. She began each morning with 500 milliliters of electrolyte water before getting out of bed (the "pre-loading" strategy). She prepared a batch of homemade electrolyte drink each morning using the following recipe: 1 liter of water, 1/2 teaspoon of table salt (approximately 1,150 milligrams of sodium), 1/4 teaspoon of potassium-based salt substitute (approximately 350 milligrams of potassium), and 1 tablespoon of honey (providing the glucose for co-transport). This cost approximately $0.08 per liter compared to $1.50 per serving for her preferred commercial brand. She carried a water bottle with measured markings and set phone alarms every two hours to drink.

Outcome

Within two weeks, Faustina reported noticeable improvement in afternoon brain fog and fewer episodes of lightheadedness. After one month, she described the change as "like upgrading from a dial-up connection to broadband in my brain." Her total daily fluid intake stabilized at 2.5 liters, and her sodium intake reached approximately 5,000 milligrams through the combination of electrolyte drinks, salted foods, and liberal use of salt during cooking.

Teaching Points

- Vague instructions to "drink more water and eat more salt" are insufficient. POTS patients need specific numerical targets and practical implementation strategies
- Homemade electrolyte solutions can be as effective as commercial products at a fraction of the cost
- The morning pre-loading strategy (drinking before standing) leverages the physiology of blood volume expansion during the highest-risk period of the day

4.6 Comparing Electrolyte Needs

Sodium gets the most attention in POTS management, but it is not the only electrolyte that matters. **Potassium**, **magnesium**, and **calcium** each play distinct roles in cardiovascular and neuromuscular function.

Potassium works in opposition to sodium to regulate fluid balance, nerve signals, and muscle contractions, including the heart muscle. POTS patients taking fludrocortisone (a medication that increases sodium retention) are particularly vulnerable to potassium depletion because this drug causes the kidneys to excrete extra potassium (Raj, 2013). Signs of low potassium include muscle weakness, cramping, constipation, and heart palpitations, symptoms that overlap with POTS itself.

Magnesium is essential for muscle relaxation, nerve function, and maintaining a steady heart rhythm. Deficiency contributes to muscle cramps, headaches, anxiety, and irregular heartbeat. Many POTS patients report improvement in cramping and headache frequency with magnesium supplementation, though formal trials specific to POTS are limited (Blitshteyn, 2018). The form of magnesium matters: magnesium glycinate is generally well tolerated and less likely to cause diarrhea than magnesium citrate or oxide.

Calcium supports muscle contraction, nerve transmission, and bone health. EDS patients are at particular risk for bone density concerns because of their connective tissue disorder and frequent vitamin D deficiency (Tinkle et al., 2017). Adequate calcium intake, either through diet or supplementation, supports skeletal health in a population that is already at structural disadvantage.

4.7 Commercial Versus Homemade Products

The electrolyte supplement market has exploded in recent years, driven partly by the POTS community's demand. Products range from $0.22 per serving (generic salt capsules) to over $1.50 per serving (premium electrolyte powders with added vitamins). Here is a practical comparison framework:

High-sodium options (500+ milligrams sodium per serving): LMNT (1,000 milligrams sodium, zero sugar, approximately $1.50 per stick), Vitassium capsules (500 milligrams sodium per two capsules, approximately $0.38 per serving), and NormaLyte (approximately 680 milligrams sodium, WHO-based ORS formula, approximately $0.90 per stick on subscription).

Moderate-sodium options (200 to 500 milligrams sodium per serving): Liquid IV (500 milligrams sodium, 11 grams sugar, approximately $1.25 per stick), DripDrop (670 milligrams sodium for the 16-ounce pack, approximately $1.00 per stick), and Thorne Catalyte (485 milligrams sodium, includes methylated folate and B vitamins, approximately $0.79 per scoop).

Budget alternative: Table salt dissolved in water. One-quarter teaspoon of table salt provides approximately 575 milligrams of sodium at a cost of less than one cent. Adding a pinch of potassium-based salt substitute and a tablespoon of honey or sugar creates a functional ORS-style drink for approximately $0.05 to $0.10 per liter.

The bottom line is this: there is no evidence that expensive electrolyte products hydrate better than properly formulated homemade solutions. The advantage of commercial products is convenience, consistent dosing, palatability, and portability. The advantage of homemade solutions is cost savings, which can be substantial given that POTS patients may need three to five servings daily, 365 days per year.

4.8 Fluid Rich Food Sources

Many patients struggle to drink the recommended 2 to 3 liters of fluid daily. One underused strategy is counting **fluid-rich foods** toward the daily total. All beverages and many foods contribute to hydration. The UK PoTS guidelines specifically recommend increasing fluid in foods as a strategy for patients who find it difficult to drink enough volume (PoTS UK, 2023).

Foods with high fluid content include soups and broths (an excellent vehicle for both sodium and fluid), yogurt and custard, ice cream and sorbet, ice pops and ice lollies, jelly (gelatin-based desserts), smoothies, sauces and gravies, and watermelon, cucumber, and other high-water-content produce. A bowl of broth-based soup can contribute 300 to 400 milliliters of fluid along with 800 to 1,200 milligrams of sodium, accomplishing both hydration and sodium targets simultaneously.

Caffeine deserves specific mention. The evidence on caffeine in POTS is mixed. Caffeine is a mild diuretic, which could theoretically worsen dehydration. However, some studies suggest that caffeine may improve alertness and vasoconstriction in patients with orthostatic hypotension (Gibbon et al., 2021). The practical recommendation is moderation. If caffeine is tolerated, it does not need to be eliminated, but it should not be counted as the primary fluid source, and it should be balanced with non-caffeinated fluids.

4.9 Marius's Morning Protocol

Background

Marius, a 41-year-old accountant with POTS and MCAS, experienced his worst symptoms each morning. He described "feeling like my body forgot how to pump blood overnight" and typically needed 30 to 45 minutes of lying in bed before he could stand without severe dizziness. He had been late to work repeatedly and was facing disciplinary action.

Presentation

Overnight, the body naturally reduces blood volume through urine production and insensible fluid loss (perspiration and respiration). For a POTS patient who already has marginal blood volume, this overnight depletion can bring them below their symptomatic threshold by morning. Marius had been getting out of bed immediately upon waking, taking a hot shower (which dilated blood vessels further), and eating nothing until he reached the office.

Analysis

Marius's morning routine was inadvertently maximizing his POTS symptoms. Overnight dehydration, immediate standing, and heat exposure from the shower created a triple challenge for his cardiovascular system. By the time he arrived at work, he was symptomatic, fatigued, and unable to concentrate.

Intervention

Marius adopted a structured morning hydration protocol. He placed a 500-milliliter bottle of electrolyte water on his bedside table each night. Upon waking, before any change in position, he drank the entire bottle while still lying down. He then waited 15 minutes for the fluid to begin absorbing. He sat up slowly, pausing at the edge of the bed for five minutes. He switched from hot showers to lukewarm ones. He ate a small, salted breakfast before leaving home.

Outcome

Within one week, Marius's morning symptoms improved by approximately 50% by his own assessment. He was able to get ready for work within a normal timeframe. He described the pre-loading strategy as "the single most useful thing anyone has ever told me about managing POTS." His afternoon symptoms also improved modestly, likely because starting the day with adequate hydration provided a better baseline for the rest of the day.

Teaching Points

- Overnight fluid loss creates a predictable daily vulnerability for POTS patients, and the morning pre-loading strategy directly addresses this
- Environmental factors like shower temperature and position changes interact with hydration status to determine symptom severity
- Simple behavioral changes (bedside water, delayed standing, temperature modification) can produce clinically meaningful improvement without medication

4.10 Heat and Exercise Strategies

Heat intolerance is one of the most common complaints among POTS patients. Heat causes peripheral vasodilation (blood vessels in the skin and extremities expand), which further reduces the effective circulating blood volume available for the brain and heart. During hot weather or exercise, sweat losses compound the problem by depleting both fluid and sodium.

The practical implications for hydration are straightforward but often underappreciated. On hot days or during exercise, fluid and sodium needs increase beyond the already elevated baseline. A POTS patient who maintains adequate hydration at 2.5 liters per day in a climate-controlled environment may need 3.5 liters or more on a hot day or during even moderate physical activity.

Pre-hydration before exercise is essential. Consuming 500 milliliters of electrolyte water 30 to 60 minutes before physical activity helps ensure adequate blood volume at the start of exercise. During activity, sipping electrolyte fluids every 15 to 20 minutes maintains hydration. Post-exercise, replacement should account for sweat losses. A practical rule of thumb is to drink an additional 500 milliliters of electrolyte water for every 30 minutes of moderate exercise (Cleveland Clinic, 2022).

Compression garments (graduated compression stockings or abdominal binders) work synergistically with hydration during exercise by preventing blood pooling in the lower extremities, effectively keeping more of the expanded blood volume available for circulation. The combination of adequate pre-hydration and compression often allows POTS patients to tolerate exercise that would otherwise trigger near-syncope.

4.11 Putting Knowledge Into Practice

Hydration and sodium management is the single most universally recommended non-pharmacological intervention for POTS. The evidence supporting 2 to 3 liters of daily fluid and 3 to 10 grams of sodium is grounded in expert consensus from the Heart Rhythm Society, the National Institutes of Health, and the Canadian

Cardiovascular Society. These targets exceed general population guidelines by a factor of two to four because POTS patients face a physiological challenge (hypovolemia and autonomic dysfunction) that the general population does not.

The sodium-glucose co-transport system explains why adding a small amount of sugar to electrolyte solutions improves absorption efficiency. The hyperadrenergic subtype of POTS represents an important exception to blanket high-sodium recommendations. Morning pre-loading, fluid-rich foods, and structured hydration schedules are practical tools for achieving daily targets. Commercial electrolyte products offer convenience, but homemade solutions are equally effective at a fraction of the cost.

As we move into Chapter 5.0, we will examine how the same factors that make hydration challenging for trifecta patients (restricted diets, GI dysfunction, malabsorption, and bacterial overgrowth) also place them at elevated risk for micronutrient deficiencies that compound every symptom.

Chapter 5.0: Hidden Micronutrient Deficiencies

A 38-year-old woman with hEDS and POTS has been told by three different doctors that her lab work "looks fine." Her complete blood count is normal. Her basic metabolic panel is normal. Her thyroid function is normal. And yet she can barely get through the day. She is so fatigued that she naps for three hours every afternoon. Her brain fog makes it impossible to read more than a page without losing the thread. Her muscles cramp constantly. Her hair is thinning. She has been told this is "just part of her condition." But no one has checked her vitamin B1, B12, vitamin D, ferritin, magnesium, or folate levels. When a new specialist finally orders these tests, four of the six come back low. Within eight weeks of targeted supplementation, her fatigue improves by 40% and her cramping resolves entirely.

This chapter will address the following:

- Why trifecta patients are at uniquely elevated risk for multiple micronutrient deficiencies
- The specific vitamins and minerals most commonly deficient in this population, including the evidence base for each
- How to request appropriate testing and communicate effectively with healthcare providers
- The dangers of both under-supplementation and over-supplementation, including the cautionary tale of vitamin B6 toxicity

5.1 Why Deficiencies Are Common

Micronutrient deficiency in the trifecta population results from a convergence of at least four independent risk factors, each of which would be concerning on its own. Together, they create a near-guarantee that nutritional gaps will develop if proactive monitoring is not in place.

First, restricted dietary intake. As we explored in Chapter 3.0, the majority of hEDS patients alter their diets in response to GI symptoms, with 62.1% reporting dietary changes in the previous year (Topan et al., 2024). Many patients follow low-histamine, gluten-free, dairy-free, low-FODMAP, or low-oxalate diets (sometimes simultaneously), each of which eliminates food groups that serve as primary sources for specific nutrients. A patient who avoids dairy loses their most convenient source of calcium and vitamin D. A patient who avoids citrus and tomatoes (high-histamine) loses reliable sources of vitamin C. A patient who avoids red meat (often poorly tolerated or high in histamine if not extremely fresh) loses their best source of heme iron and B12.

Second, impaired absorption. Even when trifecta patients eat adequate amounts of nutrient-rich food, GI dysfunction can prevent those nutrients from being properly absorbed. Gastroparesis delays the exposure of food to absorptive surfaces in the small intestine. SIBO can actively consume nutrients (particularly B12 and fat-soluble vitamins) before the host absorbs them. Chronic intestinal inflammation from mast cell activation damages the intestinal lining, reducing its absorptive capacity (DiBaise et al., 2019). Medications commonly prescribed for trifecta patients, particularly proton pump inhibitors (PPIs) for GERD, further impair absorption of B12, magnesium, calcium, and iron (Heidelbaugh, 2013).

Third, increased utilization. Chronic illness increases the body's demand for certain nutrients. Wound healing (common in EDS due to tissue fragility) rapidly consumes vitamin C. Chronic inflammation and immune activation increase the need for antioxidants and anti-inflammatory nutrients. The elevated metabolic stress of managing autonomic dysfunction day after day depletes B vitamins and magnesium (Tseng et al., 2021).

Fourth, increased losses. POTS patients who follow high-fluid, high-sodium regimens excrete more urine, which can flush water-soluble vitamins and minerals. Patients with diarrhea-predominant IBS lose nutrients through rapid transit. Those who experience vomiting from gastroparesis lose whatever nutrients were in the vomited food.

A retrospective study at a tertiary care hospital followed 332 POTS patients for seven years. Of these, a subset of 32 patients (approximately 10%) required formal nutrition support: 66% required intravenous fluids, 59% required enteral nutrition (tube feeding), and 28% required parenteral nutrition (IV nutrition bypassing the GI tract entirely) (Tseng et al., 2021). This represents the severe end of the spectrum, but it illustrates that nutritional compromise in this population is not theoretical. It is documented, common, and sometimes dangerous.

5.2 Thiamine and Energy Metabolism

Vitamin B1 (thiamine) is a water-soluble vitamin that serves as a cofactor for enzymes involved in energy metabolism, particularly the conversion of carbohydrates into usable cellular energy (ATP). Every cell in the body requires thiamine for energy production, but the nervous system and heart are particularly dependent on it because of their high metabolic rates.

Thiamine deficiency produces symptoms that directly overlap with dysautonomia: fatigue, weakness, irritability, poor memory, tachycardia, and peripheral neuropathy (Blitshteyn, 2018). In severe cases, thiamine deficiency causes beriberi, which presents as either "wet" beriberi (cardiovascular symptoms including tachycardia, edema, and heart failure) or "dry" beriberi (neurological symptoms including neuropathy and muscle wasting). The overlap between wet beriberi symptoms and POTS symptoms is striking enough that Blitshteyn (2018) specifically studied B1 levels in POTS patients and found deficiency rates warranting supplementation.

The practical implication is that some portion of POTS patients may be experiencing worse symptoms than necessary because of unrecognized thiamine deficiency. Since thiamine is a water-soluble vitamin with a very wide safety margin, empirical supplementation at 100 to 300 milligrams daily is considered low-risk and is recommended by several dysautonomia specialists pending formal deficiency testing. The preferred form is **benfotiamine** or **thiamine mononitrate**, which have better bioavailability than thiamine hydrochloride (Lonsdale, 2015).

5.3 B12 and Orthostatic Function

Vitamin B12 (cobalamin) is necessary for the formation of red blood cells, the maintenance of nerve myelin sheaths, DNA synthesis, and the proper functioning of the nervous system. B12 deficiency causes a specific type of anemia (megaloblastic anemia) and can produce neurological symptoms including numbness, tingling, balance problems, cognitive impairment, and autonomic dysfunction.

Research has demonstrated that B12 levels are lower in children and adolescents with POTS compared to healthy controls (Oner et al., 2014). This finding is clinically relevant because B12 deficiency can independently cause orthostatic intolerance, meaning that a POTS patient with concurrent B12 deficiency may have worse orthostatic symptoms than their POTS alone would explain. Supplementation in deficient patients has been associated with improvement in orthostatic symptoms, though controlled trials specific to POTS remain limited.

B12 deficiency in trifecta patients can result from several mechanisms. SIBO bacteria in the small intestine can consume dietary B12 before the host absorbs it. Proton pump inhibitors reduce the stomach acid necessary for B12 liberation from food proteins. Patients who avoid or limit animal products (meat, fish, eggs, dairy) remove the only natural dietary sources of B12. Additionally, the intrinsic factor pathway (the specialized absorption mechanism for B12 in the terminal ileum) can be impaired by intestinal inflammation.

Testing for B12 deficiency should include serum B12 levels and **methylmalonic acid (MMA)**, which is a more sensitive indicator. A normal serum B12 with an elevated MMA suggests functional B12 deficiency at the cellular level, a condition that standard B12 testing alone would miss.

5.4 Jessamine's Hidden Deficiency

Background

Jessamine, a 44-year-old librarian with hEDS, POTS, and MCAS, had been managing her conditions for six years. She followed a strict low-histamine, dairy-free, gluten-free diet and took cromolyn sodium, a beta-blocker, and daily electrolyte supplementation. Despite stable MCAS control and consistent POTS management, she noticed progressive worsening of fatigue, increasing numbness in her feet, and difficulty remembering words during conversations. She attributed these symptoms to "getting older with chronic illness."

Presentation

Jessamine's primary care physician had ordered annual basic metabolic panels and complete blood counts for the past three years, all of which returned normal. Her hemoglobin was 13.2 g/dL (normal). Her MCV (mean corpuscular volume) was 96 fL, at the high end of normal but not flagged. She had never been tested for B12, folate, vitamin D, thiamine, iron studies (ferritin), or magnesium.

Analysis

Jessamine's dairy-free, gluten-free, low-histamine diet eliminated most of the dietary sources of B12 (she ate little red meat due to histamine concerns, avoided aged cheeses and yogurt, and consumed limited eggs). She had been taking a PPI for GERD for two years, further impairing B12 absorption. Her peripheral neuropathy (numbness in feet) and cognitive symptoms (word-finding difficulty) were classic presentations of B12 deficiency. Her borderline-high MCV was a subtle clue that red blood cells were larger than optimal, an early sign of megaloblastic changes.

When her new specialist ordered a full micronutrient panel, the results revealed serum B12 at 189 pg/mL (low-normal range starts at 200), MMA elevated at 0.41 µmol/L (confirming functional deficiency), vitamin D at 18 ng/mL (deficient, optimal is 30 to 50), and ferritin at 12 ng/mL (low, optimal is above 30 for symptomatic patients).

Intervention

Jessamine began weekly B12 injections (since oral absorption was compromised by PPI use and potential intestinal inflammation), vitamin D3 supplementation at 5,000 IU daily, and an iron bisglycinate supplement at 25 milligrams every other day (the alternate-day protocol improves absorption). Her PPI was tapered with her gastroenterologist's guidance, and alternative GERD management strategies were implemented.

Outcome

After three months, Jessamine's B12 had risen to 650 pg/mL, her MMA normalized, her vitamin D reached 42 ng/mL, and her ferritin climbed to 35 ng/mL. The numbness in her feet resolved. Her word-finding difficulty improved substantially. Her overall fatigue decreased to a level she described as "back to my baseline, not better than my illness, but not worse from something fixable." She expressed frustration that no one had tested these levels for six years while she assumed her worsening symptoms were inevitable.

Teaching Points

- Standard lab work (CBC, BMP) does not screen for the micronutrient deficiencies most common in the trifecta population; specific testing must be requested
- Dietary restrictions and medication interactions (particularly PPIs) create compounding risk factors for deficiency that may not be obvious to primary care providers unfamiliar with these conditions
- Some symptoms attributed to "just living with chronic illness" may be partially or fully correctable through targeted nutrient repletion

5.5 Vitamin D and Bone Health

Vitamin D functions as both a nutrient and a hormone precursor in the body. It is essential for calcium absorption, bone mineralization, immune system regulation, and cardiovascular function. Low vitamin D levels have been linked to increased orthostatic intolerance and cardiac autonomic dysfunction in multiple studies (Antiel et al., 2011). EDS patients are known to have low vitamin D serum levels at rates exceeding those of the general population (Gensemer et al., 2021).

The recommended supplementation for EDS patients is 5,000 IU of vitamin D3 (cholecalciferol) daily year-round, or at minimum during non-summer months (DiBaise et al., 2019). This exceeds the standard Recommended Dietary Allowance of 600 to 800 IU for the general population, reflecting the elevated needs and frequently documented deficiency in this group. Vitamin D3 is preferred over vitamin D2 (ergocalciferol) because it is more effective at raising and maintaining serum 25-hydroxyvitamin D levels (Tripkovic et al., 2012).

Because vitamin D is fat-soluble, patients with fat malabsorption (common in gastroparesis and SIBO) may have difficulty absorbing oral supplements. Taking vitamin D with a meal containing fat improves absorption. In cases of severe deficiency (serum levels below 20 ng/mL), a loading protocol of 50,000 IU weekly for 8 to 12 weeks may be prescribed before transitioning to a maintenance dose. Monitoring serum 25-hydroxyvitamin D levels every three to six months is advisable during repletion.

5.6 Vitamin C's Multiple Roles

Vitamin C (ascorbic acid) occupies a unique position in trifecta nutrition because it serves three distinct functions relevant to these conditions.

First, vitamin C is a required cofactor in collagen synthesis. Without adequate vitamin C, the body cannot produce properly structured collagen fibers. For EDS patients whose collagen is already structurally compromised, inadequate vitamin C compounds an existing problem. The recommendation for EDS patients is 750 to 1,000 milligrams daily, well above the general RDA of 75 to 90 milligrams (DiBaise et al., 2019). This supports ongoing tissue repair and wound healing.

Second, vitamin C functions as a mast cell stabilizer. Research has shown that vitamin C can reduce histamine levels in the blood and may decrease mast cell degranulation (Hagel et al., 2013). For MCAS patients, this means that vitamin C supplementation may provide a modest anti-histamine effect alongside dietary strategies.

Third, vitamin C is a potent antioxidant that reduces oxidative stress and supports immune function. Chronic illness generates increased oxidative stress, and the anti-inflammatory benefits of vitamin C are well-documented across multiple disease states.

For trifecta patients following a low-histamine diet that restricts citrus fruits, tomatoes, and strawberries (all of which are among the richest dietary sources of vitamin C), supplementation becomes especially important because dietary intake is often inadequate. Buffered vitamin C or sodium ascorbate may be better tolerated than straight ascorbic acid for patients with sensitive stomachs.

5.7 Iron Folate and Magnesium

Three additional micronutrients deserve specific attention in the trifecta population.

Iron is necessary for oxygen transport in hemoglobin and for energy production in mitochondria. Iron deficiency, even in the absence of frank anemia (a condition called **iron deficiency without anemia**), produces fatigue, dizziness, weakness, and exercise intolerance, all of which overlap with POTS symptoms (Raj, 2013). Studies have found that adolescents with POTS are at higher risk for low iron stores. The key marker is **serum ferritin**, which reflects the body's iron storage. A ferritin level below 30 ng/mL in a symptomatic POTS patient warrants supplementation, even if hemoglobin is technically normal. Iron bisglycinate is the preferred form because it causes less GI distress than ferrous sulfate. Alternate-day dosing (taking iron every other day rather than daily) has been shown to improve fractional absorption (Stoffel et al., 2017).

Folate (vitamin B9) supports DNA synthesis, red blood cell formation, and nerve function. Deficiency contributes to fatigue, weakness, and cognitive difficulties. Some trifecta patients carry **MTHFR polymorphisms**, genetic variants that impair the body's ability to convert dietary folate into its active form (methylfolate). For these individuals, supplementing with **methylated folate** (5-MTHF) rather than folic acid is recommended. Several electrolyte products formulated for POTS patients (such as Thorne Catalyte) include methylated folate for this reason.

Magnesium plays a role in over 300 enzymatic reactions in the body, including muscle and nerve function, blood sugar regulation, blood pressure management, and energy production. Magnesium deficiency contributes to muscle cramps, headaches, anxiety, irregular heartbeat, and constipation. POTS patients who drink large volumes of fluid may excrete more magnesium through urine. The preferred supplemental forms are **magnesium glycinate** (well-absorbed, less likely to cause diarrhea, calming effect) and **magnesium threonate** (may support cognitive function by crossing the blood-brain barrier). Magnesium oxide is poorly absorbed and primarily useful as a laxative (Schwalfenberg & Genuis, 2017).

5.8 Cyril's Supplement Overload

Background

Cyril, a 52-year-old retired firefighter, was diagnosed with POTS after a COVID-19 infection in 2022. Frustrated by slow progress with conventional treatment, he began researching supplements online. Over the following 18 months, he accumulated a regimen of 23 daily supplements, including high-dose B complex (containing 100 milligrams of vitamin B6), vitamin D (10,000 IU daily without monitoring), multiple magnesium products (totaling 1,200 milligrams daily), iron (65 milligrams daily without confirmed deficiency), quercetin, NAC, alpha-lipoic acid, CoQ10, fish oil, turmeric, collagen peptides, and several others.

Presentation

Cyril presented to his neurologist with new symptoms: progressive numbness and tingling in his hands and feet, unsteadiness when walking, and burning sensations in his legs. He assumed these were new manifestations of his POTS. Nerve conduction studies revealed a sensory neuropathy.

Analysis

Cyril's neuropathy was traced to **vitamin B6 toxicity (pyridoxine neuropathy)**. His B complex supplement contained 100 milligrams of B6 per dose, and he was taking it twice daily for a total of 200 milligrams. The tolerable upper intake level for B6 is 100 milligrams daily. Chronic intake above this level is well-documented to cause peripheral sensory neuropathy that can be severe and sometimes irreversible (Gdynia et al., 2008). His high-dose iron supplementation without confirmed deficiency risked iron overload. His unsupervised vitamin D at 10,000 IU daily without monitoring risked hypercalcemia. His total magnesium intake exceeded the tolerable upper limit from supplements (350 milligrams), though he had not yet developed symptoms from this.

Intervention

Cyril's B6-containing supplements were immediately discontinued. His vitamin D was reduced to 5,000 IU daily with quarterly monitoring. Iron was stopped pending ferritin testing (which returned at 285 ng/mL, elevated). His magnesium was consolidated to a single product at 400 milligrams daily. His supplement regimen was reduced from 23 products to 8, each with a specific evidence-based rationale tied to his diagnosed conditions.

Outcome

Over six months, Cyril's neuropathy partially improved but did not fully resolve, consistent with the known trajectory of pyridoxine neuropathy, which can leave permanent nerve damage in severe cases. His ferritin normalized after iron cessation. He described the experience as "a wake-up call that more is not better, and that supplements are real medicine with real side effects."

Teaching Points

- Vitamin B6 toxicity is a well-documented cause of peripheral neuropathy that can mimic or worsen the neurological symptoms of dysautonomia; any B-complex supplement should be evaluated for its B6 content

- Unsupervised high-dose supplementation of fat-soluble vitamins (D, A, E, K) and minerals (iron) carries risks of accumulation and toxicity that water-soluble vitamins do not
- Supplement regimens should be built on confirmed deficiencies or evidence-based indications, not on the assumption that more supplementation provides more benefit

5.9 Testing and Doctor Communication

Getting appropriate micronutrient testing can be challenging. Many primary care physicians are accustomed to ordering basic labs (CBC, BMP, thyroid panel) and may not spontaneously think to check the specific micronutrients most relevant to the trifecta. Patients often need to advocate for specific tests.

The following panel represents a reasonable starting point for trifecta patients:

- **Serum B12 and methylmalonic acid (MMA):** Together, these confirm or rule out B12 deficiency more reliably than serum B12 alone
- **Serum folate:** Assesses folate status; low levels warrant supplementation with methylated folate
- **25-hydroxyvitamin D:** The standard test for vitamin D status; optimal levels for trifecta patients are 30 to 50 ng/mL
- **Serum ferritin and total iron-binding capacity (TIBC):** Ferritin reflects iron stores; TIBC provides context about iron metabolism
- **Whole blood thiamine (B1):** More accurate than serum thiamine; deficiency is underrecognized in POTS
- **Serum magnesium or red blood cell (RBC) magnesium:** RBC magnesium is more accurate than serum magnesium because the body maintains serum levels at the expense of intracellular stores
- **Vitamin B6 level:** Especially important if taking B-complex supplements, to screen for both deficiency and excess

When requesting these tests, a straightforward approach works well. You might say: "I have POTS and EDS, and the research literature identifies several micronutrient deficiencies that are common in my conditions and that can worsen my symptoms. I'd like to check B12 with methylmalonic acid, vitamin D, ferritin with TIBC, whole blood thiamine, RBC magnesium, and folate. If any of these are low, targeted supplementation could help my symptoms without adding another medication."

Most physicians will order these tests when presented with a clear, evidence-based rationale. If a provider declines, requesting the reason for refusal in writing often opens the conversation.

5.10 Core Concepts Recap

Trifecta patients face micronutrient deficiency risk from four converging factors: restricted dietary intake, impaired GI absorption, increased metabolic demand from chronic illness, and increased losses through high-volume fluid intake and GI symptoms. Standard lab panels do not screen for the most commonly deficient nutrients in this population. Specific testing for B1, B12 (with MMA), vitamin D, ferritin, folate, and magnesium should be requested proactively.

Thiamine deficiency mimics dysautonomia symptoms and may contribute to POTS severity. B12 deficiency is documented at higher rates in POTS patients and can independently worsen orthostatic intolerance. Vitamin D deficiency is common in EDS and affects bone health, immune function, and cardiovascular regulation. Vitamin C serves triple duty as a collagen synthesis cofactor, mast cell stabilizer, and antioxidant. Iron deficiency without anemia causes fatigue and dizziness that amplify POTS symptoms. Magnesium deficiency contributes to cramping, headaches, and cardiac irritability.

The danger of unsupervised supplementation is real. Vitamin B6 toxicity causes peripheral neuropathy. Iron overload damages the liver. Excessive vitamin D causes hypercalcemia. Supplements are tools, and like any tool, they require informed use. In Chapter 6.0, we will begin building the practical dietary framework that integrates the physiological principles from Chapters 3.0 through 5.0 into a workable daily eating plan.

PART TWO: THE TRIFECTA DIETARY FRAMEWORK

Chapter 6.0: Low Histamine Dietary Foundation

A woman eats a salad for lunch: spinach, cherry tomatoes, avocado, leftover grilled chicken from two days ago, balsamic vinaigrette, and a squeeze of lemon. Every single ingredient in that "healthy" meal is either high in histamine, a histamine liberator, or a DAO enzyme blocker. Within 45 minutes, she develops flushing across her chest, abdominal cramping, diarrhea, and a pounding headache. She has no food allergies. Her IgE testing is clean. But her mast cells have just been flooded with histamine from every direction at once, and her body's primary enzyme for clearing it has been blocked by the alcohol in the vinaigrette. For patients with mast cell activation syndrome, this scenario is not unusual. It is Tuesday.

This chapter will cover the following:

- How histamine accumulates in food through fermentation, aging, and bacterial activity
- The freshness principle and why frozen foods can be safer than supermarket "fresh" foods
- How to identify high-histamine foods, histamine liberators, and DAO enzyme blockers
- Building a low-histamine pantry with safe options across all food groups
- The three-phase elimination and reintroduction protocol
- Why MCAS and histamine intolerance are different conditions requiring different approaches

6.1 How Histamine Forms in Food

Histamine is a biogenic amine produced when bacteria convert the amino acid histidine into histamine through a process called decarboxylation (Maintz & Novak, 2007). This conversion happens naturally during fermentation, aging, curing, smoking, and spoilage. The longer a food sits, the more opportunity bacteria have to produce histamine. Once histamine forms in food, cooking cannot destroy it. Histamine is heat-stable, meaning that boiling, frying, or baking a high-histamine food does not reduce its histamine content (Kovacova-Hanuskova et al., 2015).

This fact carries enormous practical weight. It means that the histamine content of a food is not fixed. A piece of fresh salmon purchased and cooked within hours of being caught contains minimal histamine. That same piece of salmon, left in the refrigerator for three days, may contain enough histamine to trigger symptoms in a sensitive individual. The fish itself hasn't changed. The bacterial activity on its surface has.

Understanding this mechanism reframes the entire approach to food selection for MCAS patients. The question is not simply "is this food high in histamine?" but rather "how much histamine has accumulated in this particular piece of food based on how it was handled, stored, and prepared?" This is what makes dietary histamine management fundamentally different from managing a food allergy, where the problem is the food itself regardless of preparation.

6.2 The Freshness Principle

The freshness principle is the single most useful concept in low-histamine eating. It states that histamine content in food is primarily a function of time and temperature exposure after harvest, slaughter, or preparation (Comas-Basté et al., 2020). Foods that are processed quickly after harvest and stored at very low temperatures contain less histamine than foods that sit at room temperature or in standard refrigeration for extended periods.

This principle produces a counterintuitive conclusion: commercially frozen foods are often safer than "fresh" supermarket foods for histamine-sensitive individuals. A package of flash-frozen salmon fillets that was processed and frozen within hours of being caught contains far less histamine than a "fresh" salmon fillet that traveled for two days in a refrigerated truck, sat in the store's display case for another day, and then spent an additional day in the buyer's refrigerator before cooking. The "fresh" label is misleading because freshness, in the histamine sense, refers to time since biological activity began, not time since the product appeared in the store.

The same logic applies to leftovers. Refrigeration slows bacterial activity but does not stop it. A meal cooked on Monday evening and eaten as leftovers on Wednesday has been accumulating histamine for roughly 48 hours at refrigerator temperature (Sánchez-Pérez et al., 2018). For many MCAS patients, this is enough to push them over their symptomatic threshold. Practical strategies include eating meals immediately after cooking, freezing individual portions within one to two hours of cooking (rather than refrigerating for later consumption), and defrosting only what will be eaten at that meal.

6.3 High Histamine Foods

Certain food categories are consistently high in histamine due to their production methods. Understanding the categories (rather than memorizing long lists) makes the principle portable across cuisines and situations.

Fermented foods are among the highest histamine sources because fermentation is, by definition, controlled bacterial activity. Sauerkraut, kimchi, kombucha, kefir, miso, tempeh, and traditional sourdough all undergo bacterial fermentation that produces substantial histamine (Comas-Basté et al., 2020). This creates a direct conflict with the POTS literature, which often recommends fermented foods for gut health (as discussed in Chapter 2.0). For trifecta patients, this tension must be resolved individually based on tolerance.

Aged cheeses accumulate histamine during the aging process. Parmesan, cheddar, Gouda, blue cheese, and Gruyère can contain very high histamine levels. Fresh cheeses (ricotta, fresh mozzarella, cream cheese, cottage cheese) are generally lower in histamine because they have not undergone extended aging (Maintz & Novak, 2007).

Processed and smoked meats including salami, pepperoni, ham, bacon, hot dogs, and smoked sausage are high in histamine due to curing and smoking processes. Fresh, unprocessed meat that is cooked and consumed promptly is significantly lower in histamine.

Canned fish (tuna, sardines, anchovies, mackerel) tends to be very high in histamine because the fish undergoes processing, storage, and canning over an extended period. Fresh or flash-frozen fish is a substantially safer option (Kovacova-Hanuskova et al., 2015).

Alcohol is problematic for multiple reasons. Wine and beer are fermented products. Red wine contains high levels of histamine itself. Alcohol also blocks DAO enzyme activity, reducing the body's ability to clear histamine from the bloodstream (Maintz & Novak, 2007). For trifecta patients, alcohol combines histamine, DAO blockade, vasodilation (worsening POTS), and dehydration into a single beverage.

Certain vegetables and fruits contain either histamine itself or compounds that trigger histamine release. Spinach, tomatoes, eggplant, and avocado contain histamine. Strawberries, citrus fruits, pineapple, and papaya are classified as histamine liberators. Vinegar (found in most condiments, dressings, and sauces) is a fermented product with high histamine content.

6.4 Liberators and DAO Blockers

Two additional categories of foods cause problems for histamine-sensitive individuals even though the foods themselves may be low in histamine.

Histamine liberators are foods that trigger mast cells to release their stored histamine, independently of the histamine content of the food itself. Citrus fruits, strawberries, pineapple, papaya, tomatoes, egg whites, chocolate, certain food additives (tartrazine, benzoates, sulfites), and some spices fall into this category (Reese et al., 2017). The mechanism is direct mast cell degranulation rather than dietary histamine intake. This means that a person could eat a meal with zero dietary histamine and still experience a histamine-mediated reaction if the meal contains liberators.

Diamine oxidase (DAO) blockers interfere with the body's primary enzyme for breaking down ingested histamine. **DAO** (diamine oxidase) is an enzyme produced primarily in the intestinal lining that metabolizes histamine in the gut before it enters the bloodstream (Comas-Basté et al., 2020). When DAO activity is blocked, even modest amounts of dietary histamine can overwhelm the body's clearance capacity. Known DAO blockers include alcohol, black tea, green tea, energy drinks, and certain medications (NSAIDs, some antibiotics, and some antidepressants). The woman in our opening scenario consumed alcohol (in vinaigrette) alongside multiple high-histamine foods and liberators, effectively disabling her body's ability to process the histamine flood.

6.5 Apollonia's Histamine Discovery

Background

Apollonia, a 27-year-old veterinary technician, was diagnosed with MCAS at age 25 after two years of episodic flushing, hives, abdominal pain, and diarrhea that her gastroenterologist could not explain through standard allergy testing. She had read about low-histamine diets online and attempted to follow one, but found the conflicting food lists on different websites confusing and contradictory. Some sources listed blueberries as safe while others flagged them. Some included chicken as low-histamine while others warned against it.

Presentation

Apollonia arrived at her dietitian appointment with a list of 47 foods she had eliminated. She was eating primarily white rice, boiled zucchini, peeled pears, and chicken breast cooked fresh daily. Despite these severe restrictions, she still experienced symptoms two to three times per week. Her food journal showed no consistent pattern between specific foods and reactions, which increased her frustration and led her to eliminate additional foods each week.

Analysis

The dietitian identified two issues. The first was that Apollonia was not applying the freshness principle consistently. She was buying chicken breast in bulk, storing it in her refrigerator for up to four days, and cooking it on different days. By day three or four, the chicken had accumulated enough histamine from refrigerator storage to trigger symptoms, even though fresh chicken is typically well-tolerated. Her second issue was the inconsistency between online food lists. The dietitian explained that most low-histamine food lists are based on expert opinion rather than standardized laboratory testing, and that individual tolerance varies substantially (Reese et al., 2017). The goal is not to find the "correct" list but to identify personal tolerance through structured elimination and reintroduction.

Intervention

Apollonia adopted a strict freshness protocol: buying protein in smaller quantities, cooking within 24 hours of purchase, freezing individual portions immediately after cooking, and defrosting only what she would eat at that meal. She stopped trying to follow multiple conflicting online lists and instead worked with her dietitian to establish a baseline of consistently tolerated foods using a structured elimination protocol.

Outcome

Within three weeks, Apollonia's symptom frequency dropped from two to three episodes weekly to approximately one every 10 days. More importantly, she identified that her residual symptoms correlated with freshness violations (eating day-old leftovers, using chicken stored for more than 48 hours) rather than with specific foods. She successfully reintroduced blueberries, carrots, sweet potatoes, and fresh mozzarella without incident.

Teaching Points

- Low-histamine food lists from online sources conflict with each other because they are based on varying levels of evidence, making dietitian guidance essential for individualized application
- The freshness principle often accounts for more symptom variability than specific food choices, and applying it consistently can be more effective than eliminating additional foods
- Bulk purchasing and multi-day refrigerator storage of proteins is a common, overlooked source of histamine accumulation

6.6 The Low Histamine Pantry

Building a functional low-histamine pantry requires identifying reliably tolerated options across all macronutrient categories. The following lists represent foods that are generally lower in histamine when purchased fresh and prepared promptly. Individual tolerance will vary, and these lists should be used as starting points rather than absolute rules (Joneja, 2017).

Lower-histamine proteins include fresh or flash-frozen chicken, turkey, lamb, and most fresh-caught or flash-frozen white fish (cod, halibut, sole, tilapia). Eggs are tolerated by many individuals, though egg whites can act as histamine liberators in some. Fresh, unprocessed beef is generally tolerated if cooked within 24 hours of purchase.

Lower-histamine vegetables include zucchini, yellow squash, carrots, sweet potatoes, broccoli, cauliflower, asparagus, lettuce (romaine, butter), cucumber, green beans, and bell peppers (though some individuals react to peppers as nightshades).

Lower-histamine fruits include blueberries, blackberries, apples, pears, peaches, mangoes, grapes, cherries, and watermelon. Citrus fruits, strawberries, and pineapple should be avoided or tested individually.

Lower-histamine grains include rice (white and brown), quinoa, oats, millet, and amaranth. Most gluten-free flours (rice flour, tapioca, arrowroot) are well tolerated from a histamine perspective, though gluten-containing grains may need separate evaluation as discussed in Chapter 7.0.

Lower-histamine fats and oils include olive oil, coconut oil, ghee (clarified butter), and most seed oils (sunflower, safflower). Butter is generally tolerated. Avocado and avocado oil are higher in histamine and should be tested individually.

Lower-histamine seasonings include fresh herbs (basil, oregano, thyme, rosemary, parsley, cilantro), salt, garlic (fresh), ginger (fresh), turmeric, and black pepper in small amounts. Vinegar, soy sauce, fish sauce, and pre-made spice blends (which often contain unstated ingredients) should be avoided.

6.7 Beyond Histamine Alone

Some trifecta patients find that a low-histamine diet improves but does not resolve their symptoms. In these cases, additional food sensitivities may be layering on top of histamine intolerance. The most common overlapping sensitivities include oxalates, salicylates, lectins, and FODMAPs (Beckers et al., 2021).

Oxalates are compounds found in many plant foods (spinach, beet greens, rhubarb, sweet potatoes, almonds, chocolate) that can accumulate in tissues and cause pain, kidney stones, and inflammation in sensitive individuals. Some MCAS patients report worsening with high-oxalate foods, though the research connecting oxalate sensitivity to mast cell activation specifically is limited.

Salicylates are naturally occurring chemicals in many fruits, vegetables, herbs, and spices that can trigger reactions in susceptible individuals. Salicylate sensitivity overlaps with MCAS in symptom presentation (flushing, GI symptoms, respiratory symptoms) and can confuse diagnostic efforts (Raithel et al., 2005).

FODMAPs (fermentable oligosaccharides, disaccharides, monosaccharides, and polyols) are short-chain carbohydrates that are poorly absorbed in the small intestine and fermented by gut bacteria, producing gas, bloating, and altered bowel habits. As discussed in section 3.3, up to 62% of hEDS patients meet IBS criteria (Choudhary et al., 2021), making FODMAP sensitivity common in this population.

The critical caution here is against layering multiple restrictive diets simultaneously without professional guidance. As we saw with Dorothea in section 3.9, stacking low-histamine, low-oxalate, low-FODMAP, and gluten-free restrictions can rapidly lead to caloric and nutritional inadequacy. Each additional restriction should be tested individually, with clear evidence of benefit before it becomes permanent.

6.8 MCAS Versus Histamine Intolerance

A distinction that is frequently overlooked, even in some clinical settings, is the difference between **histamine intolerance** and **mast cell activation syndrome**. These are not the same condition, and they do not respond identically to dietary intervention.

Histamine intolerance is a condition in which the body cannot adequately break down ingested histamine, typically due to reduced DAO enzyme activity. The problem is primarily in the gut, and the solution is primarily dietary: reduce histamine intake, avoid DAO blockers, and possibly supplement with DAO enzyme capsules before meals (Maintz & Novak, 2007). Patients with pure histamine intolerance tend to respond predictably to low-histamine diets.

MCAS is a systemic condition in which mast cells throughout the body release excessive amounts of histamine and over 1,000 other chemical mediators (tryptase, prostaglandins, leukotrienes, cytokines, heparin, and others) in response to a wide range of triggers (Afrin et al., 2016). As discussed in section 3.5, only 3.4% of self-reported food reactions in mastocytosis patients were confirmed as IgE-mediated allergies (Vlieg-Boerstra et al., 2005). The remaining reactions involve nonimmunological mast cell activation that can be triggered by stress, temperature changes, hormonal fluctuations, medications, infections, and physical exertion in addition to dietary histamine.

This distinction matters for dietary management because not all MCAS patients will benefit from a strict low-histamine diet. If a patient's primary mast cell triggers are heat, stress, and hormonal changes rather than dietary histamine, restricting food may accomplish little beyond reducing nutritional adequacy and quality of life. The three-phase protocol described in the next sections helps determine if dietary histamine is a meaningful trigger for each individual patient.

6.9 The Three Phase Protocol

The structured elimination and reintroduction protocol consists of three phases designed to establish a baseline, stabilize symptoms, and systematically identify individual triggers (Reese et al., 2017).

Phase 1: Elimination (two to four weeks). During this phase, the patient removes all known high-histamine foods, histamine liberators, and DAO blockers from their diet. The goal is to reduce the overall histamine load to the lowest practical level and observe if symptoms improve. This phase should not last longer than four weeks, as prolonged elimination increases the risk of nutritional deficiency (as discussed in Chapter 5.0) and can make reintroduction psychologically more difficult. During elimination, the patient eats only from the lower-histamine food lists described in section 6.6, applies the freshness principle rigorously, and maintains a daily food and symptom journal.

Phase 2: Stabilization and symptom tracking (one to two weeks). Once symptom improvement is observed (or if no improvement occurs after four weeks, which is itself useful diagnostic information), the patient holds steady on the elimination diet while carefully tracking symptom patterns. The purpose of this phase is to establish a reliable symptom baseline against which reintroductions can be measured. A symptom scoring system helps quantify daily symptom burden using a standardized scale.

Phase 3: Systematic reintroduction (four to eight weeks or longer). One food or food category is reintroduced at a time. The patient eats a moderate portion of the test food on day one, then waits 48 to 72 hours while monitoring for symptom changes. Some mast cell reactions are delayed by 24 to 48 hours, making this waiting period essential (Joneja, 2017). If no symptoms occur, the food is added to the "tolerated" list. If symptoms occur, the food is removed and the patient returns to baseline for several days before testing the next food. Keeping a detailed food journal during this phase allows patterns to emerge over weeks that would be invisible on a day-to-day basis.

6.10 Gawain's Reintroduction Protocol

Background

Gawain, a 36-year-old software developer with MCAS and hEDS, had been on a strict low-histamine elimination diet for 11 months. His initial elimination period had produced noticeable symptom improvement, and he had never moved beyond Phase 1. He was eating approximately 12 foods and experienced significant social isolation because he could not eat at restaurants, attend social gatherings involving food, or travel comfortably.

Presentation

Gawain's dietitian expressed concern that 11 months of uninterrupted elimination was excessive and carried nutritional risks. His vitamin D was low, his protein intake was borderline, and his caloric intake hovered around 1,400 calories daily. He had developed anxiety about reintroduction, describing a fear that "if I add anything back and react, I'll lose all the progress I've made." His MCAS specialist confirmed that his mast cell symptoms were well-controlled on medication (H1 and H2 antihistamines plus cromolyn sodium).

Analysis

Gawain's case illustrates the phenomenon of elimination diet entrenchment, where the psychological comfort of symptom control during elimination creates resistance to moving forward to reintroduction. The longer a patient remains in elimination, the more the diet becomes an identity rather than a diagnostic tool. Meanwhile, his nutritional status deteriorated and his social functioning suffered. The mast cell stabilizing medications had been addressing much of his baseline mast cell activity, meaning that many foods he was avoiding might now be tolerated.

Intervention

A structured reintroduction schedule was created, starting with foods most likely to be tolerated (fresh fruits like peaches, additional vegetables like sweet potatoes and carrots) before testing higher-risk categories (aged cheese, tomatoes). Reintroductions occurred on Saturdays so Gawain could monitor symptoms over the weekend without work stress confounding the results. His dietitian met with him weekly to review the food journal and adjust the schedule.

Outcome

Over eight weeks, Gawain successfully reintroduced 15 foods, expanding his diet to 27 items. He tolerated peaches, sweet potatoes, carrots, fresh mozzarella, blueberries, grapes, broccoli, asparagus, lamb, turkey, ghee, fresh ginger, and quinoa. He did not tolerate aged cheddar (flushing and GI symptoms within four hours), canned tuna (headache and nausea), or strawberries (hives within two hours). His caloric intake increased to 1,900 calories, and his protein intake reached target levels. He attended a dinner party for the first time in a year.

Teaching Points

- Elimination diets are diagnostic tools with defined timelines, not permanent dietary states, and should always progress to reintroduction
- Mast cell stabilizing medications can expand dietary tolerance by reducing baseline mast cell reactivity, making reintroduction possible for foods previously not tolerated
- Structured reintroduction with 48 to 72 hour observation windows and detailed journaling produces actionable data about individual tolerance patterns

6.11 Food Journal and Scoring

A food and symptom journal is the most useful tool in the three-phase protocol. Without systematic tracking, patterns remain invisible because MCAS reactions can be delayed by 24 to 48 hours and because multiple variables (stress, sleep, hormonal cycles, weather, exercise) interact with dietary triggers (Afrin et al., 2016).

An effective food journal captures the following for each eating occasion: the time of the meal, all foods consumed (including brands for packaged items), how the food was prepared (fresh, frozen, leftover, number of days since cooking), estimated portion size, and any symptoms that follow within the next 24 to 48 hours. A simple symptom scoring system assigns a severity rating from 0 (no symptoms) to 3 (severe, interfering with function) across key categories: skin (flushing, hives, itching), GI (nausea, cramping, diarrhea, bloating), neurological (headache, brain fog, dizziness), cardiovascular (tachycardia, blood pressure changes), and respiratory (nasal congestion, throat tightness).

Over time, patterns emerge. A patient might discover that they tolerate chicken breast cooked and eaten immediately but react when eating it as next-day leftovers. They might find that tomatoes trigger symptoms when eaten in combination with other moderate-histamine foods but are tolerated in isolation when total histamine load is low. These nuanced patterns are impossible to detect without systematic tracking and impossible to predict from generic food lists alone.

6.12 Chapter Conclusions

Dietary histamine management in MCAS is governed by the freshness principle: histamine accumulates in food as a function of time and bacterial activity, and managing that accumulation matters more than memorizing fixed food lists. High-histamine foods, histamine liberators, and DAO blockers represent three distinct categories that each contribute to the total histamine load through different mechanisms. A low-histamine pantry can be built from reliably tolerated foods across all macronutrient categories, but individual tolerance varies and must be determined through structured testing.

The three-phase protocol (elimination, stabilization, reintroduction) transforms the low-histamine diet from a permanent restriction into a diagnostic tool that produces actionable information about individual triggers. MCAS and histamine intolerance are distinct conditions, and not all MCAS patients will benefit equally from dietary histamine restriction. Food journals with standardized symptom scoring provide the data necessary to distinguish genuine dietary triggers from coincidental symptom fluctuation. In Chapter 7.0, we will address the challenge of achieving high sodium intake for POTS management while remaining compatible with the low-histamine foundation established here.

Chapter 7.0: High Sodium POTS Strategy

A 31-year-old man newly diagnosed with POTS sits across from his cardiologist, who has just told him to eat 8 to 10 grams of salt every day. He stares at the doctor as if she has suggested he drink motor oil. For his entire adult life, he has been told that salt causes high blood pressure, heart disease, and stroke. He has been choosing low-sodium options at the grocery store, avoiding salting his food, and feeling virtuous about it. Now he is being told that everything he believed about salt is, for his specific condition, exactly backwards. And he needs to make that mental shift while simultaneously learning which salty foods are compatible with his MCAS and which ones are not. This chapter addresses both the psychological barrier and the practical strategy.

This chapter will cover the following:

- How to overcome the ingrained belief that salt is harmful and reframe sodium as a medical intervention
- Practical strategies for achieving 3 to 10 grams of sodium daily through food and supplements
- A curated list of high-sodium foods that are also trifecta-compatible (low-histamine and GI-friendly)
- Why smaller, frequent meals prevent postprandial blood pooling
- The relationship between blood sugar, POTS symptoms, and histamine release
- Evidence on gluten, caffeine, and alcohol in the POTS population

7.1 Reframing Salt as Medicine

The psychological barrier to high-sodium eating is real and should not be dismissed. Decades of public health messaging have established a deep association between salt and cardiovascular disease. The Dietary Guidelines for Americans recommend limiting sodium to 2,300 milligrams daily, and many health-conscious individuals aim even lower (U.S. Department of Agriculture, 2020). For a person who has internalized these messages, being told to consume three to five times the recommended amount feels wrong at a visceral level.

The reframing begins with understanding that public health recommendations are designed for the general population, the majority of whom do not have autonomic dysfunction or chronic hypovolemia. POTS patients occupy a specific physiological niche in which the standard rules do not apply. As discussed in section 4.2, the 2021 Expert Consensus Review (Vernino et al., 2021), the 2015 Heart Rhythm Society Expert Consensus Statement (Sheldon et al., 2015), and the

Canadian Cardiovascular Society Position Statement (Raj et al., 2020) all endorse elevated sodium intake for POTS patients. These are not fringe recommendations. They represent the consensus of the world's leading autonomic medicine specialists.

A practical way to think about it: sodium for POTS functions like insulin for diabetes. No one would tell a diabetic person that they shouldn't take insulin because insulin is "dangerous" for people without diabetes. The same logic applies to sodium in POTS. The therapeutic target exists because the underlying condition creates a specific physiological need.

7.2 Achieving Sodium Through Food

Supplements and electrolyte drinks (discussed in section 4.7) are useful tools, but food remains the most palatable and sustainable vehicle for sodium intake. Achieving 3,000 to 10,000 milligrams of sodium daily through food requires both deliberate food selection and cooking strategies.

Cooking with salt. The simplest approach is to salt food liberally during cooking and again at the table. One-quarter teaspoon of table salt contains approximately 575 milligrams of sodium. Adding half a teaspoon of salt to each of five or six daily eating occasions contributes approximately 3,450 milligrams before counting the sodium already present in the foods themselves. Sea salt, kosher salt, and Himalayan pink salt all provide sodium in roughly equivalent amounts per gram; the differences in trace minerals are nutritionally negligible (Harris, 2022).

Broth and soup. A single cup of commercially prepared chicken broth contains 800 to 1,000 milligrams of sodium. Drinking two cups of broth daily contributes 1,600 to 2,000 milligrams. For MCAS patients, homemade broth using fresh chicken or turkey bones (cooked for a shorter duration of two to four hours rather than the 24-hour bone broth popular in wellness circles) is safer from a histamine perspective because shorter cooking times produce less histamine accumulation (Comas-Basté et al., 2020). The broth should be consumed immediately or frozen in portions rather than stored in the refrigerator.

Salted snacks and condiments. Salted rice cakes, salted nuts (if tolerated), pretzels (if gluten is tolerated), salted popcorn, and salted roasted chickpeas provide sodium between meals. Olives provide excellent sodium content but may be problematic for some MCAS patients due to the brining process. Pickles are high in sodium but are fermented, creating a histamine concern.

7.3 Trifecta Compatible Salty Foods

The challenge unique to trifecta patients is that many traditional high-sodium foods are also high in histamine, making them unsuitable. Deli meats, aged cheeses, soy sauce, fish sauce, and many canned soups fall into both categories simultaneously. The following foods are both high in sodium and generally compatible with a low-histamine, GI-friendly approach:

Fresh chicken or turkey breast seasoned generously with salt and herbs; salted rice (prepared with added salt and butter or ghee); salted sweet potato wedges; salted roasted root vegetables (carrots, parsnips, turnips); homemade broth (short-cooked, from fresh ingredients); salted nut butters (almond butter, sunflower seed butter with added salt); salted rice cakes; salted popcorn (air-popped with added salt and oil); saltine or rice crackers; cottage cheese (fresh, not aged); miso paste in small amounts (fermented but tolerated by some at low doses); celery with salt and nut butter; baked potato with salt, butter, and fresh herbs; scrambled eggs with added salt; oatmeal with salt and maple syrup; roasted chickpeas with salt.

These 15 options span breakfast, lunch, dinner, and snack occasions. Each can be seasoned with additional salt beyond what a typical recipe would call for. The goal is to make every eating occasion contribute to the daily sodium target rather than relying solely on supplements or dedicated "salt loading" moments.

7.4 Meal Timing and Blood Pooling

The autonomic nervous system coordinates the redistribution of blood flow during digestion. After eating, blood flow increases to the splanchnic circulation (the blood vessels supplying the stomach, intestines, liver, and spleen) to support nutrient absorption. In a healthy person, compensatory vasoconstriction elsewhere in the body maintains blood pressure. In POTS patients, this compensation is impaired, leading to **postprandial hypotension**, a drop in blood pressure after eating that triggers tachycardia, dizziness, and fatigue (Mehr et al., 2018).

Larger meals require more splanchnic blood flow than smaller meals. This is why smaller, more frequent meals (four to six eating occasions per day rather than two or three large ones) are consistently recommended for POTS patients (Ganesh et al., 2020). Dividing the same total caloric intake across more eating occasions reduces the hemodynamic challenge at any single meal. A practical framework involves three smaller main meals plus two to three snacks, with each eating occasion contributing to fluid, sodium, and protein targets.

Post-meal positioning also matters. Lying flat after eating increases blood pooling in the splanchnic vessels. Sitting upright or reclining at a 30 to 45 degree angle for 20 to 30 minutes after eating helps maintain cerebral blood flow during the postprandial period. This recommendation overlaps with GERD management advice, as upright positioning also reduces acid reflux (discussed further in section 8.2).

7.5 Berenice's Salt Transition

Background

Berenice, a 45-year-old high school biology teacher, was diagnosed with POTS after developing post-COVID dysautonomia in 2023. For 20 years, she had followed a low-sodium diet due to a family history of hypertension. Her father had died of a stroke at 62, and her mother had been on blood pressure medication since age 50. When her cardiologist prescribed 6 to 8 grams of sodium daily, Berenice experienced intense anxiety. She described feeling like she was "poisoning myself with every pinch of salt."

Presentation

Three weeks into her POTS treatment, Berenice's sodium intake remained at approximately 2,800 milligrams daily, well below her prescribed target. She was drinking electrolyte water but diluting it to half concentration because the salty taste made her anxious. She was not adding salt to her cooking. Her POTS symptoms remained severe: near-syncope episodes twice daily, resting heart rate of 112, and inability to stand for more than five minutes.

Analysis

Berenice's case demonstrates the clash between lifelong health messaging and condition-specific medical needs. Her fear was not irrational. In the general population, high sodium intake does correlate with elevated blood pressure. But Berenice did not have hypertension. She had POTS with documented hypovolemia. Her blood pressure was typically 90/58 mmHg supine and dropped further upon standing. The sodium prescription was addressing her actual physiological deficit, not working against it. Her cardiologist explained that patients with autonomic dysfunction and low blood volume process sodium differently than the general population (Garland et al., 2021).

Intervention

A graded approach helped Berenice adjust psychologically and physically. Week one: add a half-teaspoon of salt to each meal (additional 1,725 milligrams). Week two: begin full-concentration electrolyte drinks twice daily (additional 1,000 to 2,000 milligrams). Week three: introduce salted snacks between meals (additional 500 to 1,000 milligrams). Her blood pressure and heart rate were monitored weekly to demonstrate that sodium was improving rather than worsening her cardiovascular parameters.

Outcome

By week four, Berenice's sodium intake reached approximately 5,500 milligrams daily. Her standing heart rate dropped from 142 to 118. Her blood pressure improved to 100/65 supine. Near-syncope episodes decreased from twice daily to two to three times weekly. She described the psychological shift as "the hardest part of the whole diagnosis, harder than accepting I was sick."

Teaching Points

- The psychological barrier to high-sodium eating is a legitimate clinical challenge, especially for patients with family histories of hypertension or cardiovascular disease
- Graded sodium increases with concurrent blood pressure and heart rate monitoring help patients see objective evidence that sodium is therapeutic for their condition
- POTS patients with hypovolemia and low blood pressure metabolize sodium differently than the general population, and general dietary guidelines do not apply to their situation

7.6 Blood Sugar and POTS

High-glycemic foods (those that cause rapid blood sugar spikes) worsen POTS symptoms through several interconnected mechanisms. When blood sugar rises rapidly, the body releases insulin to drive glucose into cells. If insulin overshoots (reactive hypoglycemia), blood sugar drops below baseline, triggering an adrenergic response: the sympathetic nervous system releases catecholamines (adrenaline and norepinephrine) to raise blood sugar (Shibao et al., 2005). In POTS patients, this adrenergic surge amplifies existing sympathetic overdrive, worsening tachycardia, tremor, and anxiety.

Additionally, high-carbohydrate meals increase splanchnic blood flow more than protein-rich or fat-rich meals, exacerbating postprandial blood pooling (Mehr et al., 2018). There is also emerging evidence that rapid blood sugar fluctuations may trigger mast cell degranulation in some individuals, linking glycemic instability to MCAS symptom flares (Theoharides et al., 2019).

Protein-forward eating addresses this by stabilizing blood sugar and reducing postprandial blood pooling. Including 15 to 25 grams of protein at each eating occasion (a palm-sized portion of chicken, a serving of cottage cheese, two eggs, or a scoop of collagen peptides in a smoothie) slows gastric emptying, blunts blood sugar spikes, and provides the amino acids necessary for tissue repair in EDS. This approach aligns with the smaller, more frequent meals strategy: six eating occasions with 15 to 20 grams of protein each produces 90 to 120 grams of daily protein, meeting the needs of most adults (Ganesh et al., 2020).

7.7 The Gluten Question

Research suggests that POTS patients have higher rates of both celiac disease and non-celiac gluten sensitivity than the general population. A study by Penny et al. (2016) found that 4% of POTS patients tested positive for celiac disease compared to approximately 1% background prevalence, a fourfold increase. Even more striking, 42% of POTS patients reported gluten intolerance compared to 19% in the comparison group.

A separate study by Zha et al. (2022) surveyed 20 POTS patients who had voluntarily adopted a gluten-free diet and found that 45% reported symptom reduction. While this was a small, uncontrolled survey (and self-reported data should be interpreted cautiously), it adds to the accumulating evidence that gluten may be a contributing factor for a meaningful subset of POTS patients.

The practical recommendation is not that all POTS patients should adopt a gluten-free diet. Rather, patients who continue to experience GI symptoms, brain fog, or fatigue despite adequate hydration, sodium, and other interventions should consider a structured gluten trial: eliminating gluten for four to six weeks and monitoring symptoms systematically. If symptoms improve, a deliberate reintroduction (eating gluten-containing foods for one to two weeks) can confirm the connection. If symptoms return, the data supports ongoing gluten avoidance.

7.8 Caffeine and Alcohol Evidence

Caffeine presents a genuinely mixed picture for POTS patients. On one hand, caffeine is a vasoconstrictor that can temporarily increase blood pressure and reduce orthostatic symptoms in some patients (Gibbon et al., 2021). On the other hand, caffeine is a stimulant that can worsen tachycardia, anxiety, and sleep disruption. It is also a mild diuretic that could theoretically counteract hydration efforts, though the diuretic effect of habitual caffeine consumption is modest (Killer et al., 2014).

The evidence does not support a blanket recommendation for or against caffeine in POTS. Individual response varies. Some patients find that a morning coffee improves alertness and reduces morning orthostatic symptoms. Others find that caffeine triggers palpitations and anxiety. Caffeine can also trigger mast cell degranulation in some MCAS patients (Theoharides et al., 2019). A reasonable approach is to maintain existing caffeine habits if they are not causing problems, to reduce or eliminate caffeine if symptoms suggest it is a trigger, and to avoid using caffeine as a substitute for adequate hydration.

Alcohol is a different story. The evidence against alcohol consumption in trifecta patients is consistent and multi-directional. Alcohol causes vasodilation, directly worsening POTS symptoms by dilating blood vessels and reducing effective circulating volume (Vernino et al., 2021). Alcohol is a fermented product containing histamine, triggering MCAS symptoms. Alcohol blocks DAO enzyme activity, reducing the body's ability to clear histamine (Maintz & Novak, 2007). Alcohol causes dehydration by suppressing antidiuretic hormone. And alcohol impairs proprioception and balance, which is already compromised in EDS patients with joint instability. The combination of vasodilation, histamine, DAO blockade, and dehydration in a single substance makes alcohol one of the few dietary categories where a clear recommendation against consumption is supported by convergent evidence.

7.9 Simeon's Meal Restructuring

Background

Simeon, a 39-year-old construction foreman, was diagnosed with POTS and suspected MCAS following a bout of COVID-19. He had been eating two large meals daily (a late breakfast and an evening dinner) with no snacks. His meals were typically high in carbohydrates: large bowls of pasta, sandwiches on white bread, or takeout pizza. He had been told to eat more salt but found it difficult to integrate into his existing eating pattern.

Presentation

Simeon reported severe postprandial symptoms after both meals: tachycardia (heart rate spiking to 140 after dinner), lightheadedness, brain fog lasting one to two hours after eating, and afternoon fatigue so severe he sometimes had to sit in his truck for 30 minutes before driving home. His sodium intake was approximately 3,200 milligrams (mostly from processed foods), and his fluid intake was about 1.5 liters including coffee.

Analysis

Simeon's two-meal pattern created enormous postprandial hemodynamic stress. Each meal was large enough to require substantial splanchnic blood flow redistribution. His high-carbohydrate food choices amplified postprandial blood pooling and likely produced reactive hypoglycemia contributing to afternoon crashes. His sodium intake, while above general population recommendations, was well below his POTS target. His fluid intake was half the minimum recommendation.

Intervention

The dietitian restructured Simeon's eating into six occasions: a small breakfast, a mid-morning snack, lunch, an afternoon snack, dinner, and an evening snack. Each occasion included a protein source and was salted generously. His carbohydrate sources shifted from high-glycemic (white bread, pasta) to lower-glycemic (sweet potatoes, rice with protein, oatmeal with nut butter). His fluid intake increased to 2.5 liters with three electrolyte servings per day. His processed food intake was reduced (eliminating high-histamine deli meats and aged cheese) and replaced with freshly cooked proteins.

Outcome

Within two weeks, Simeon's postprandial tachycardia decreased from peaks of 140 to peaks of 115. His afternoon crashes became significantly less severe. His brain fog after meals shortened from one to two hours to approximately 20 minutes. He described the transition as "eating like a hobbit" (six meals a day) and initially resisted it, but the rapid symptom improvement motivated compliance.

Teaching Points

- Large, infrequent meals create disproportionate postprandial hemodynamic stress in POTS patients compared to smaller, more frequent eating occasions
- Shifting from high-glycemic carbohydrate sources to lower-glycemic options with protein reduces reactive hypoglycemia and sympathetic nervous system activation
- Meal restructuring can produce measurable cardiovascular improvement within days, making it one of the fastest-acting dietary interventions for POTS

7.10 Essential Points to Remember

High sodium intake for POTS patients is a medical intervention supported by multiple expert consensus statements, not a dietary indulgence. The psychological barrier to eating "too much salt" is real, especially for patients with family histories of cardiovascular disease, and should be addressed through education and gradual exposure with objective monitoring. Achieving 3 to 10 grams of sodium daily works through a combination of liberal cooking salt, broth, salted snacks, and electrolyte products.

Smaller, more frequent meals (four to six daily eating occasions) reduce postprandial blood pooling and its associated symptoms. Protein-forward eating stabilizes blood sugar and reduces reactive hypoglycemia. POTS patients have elevated rates of celiac disease and gluten sensitivity, warranting a structured trial for symptomatic patients. Caffeine effects are individually variable and require personal assessment. Alcohol combines vasodilation, histamine, DAO blockade, and dehydration, making it the clearest dietary restriction for trifecta patients. In Chapter 8.0, we will address the specific GI challenges of eating with EDS, including gastroparesis, reflux, and the practical difficulties of food preparation with joint hypermobility and fatigue.

Chapter 8.0: Eating with EDS

A 33-year-old woman with hypermobile EDS stands in her kitchen at 6 PM, exhausted after a day of managing joint pain and fatigue. She needs to cook dinner, but her hands ache and her grip strength has faded after using her computer all day. She reaches for a can of soup (easy to prepare, minimal effort) but stops. The canned soup is high in histamine. She considers making a salad but knows the raw vegetables will aggravate her gastroparesis. She thinks about ordering takeout but the restaurant food will be reheated (histamine accumulation) and likely high in fat (worsening reflux). She eventually eats a handful of crackers and goes to bed hungry. This is not a failure of motivation. It is the collision of GI dysfunction, dietary restrictions, physical limitations, and fatigue that defines eating with EDS.

This chapter will cover the following:

- Gastroparesis-friendly eating strategies adapted for trifecta patients
- Dietary management of GERD and functional dyspepsia in the EDS population
- How IBS interacts with low-histamine and high-sodium requirements
- Why protein intake is particularly important (and particularly challenging) in EDS
- Nutrients that support collagen synthesis and connective tissue health
- Adaptive kitchen strategies for managing food preparation with hypermobility, pain, and fatigue
- When to discuss enteral nutrition or supplemental feeding with your medical team

8.1 Gastroparesis Friendly Eating

As we established in section 3.2, EDS patients have a 12.26 times higher odds ratio for gastroparesis compared to the general population (Thwaites et al., 2022). For these patients, the stomach functions as a bottleneck: food enters but does not exit at a normal rate. Everything that follows in the digestive process is affected by this initial delay. Gastroparesis-friendly eating addresses this bottleneck through several coordinated strategies.

Meal volume reduction is the first line of defense. A gastroparetic stomach that struggles to process 500 milliliters will often handle 200 to 250 milliliters without triggering nausea, vomiting, or severe bloating. This means splitting caloric intake across six or more smaller eating occasions rather than concentrating it in two or three meals. Each occasion should be small enough to feel comfortable, even if that means eating every two to three hours (Steiner et al., 2023).

Texture modification can dramatically affect tolerability. Liquids and purees empty from the stomach faster than solid foods, and soft solids empty faster than raw, crunchy, or fibrous foods. On days when gastroparesis is severe, shifting toward smoothies (with protein powder, nut butter, and tolerated fruits), soups (short-cooked broth with soft vegetables and shredded protein), and well-cooked grains (oatmeal, congee, soft rice) maintains nutrition while reducing the mechanical work the stomach must perform. On better days, softer solid foods can be reintroduced.

Fiber management requires nuance. In a normally functioning GI tract, fiber promotes healthy motility and supports the gut microbiome. In a gastroparetic stomach, insoluble fiber (found in raw vegetable skins, whole grain husks, and fruit peels) can form obstructive masses called bezoars. This does not mean eliminating all fiber. Soluble fiber (found in oatmeal, peeled fruits, cooked vegetables, and chia seeds when fully hydrated) is generally better tolerated because it absorbs water and forms a gel rather than remaining as rigid particles (Thwaites et al., 2022). Peeling fruits and vegetables, cooking them thoroughly, and avoiding raw salads on bad gastroparesis days are practical adjustments.

Fat distribution matters because fat is the macronutrient that most slows gastric emptying. This does not mean avoiding fat (which would compromise caloric intake and nutrient absorption). Rather, it means distributing fat intake across multiple small meals rather than concentrating it in one large, fat-rich meal. A tablespoon of olive oil on each of five small meals is better tolerated than five tablespoons in a single dinner.

8.2 GERD Dietary Management

Gastroesophageal reflux disease (GERD) is common in EDS patients because the lower esophageal sphincter (the muscular valve that prevents stomach acid from flowing back into the esophagus) is composed of smooth muscle and connective tissue that may be laxer than normal (Thwaites et al., 2022). Gastroparesis compounds the problem by increasing gastric pressure against this weakened valve.

Dietary GERD management in trifecta patients involves timing, positioning, and trigger identification rather than blanket food avoidance. The traditional list of "GERD foods to avoid" (chocolate, coffee, spicy food, citrus, tomatoes, mint) was developed for the general population, and many of these foods are already restricted on a low-histamine diet (citrus, tomatoes). For trifecta patients who are already following a low-histamine protocol, additional GERD-specific restrictions may be unnecessary (Duncanson et al., 2021).

Timing and positioning strategies include: eating the last meal or snack at least two to three hours before lying down; remaining upright or reclined at 30 to 45 degrees for 30 minutes after eating; elevating the head of the bed by six to eight inches for nighttime reflux; and avoiding drinking large volumes of fluid during meals (which increases gastric volume and pressure), instead sipping fluid between meals. These strategies are compatible with POTS hydration targets because they redirect fluid intake to between-meal periods rather than eliminating it.

8.3 IBS Compatible Strategies

The **low-FODMAP diet** was developed at Monash University in Australia as a treatment for IBS and has shown efficacy in reducing bloating, gas, and abdominal pain in 50 to 80% of IBS patients (Halmos et al., 2014). For the 62% of hEDS patients who meet IBS criteria (Choudhary et al., 2021), it represents a potential tool, but it requires careful integration with the other dietary considerations already in play.

The low-FODMAP protocol involves a two- to six-week elimination of high-FODMAP foods (onions, garlic, wheat, certain fruits, beans, lactose-containing dairy) followed by systematic reintroduction of each FODMAP category to identify specific triggers. The critical point is that the low-FODMAP diet is designed as a short-term diagnostic tool, not a permanent dietary pattern. Long-term FODMAP restriction can harm the gut microbiome by starving beneficial bacteria of the prebiotic fibers they need to thrive (Staudacher et al., 2017).

For trifecta patients, the challenge is layering FODMAP restrictions on top of existing low-histamine and high-sodium requirements without creating an impossibly narrow diet. A dietitian experienced in managing multiple simultaneous dietary modifications should coordinate this process. In many cases, it is more practical to test one dietary intervention at a time (low-histamine first, then FODMAP if needed) rather than implementing both simultaneously.

8.4 Protein and Bone Density

Protein intake deserves special attention in the EDS population. A 2024 cross-sectional study of 680 hEDS patients found that decreased protein intake correlated with lower bone mineral density (Topan et al., 2024). This finding is concerning because EDS patients already face skeletal challenges from defective collagen, and adding protein malnutrition to the equation accelerates bone loss. The same study found that 62.3% of patients regularly skipped meals, making protein intake even more precarious.

The mechanism is straightforward: protein provides the amino acids that serve as building blocks for collagen, bone matrix, muscle tissue, and connective tissue repair. When protein intake drops below the body's needs, the body begins breaking down existing muscle and bone to supply amino acids for essential metabolic functions. For EDS patients whose connective tissues are already structurally compromised, this catabolism accelerates tissue degradation.

Current evidence supports a protein target of 1.0 to 1.2 grams per kilogram of body weight daily for patients with chronic illness and connective tissue disorders, compared to the general population recommendation of 0.8 grams per kilogram (DiBaise et al., 2019). For a 70-kilogram (154-pound) individual, this translates to 70 to 84 grams of protein daily. Distributing this across five to six eating occasions (approximately 12 to 17 grams per meal or snack) is more practical and better tolerated with gastroparesis than consuming it in two or three large protein-heavy meals.

8.5 Collagen Supporting Nutrition

While no food or supplement can fix the underlying genetic defect in EDS collagen, specific nutrients support the body's collagen synthesis and may improve wound healing, skin integrity, and tissue resilience (DiBaise et al., 2019).

Vitamin C is the most critical nutrient for collagen synthesis. It serves as a required cofactor for the enzymes prolyl hydroxylase and lysyl hydroxylase, which stabilize the triple-helix structure of collagen fibers. Without adequate vitamin C, the body produces structurally weak collagen. The recommended intake for EDS patients is 750 to 1,000 milligrams daily, as discussed in section 5.6 (Steiner et al., 2023).

Proline and glycine are the two amino acids most abundant in collagen. While the body can synthesize both, dietary sources provide additional substrate. Bone broth (short-cooked for histamine compatibility) is a natural source of both. Collagen peptide supplements (hydrolyzed collagen powder) provide proline and glycine in a form that is easily absorbed and can be added to smoothies, soups, or beverages. A 2019 review suggested that oral collagen supplementation may improve skin elasticity and joint comfort, though studies specific to EDS are limited (de Miranda et al., 2021).

Copper is a cofactor for lysyl oxidase, the enzyme that cross-links collagen fibers for strength. Dietary sources include sunflower seeds, cashews, mushrooms, and dark chocolate (if tolerated from a histamine and MCAS perspective). **Zinc** supports wound healing and immune function, with dietary sources including pumpkin seeds, poultry, and legumes (if tolerated from a FODMAP perspective).

8.6 Honora's Adaptive Kitchen

Background

Honora, a 41-year-old single mother of two, had been diagnosed with hEDS at age 35 and POTS at age 37. She experienced daily joint pain in her hands, wrists, and shoulders, chronic fatigue that worsened throughout the day, and frequent joint subluxations in her fingers while gripping kitchen tools. She had largely stopped cooking and was relying on processed convenience foods (many of which were high in histamine) and takeout.

Presentation

Honora's diet consisted primarily of frozen pizzas, canned soup, deli sandwiches, and fast food. She wanted to cook fresh, low-histamine, high-sodium meals but described the physical barriers as insurmountable: "By 5 PM, I can barely hold a knife. My hands hurt too much to chop vegetables or grip a pan. And I'm so tired that standing at the stove for 30 minutes feels like running a marathon." Her weight had increased by 18 pounds over two years due to the calorie density of processed foods combined with her inability to exercise.

Analysis

Honora's situation illustrates a reality that dietary advice for EDS patients often overlooks: the physical act of food preparation is itself a challenge when you have joint hypermobility, chronic pain, and fatigue. Recommending fresh, home-cooked meals to a patient who cannot safely grip a knife by evening is unhelpful without also addressing the practical barriers to cooking.

Intervention

An occupational therapist specializing in hypermobility worked with Honora to redesign her kitchen workflow. Adaptive tools included ergonomic knives with large, padded handles; electric can openers; jar openers mounted under the cabinet; lightweight pots and pans; a perching stool to allow cooking while seated; and silicone grip aids for utensils. Batch-cooking strategies included preparing large quantities on her best-energy day (typically Saturday morning), portioning into single-serving containers, and freezing immediately (preventing histamine accumulation from refrigerator storage). A slow cooker allowed her to combine ingredients in the morning when her energy and hand function were best, with the meal ready by evening without further intervention.

Outcome

Over two months, Honora transitioned approximately 70% of her meals from processed or takeout food to home-prepared meals. Her histamine intake decreased substantially. Her sodium intake became more controlled (she could add specific amounts of salt rather than relying on the unpredictable sodium content of restaurant food). She lost four pounds in the first month without intentionally restricting calories. She described the perching stool as "the single best purchase I've ever made for my kitchen."

Teaching Points

- Dietary recommendations for EDS patients must account for the physical challenges of food preparation, including joint pain, hypermobility, grip weakness, and fatigue
- Adaptive kitchen tools and modifications recommended by occupational therapists can make home cooking accessible for patients who would otherwise depend on processed foods
- Batch cooking with immediate freezing addresses both the energy conservation needs of EDS patients and the histamine management needs of MCAS patients

8.7 When Oral Intake Falls Short

For some trifecta patients, GI dysfunction becomes severe enough that oral intake alone cannot meet nutritional needs. This is a clinical reality that affects approximately 10% of POTS patients at tertiary care centers, with 59% of those requiring enteral nutrition (tube feeding) and 28% requiring parenteral nutrition (IV nutrition) at some point (Tseng et al., 2021).

Indicators that oral intake may be insufficient include: unintentional weight loss exceeding 5% of body weight over three months; inability to consume more than 1,000 calories daily despite dietary modifications; persistent dehydration despite aggressive oral fluid and sodium management; laboratory evidence of protein malnutrition (low serum albumin, low prealbumin); and functional decline attributable to malnutrition.

When these indicators are present, the conversation with the medical team should shift from "how can I eat better?" to "do I need supplemental nutritional support?" Options include oral nutritional supplements (such as Ensure, Kate Farms, or Orgain), which provide concentrated calories and protein in a liquid form that empties from the stomach faster than solid food. If oral supplements are insufficient, nasogastric or gastrojejunal tube feeding may be discussed. These decisions are made collaboratively between the patient, gastroenterologist, and dietitian.

8.8 Managing Weight Changes

Weight changes in trifecta patients can go in either direction, and both unintentional weight loss and unintentional weight gain require specific dietary strategies.

Unintentional weight loss typically results from inadequate caloric intake due to nausea, early satiety, food avoidance, and gastroparesis. Strategies for increasing caloric intake without increasing meal volume include: adding calorie-dense fats to foods (olive oil, ghee, coconut oil, nut butters); choosing calorie-dense carbohydrates (sweet potatoes, rice, oats with toppings); drinking calories through smoothies, shakes, and fortified beverages; and using collagen peptide powder in beverages for additional protein without increasing food volume.

Unintentional weight gain can result from immobility (when pain, fatigue, or dysautonomia prevent exercise), medication side effects (particularly from beta-blockers, some antihistamines, and corticosteroids), and emotional eating as a coping mechanism for chronic illness. Managing weight gain in this population requires sensitivity, as standard "eat less, move more" advice ignores the physical and medical constraints these patients face. Strategies include focusing on nutrient density (choosing foods that provide maximum nutrition per calorie), structured meal timing to prevent grazing, working with a physical therapist to identify tolerable forms of movement, and addressing medication side effects with the prescribing physician.

8.9 Leocadia's Weight Recovery

Background

Leocadia, a 28-year-old graduate student with hEDS, POTS, and MCAS, had experienced progressive weight loss over eight months. She began at 135 pounds (BMI 22.5) and had dropped to 108 pounds (BMI 18.0). Her gastroparesis caused nausea after most meals, and her MCAS triggered abdominal cramping with unpredictable foods. She had developed significant anxiety around eating and was consuming approximately 900 calories daily.

Presentation

Leocadia reported eating only twice daily (a smoothie in the morning and a small portion of rice with chicken in the evening). She described constant fatigue, hair loss, bruising, and worsening POTS symptoms. Her ARFID screening was positive for the "fear of eating" subtype (recall section 3.8 on ARFID in hEDS patients).

Her dietitian calculated that she needed approximately 1,800 calories daily to halt weight loss and 2,200 calories to begin weight recovery.

Analysis

Leocadia's caloric deficit was driving a cycle of worsening: malnutrition reduced her blood volume (worsening POTS), impaired her immune function (potentially worsening MCAS flares), and weakened her connective tissue (worsening EDS symptoms). Her two-meal pattern concentrated all food intake into two large gastric challenges, maximizing gastroparesis symptoms and reinforcing her fear of eating. The ARFID component added a psychological barrier that dietary advice alone could not address.

Intervention

A multidisciplinary approach combined gastroenterology (prokinetic medication to improve gastric emptying), psychology (cognitive-behavioral therapy for food-related anxiety), and nutrition (gradual caloric increase through six small eating occasions). Calorie-dense additions were introduced first: a tablespoon of ghee on her rice added 120 calories without increasing volume. A scoop of collagen peptides in her smoothie added 70 calories and 18 grams of protein. An oral nutritional supplement between meals added 250 calories. Solid foods were introduced at textures matched to her gastroparesis severity that day.

Outcome

Over four months, Leocadia's weight increased to 121 pounds. Her caloric intake stabilized at 1,600 to 1,800 calories daily across six eating occasions. Her POTS symptoms improved as her nutritional status recovered. Her food-related anxiety decreased with CBT support, and she was able to eat in social settings again, including meals at her university cafeteria.

Teaching Points

- Unintentional weight loss in trifecta patients requires a multidisciplinary approach addressing GI dysfunction, mast cell activation, and the psychological impact of chronic food-related distress simultaneously
- Calorie-dense, low-volume additions (oils, nut butters, collagen peptides) can increase caloric intake without increasing the gastric volume that triggers gastroparesis symptoms
- ARFID in the trifecta population requires psychological intervention alongside nutritional support, as dietary modifications alone cannot address conditioned food avoidance

8.10 Summary and Applications

Eating with EDS requires adapting every meal to accommodate a GI system that is structurally and functionally compromised. Gastroparesis demands smaller, more frequent, softer, lower-fiber meals with distributed fat intake. GERD management focuses on timing and positioning rather than additional food restrictions beyond those already required by the low-histamine protocol. IBS management through the low-FODMAP diet should be approached as a short-term diagnostic tool, not a permanent dietary layer, and ideally tested separately from other restrictions.

Protein intake of 1.0 to 1.2 grams per kilogram daily supports connective tissue maintenance and prevents the bone density loss documented in protein-deficient hEDS patients. Collagen-supporting nutrients (vitamin C, proline, glycine, copper, zinc) provide the building blocks for tissue repair. The physical challenges of food preparation are a legitimate barrier requiring adaptive tools and batch-cooking strategies, not just willpower. And when oral intake becomes insufficient, supplemental nutrition support should be discussed with the medical team rather than delayed until malnutrition becomes severe. In Chapter 9.0, we will add the anti-inflammatory layer, examining how dietary patterns can reduce the systemic inflammation that drives much of the trifecta's symptom burden.

Chapter 9.0: Anti Inflammatory Dietary Strategies

A question that trifecta patients often ask their doctors is some version of: "If my body is constantly inflamed, shouldn't I be eating anti-inflammatory foods?" The answer is yes, with important qualifications. Chronic systemic inflammation drives much of the symptom burden across all three trifecta conditions. Mast cell activation generates inflammatory mediators by definition. EDS-related tissue damage triggers ongoing repair cascades that involve inflammatory pathways. Autonomic dysfunction itself is associated with elevated inflammatory markers. But "anti-inflammatory eating" has become a vague wellness buzzword applied to everything from turmeric lattes to juice cleanses. What does the evidence actually support, and how do you implement anti-inflammatory principles when you are already managing low-histamine, high-sodium, gastroparesis-friendly, and protein-adequate requirements simultaneously?

This chapter will cover the following:

- The biological basis of chronic inflammation in the trifecta and why dietary patterns matter
- The Mediterranean dietary pattern as the most evidence-supported anti-inflammatory framework
- Specific anti-inflammatory nutrients and compounds with research support
- The probiotic and prebiotic paradox for MCAS patients
- How to layer anti-inflammatory principles on top of existing trifecta dietary requirements without creating impossible restrictions

9.1 Inflammation in the Trifecta

Inflammation is the body's protective response to injury, infection, or threat. In its acute form (a cut healing, a cold being fought off), inflammation is beneficial and self-limiting. In its chronic form, inflammation becomes destructive, damaging tissues and amplifying symptoms over time. The trifecta creates conditions for chronic inflammation through at least three converging pathways.

In MCAS, mast cells release inflammatory mediators including histamine, prostaglandins, leukotrienes, cytokines (particularly interleukin-6 and tumor necrosis factor-alpha), and numerous other compounds that sustain inflammatory signaling throughout the body (Afrin et al., 2016). This is not occasional inflammation triggered by an identifiable event. It is ongoing, fluctuating, baseline inflammation driven by inappropriate mast cell activation.

In EDS, the structural weakness of connective tissue leads to chronic micro-injuries: joints that subluxate and must be repaired, skin that tears more easily, blood vessels that are more fragile. Each micro-injury activates local inflammatory cascades. Over time, the cumulative burden of these repair processes contributes to systemic inflammation (Malfait et al., 2017). Additionally, the frequent GI tissue damage in EDS (from gastroparesis, dysmotility, and reflux) creates intestinal inflammation that can increase intestinal permeability, sometimes called "leaky gut," allowing bacterial products to enter the bloodstream and activate systemic immune responses.

In POTS, research has identified elevated inflammatory markers in a subset of patients, suggesting that inflammation may contribute to autonomic nerve damage or dysfunction (Gunning et al., 2019). Post-infectious POTS (including post-COVID POTS) may involve autoimmune mechanisms in which inflammatory processes target autonomic nerve receptors.

9.2 Mediterranean Dietary Evidence

Among the many dietary patterns that claim anti-inflammatory properties, the **Mediterranean dietary pattern** has the strongest evidence base. This pattern emphasizes fruits, vegetables, whole grains, legumes, nuts, seeds, olive oil, and fish, with moderate poultry and dairy and limited red meat, processed foods, and refined sugars. Dozens of randomized controlled trials and meta-analyses have demonstrated that adherence to the Mediterranean pattern reduces markers of systemic inflammation (C-reactive protein, interleukin-6, tumor necrosis factor-alpha), cardiovascular risk, and all-cause mortality (Schwingshackl & Hoffmann, 2014).

For trifecta patients, the Mediterranean pattern offers a useful philosophical framework rather than a rigid prescription. Many traditional Mediterranean foods are problematic for MCAS patients (tomatoes, citrus, aged cheeses, wine, fermented foods, vinegar-based dressings), and strict adherence is neither possible nor necessary. The relevant principles can be extracted and applied within trifecta constraints:

Principle 1: Prioritize plant foods in the quantities you tolerate. Even if raw salads and high-histamine vegetables are off limits, cooked low-histamine vegetables (zucchini, carrots, sweet potatoes, broccoli, cauliflower) provide anti-inflammatory phytonutrients, fiber, and antioxidants. Aiming for at least three servings of tolerated vegetables daily contributes to the anti-inflammatory foundation.

Principle 2: Use olive oil as your primary cooking fat. Extra virgin olive oil contains oleocanthal, a compound with anti-inflammatory properties comparable to low-dose ibuprofen (Beauchamp et al., 2005). It is also low in histamine, well tolerated by most GI systems, and contributes to the calorie density needed by patients with gastroparesis-related weight loss.

Principle 3: Include fatty fish for omega-3 fatty acids. Omega-3 fatty acids (particularly EPA and DHA) reduce the production of inflammatory eicosanoids and cytokines (Calder, 2017). For MCAS patients, the fish must be fresh or flash-frozen (not canned, smoked, or previously thawed) to maintain low histamine levels. Fresh or flash-frozen salmon, cod, halibut, and trout are suitable options when prepared and consumed promptly.

9.3 Specific Anti Inflammatory Compounds

Several specific nutrients and compounds have demonstrated anti-inflammatory and mast cell-stabilizing properties in research settings. Their relevance to trifecta patients extends beyond general anti-inflammatory benefits because some directly address mast cell activation.

Quercetin is a flavonoid found in onions, apples, berries, broccoli, and capers. Laboratory studies have shown that quercetin inhibits mast cell degranulation and reduces histamine release (Weng et al., 2012). It also inhibits the production of pro-inflammatory cytokines by mast cells. While clinical trials in MCAS patients specifically are limited, quercetin is widely recommended by MCAS specialists as a supplemental mast cell stabilizer at doses of 500 to 1,000 milligrams twice daily (Afrin, 2016). Dietary sources contribute modest amounts, but therapeutic doses typically require supplementation.

Curcumin, the active compound in turmeric, has demonstrated anti-inflammatory properties across hundreds of studies. It inhibits NF-kB, a master regulator of inflammatory gene expression, and reduces the production of pro-inflammatory cytokines (Hewlings & Kalman, 2017). Curcumin has also shown mast cell-stabilizing activity in laboratory models. The challenge with curcumin is bioavailability: curcumin is poorly absorbed from the GI tract. Formulations that include piperine (from black pepper) or lipid-based delivery systems improve absorption substantially.

Omega-3 fatty acids (EPA and DHA) compete with arachidonic acid for incorporation into cell membranes. When omega-3s are abundant in cell membranes, the inflammatory mediators produced from those membranes are less potent than those produced from omega-6-rich membranes (Calder, 2017). This biochemical competition explains why increasing omega-3 intake relative to omega-6 intake shifts the body's inflammatory balance toward resolution rather than amplification. Food sources include fatty fish (prepared fresh or from frozen), walnuts, chia seeds, and flaxseeds. Supplementation with fish oil or algae-based omega-3 (for those who cannot tolerate fish) provides more consistent doses.

Vitamin C functions as both an antioxidant and a mast cell stabilizer, as discussed in section 5.6. Its anti-inflammatory role in the trifecta is dual: reducing oxidative stress (which contributes to inflammation) and directly reducing mast cell histamine release (Hagel et al., 2013). At 750 to 1,000 milligrams daily, vitamin C addresses EDS collagen needs, MCAS mast cell stabilization, and systemic anti-inflammatory support simultaneously.

9.4 The Probiotic Paradox

Probiotics and prebiotics occupy a complicated position in trifecta nutrition. The gut microbiome plays a well-established role in immune regulation, inflammation modulation, and gut barrier integrity (Valdes et al., 2018). Disrupted microbiome composition (dysbiosis) has been associated with increased inflammation, immune dysregulation, and GI symptoms. Theoretically, supporting the microbiome with probiotics (live beneficial bacteria) and prebiotics (fibers that feed beneficial bacteria) should help.

In practice, the situation is more nuanced for trifecta patients. Many traditional probiotic foods (yogurt, kefir, sauerkraut, kimchi, kombucha, miso) are fermented and therefore high in histamine. MCAS patients who consume fermented probiotics may experience symptom flares from the histamine content rather than benefits from the bacterial content (Comas-Basté et al., 2020). This creates a paradox: the foods most commonly recommended for gut health are the same foods most likely to trigger MCAS symptoms.

Potential workarounds include: probiotic supplements in capsule form (which bypass the histamine issue because the bacteria are freeze-dried without fermentation byproducts), specific probiotic strains that have been shown to degrade histamine rather than produce it (certain strains of *Bifidobacterium infantis*, *Lactobacillus rhamnosus GG*, and *Bifidobacterium longum*), and prebiotic fibers that feed beneficial gut bacteria without introducing histamine (partially hydrolyzed guar gum, acacia fiber, and cooked-and-cooled resistant starch from rice or potatoes) (Schnedl & Enko, 2021).

The evidence is insufficient to make blanket recommendations for or against probiotics in MCAS. Individual tolerance varies. A reasonable approach is to trial a single-strain probiotic supplement (starting at a low dose) while monitoring symptoms for two to four weeks. If symptoms worsen, discontinue. If symptoms improve or remain stable, the probiotic can be maintained.

9.5 Eudora's Anti Inflammatory Protocol

Background

Eudora, a 50-year-old librarian with long-standing hEDS, POTS, and MCAS, had been managing her trifecta for eight years. Her symptoms were partially controlled on H1/H2 antihistamines, cromolyn sodium, midodrine, and aggressive hydration. Despite this regimen, she experienced persistent low-grade joint pain, skin sensitivity, brain fog, and fatigue that she described as "the background noise of my life that never fully quiets down." Her C-reactive protein (CRP) was mildly elevated at 4.2 mg/L (normal is below 3.0), consistent with chronic low-grade inflammation.

Presentation

Eudora's diet was nutritionally adequate but not specifically anti-inflammatory. She was meeting her sodium and protein targets, following a low-histamine protocol, and managing her gastroparesis through small frequent meals. However, her dietary fat came primarily from butter and coconut oil, she ate fish rarely (due to histamine concerns about freshness), her vegetable intake consisted mainly of white potatoes and rice, and she consumed very few fruits.

Analysis

Eudora's diet, while meeting her trifecta-specific requirements, was missing the anti-inflammatory components that could address her persistently elevated CRP and background symptoms. Her fat sources, while tolerated, provided minimal omega-3 fatty acids. Her limited vegetable and fruit variety reduced her intake of phytonutrients with anti-inflammatory properties. She was not taking quercetin, curcumin, or omega-3 supplements.

Intervention

Working with her dietitian, Eudora made targeted additions to her existing diet without disrupting her established protocols. She replaced half her butter usage with extra virgin olive oil. She added flash-frozen salmon twice weekly (prepared immediately from frozen to maintain low histamine). She expanded her vegetable intake to include broccoli, carrots, and sweet potatoes (all cooked, all lower-histamine). She added blueberries and apples (peeled) as daily fruit servings. Her supplement regimen was augmented with quercetin (500 milligrams twice daily), omega-3 fish oil (2 grams EPA/DHA daily), and curcumin with piperine (500 milligrams daily).

Outcome

After three months, Eudora's CRP decreased from 4.2 to 2.1 mg/L. Her joint pain decreased by approximately 30% by self-report. Her brain fog improved modestly. She described the changes as "turning down the volume on that background noise from a 6 to about a 3 or 4." Her MCAS symptoms did not worsen with the dietary additions, confirming that the new foods were tolerated within her histamine threshold.

Teaching Points

- Anti-inflammatory dietary modifications can be layered on top of existing trifecta protocols by making targeted substitutions (olive oil for butter, flash-frozen fish for other proteins, expanded vegetable variety) rather than adding new restrictions
- Measurable inflammatory markers (CRP) can serve as objective indicators of dietary anti-inflammatory interventions, providing data beyond subjective symptom reports
- Quercetin, omega-3 fatty acids, and curcumin have both general anti-inflammatory and specific mast cell-stabilizing properties, making them particularly relevant supplements for trifecta patients

9.6 Gut Microbiome and Inflammation

The gut microbiome's relationship to systemic inflammation is mediated through several mechanisms. Beneficial bacteria produce **short-chain fatty acids (SCFAs)** including butyrate, propionate, and acetate by fermenting dietary fiber. Butyrate serves as the primary fuel source for colonocytes (the cells lining the colon), maintains gut barrier integrity, and has direct anti-inflammatory effects by inhibiting NF-kB signaling in immune cells (Valdes et al., 2018). When the microbiome is disrupted (by antibiotics, restricted diets, or SIBO), SCFA production drops, gut barrier function deteriorates, and inflammatory signaling increases.

For trifecta patients, this creates a concerning cycle. Dietary restrictions (low-histamine, possibly low-FODMAP) reduce the diversity of fibers available to gut bacteria. Reduced fiber diversity leads to reduced bacterial diversity. Reduced bacterial diversity leads to decreased SCFA production. Decreased SCFA production compromises gut barrier integrity. Compromised gut barrier allows bacterial endotoxins to enter the bloodstream, activating systemic immune responses and potentially triggering mast cell activation.

The practical implication is that anti-inflammatory eating for trifecta patients should include as much tolerated plant fiber diversity as possible, not for the traditional "roughage" benefit, but for the microbiome-mediated anti-inflammatory effects. Even small amounts of diverse plant fibers contribute to SCFA production. Cooked vegetables, peeled fruits, oatmeal, rice, quinoa, and chia seeds (well-hydrated) all provide fermentable substrate for beneficial bacteria without the histamine concerns of fermented foods.

9.7 Darian's Supplement Confusion

Background

Darian, a 34-year-old physiotherapist with MCAS and POTS, had been researching anti-inflammatory supplements online. He arrived at his appointment with a shopping list of 14 supplements he wanted to start: quercetin, curcumin, omega-3 fish oil, NAC, alpha-lipoic acid, resveratrol, boswellia, bromelain, ginger extract, vitamin D, vitamin C, zinc, selenium, and a multi-strain probiotic. His total monthly supplement cost would have exceeded $280.

Presentation

Darian was already taking five medications (two antihistamines, cromolyn sodium, a beta-blocker, and midodrine) and had stable but imperfect symptom control. He wanted to "cover all my bases" with supplements and was frustrated that his MCAS specialist had cautioned against starting everything at once. His reasoning was that "each of these has research behind it, so why wouldn't I take all of them?"

Analysis

Darian's approach illustrates a common pattern in the chronic illness community: the desire to find solutions leads to the accumulation of interventions that, while individually supported by some evidence, have not been studied in combination and can interact with each other and with existing medications. Bromelain, for instance, is derived from pineapple, a known histamine liberator, and could theoretically worsen MCAS symptoms in some patients. High-dose NAC can cause GI side effects including nausea and diarrhea, worsening existing GI dysfunction. Starting 14 new supplements simultaneously makes it impossible to identify which ones are helping, which are neutral, and which might be causing new symptoms.

Intervention

Darian's specialist recommended a staged approach: start with the three supplements with the strongest evidence and most relevance to his conditions (quercetin, omega-3 fish oil, and vitamin C). Each was introduced one at a time, two weeks apart, with symptom monitoring after each addition. If all three were tolerated and no adverse effects occurred, curcumin would be added next, followed by vitamin D (with serum level monitoring). The remaining supplements would be evaluated individually based on clinical need rather than theoretical benefit.

Outcome

Over eight weeks, Darian successfully added quercetin (well-tolerated, modest improvement in skin flushing), omega-3 fish oil (well-tolerated, no notable symptom change), and vitamin C (well-tolerated, reduced bruising frequency). Curcumin was added at week 10 and appeared to improve his joint stiffness. He decided not to add further supplements, as the improvement from four targeted additions was sufficient and manageable both financially and practically.

Teaching Points

- Multiple supplements with individual evidence support should be introduced one at a time, with monitoring periods between additions, to identify individual responses and potential interactions
- The staged approach allows clear attribution of benefits and side effects to specific supplements, preventing the confusion of polypharmacy
- Financial sustainability and practical adherence should be factored into supplement recommendations, as the cost and complexity of large supplement regimens reduce long-term compliance

9.8 Layering Anti Inflammatory Principles

The anti-inflammatory overlay is exactly that: a layer added on top of the existing trifecta dietary framework, not a replacement for it. The principles from Chapters 6.0 through 8.0 remain the foundation. Low-histamine eating (Chapter 6.0) addresses mast cell triggers. High-sodium strategy (Chapter 7.0) addresses POTS hemodynamics. Gastroparesis-friendly eating (Chapter 8.0) addresses EDS-related GI dysfunction. The anti-inflammatory layer enhances all of these by reducing the baseline inflammatory burden that amplifies symptoms across all three conditions.

Practical integration looks like this: at each eating occasion, the patient asks three questions in order. Can I tolerate this food from a histamine perspective? Does this eating occasion contribute to my sodium and protein targets? And if there is a choice between two equally tolerated options, which one provides more anti-inflammatory benefit? Choosing olive oil over butter, sweet potatoes over white potatoes, blueberries over a less-nutrient-dense snack, and fresh salmon over chicken at two meals per week are simple substitutions that do not add restrictions but shift the overall dietary pattern toward an anti-inflammatory profile.

9.9 Chapter Synthesis

Chronic systemic inflammation in the trifecta results from converging mast cell activation, connective tissue damage, and autonomic dysfunction. The Mediterranean dietary pattern provides the strongest evidence-based framework for anti-inflammatory eating, though its traditional form requires adaptation for trifecta patients who cannot tolerate fermented foods, citrus, tomatoes, and other staples. The relevant principles (prioritize plants, use olive oil, include omega-3 sources, emphasize whole foods over processed foods) can be extracted and applied within existing dietary constraints.

Quercetin, curcumin, omega-3 fatty acids, and vitamin C have both general anti-inflammatory and specific mast cell-stabilizing properties supported by peer-reviewed research. The probiotic and prebiotic question remains nuanced: fermented foods pose histamine risks, but the microbiome requires fiber diversity and may benefit from selected non-histamine-producing probiotic strains. Supplement protocols should be introduced one at a time with monitoring, not simultaneously in large batches. The anti-inflammatory overlay enhances rather than replaces the dietary foundations established in the previous chapters. In Chapter 10.0, we will bring all of these layers together into a personalized daily eating framework using the Trifecta Plate model.

Chapter 10.0: Your Personalized Trifecta Plate

You have now absorbed nine chapters of dietary science covering histamine biochemistry, sodium physiology, GI dysfunction, micronutrient deficiencies, and anti-inflammatory strategies. You understand the mechanisms. You know the research. And you are probably wondering: how do I actually eat? Because knowing that histamine accumulates in leftovers, that you need 5,000 milligrams of sodium before noon, that gastroparesis demands softer textures, and that omega-3 fatty acids stabilize mast cells does not, by itself, produce a meal. The gap between understanding dietary principles and putting food on a plate three to six times a day, every day, while managing fatigue, pain, and unpredictable symptoms, is where most trifecta patients get stuck. This chapter closes that gap.

This chapter will cover the following:

- The Trifecta Plate model for structuring meals visually and practically
- A decision tree for prioritizing dietary strategies based on your dominant condition
- The traffic light classification system for rapid food decisions
- How to build and maintain your personal safe foods master list
- Strategies for resolving conflicts between competing dietary needs
- Adapting the framework for vegetarian, vegan, and other dietary preferences
- Daily intake targets for sodium, fluid, protein, fiber, and micronutrients

10.1 The Trifecta Plate Model

The **Trifecta Plate** is a visual framework designed to translate the principles from Chapters 6.0 through 9.0 into a single, repeatable structure for every eating occasion. It is not a rigid prescription. It is a mental template that ensures each meal or snack contributes meaningfully to the multiple simultaneous nutritional targets that trifecta patients must meet.

The plate is divided into four zones. Approximately one-quarter of the plate is **protein**, which stabilizes blood sugar, prevents postprandial hypotension, and provides the amino acids necessary for connective tissue maintenance (Ganesh et al., 2020). As discussed in section 8.4, EDS patients with decreased protein intake show lower bone mineral density (Topan et al., 2024), making protein a structural priority rather than a dietary afterthought. Protein sources should be fresh or flash-frozen and prepared promptly to maintain low histamine levels (Comas-Basté et al., 2020).

Approximately one-quarter of the plate is **complex carbohydrates**, chosen for their lower glycemic index to prevent the blood sugar spikes that worsen POTS tachycardia and may trigger mast cell degranulation (Shibao et al., 2005; Theoharides et al., 2019). Sweet potatoes, rice, oats, and quinoa are examples that are generally well tolerated across all three conditions. On days when gastroparesis is more active, these carbohydrates should be well-cooked and soft rather than firm or al dente (Thwaites et al., 2022).

Approximately one-quarter of the plate is **cooked vegetables**, selected from the lower-histamine options described in section 6.6. Cooking vegetables rather than eating them raw improves gastroparesis tolerability, reduces the mechanical burden on the GI tract, and does not substantially reduce the anti-inflammatory phytonutrients discussed in Chapter 9.0 (Steiner et al., 2023). Zucchini, carrots, broccoli, cauliflower, sweet potatoes, and asparagus are reliable starting options.

The remaining quarter, represented as a smaller zone, is **healthy fats** distributed throughout the plate rather than concentrated in one item. A tablespoon of olive oil for cooking, a small amount of ghee on the carbohydrate portion, or a quarter of an avocado (if individually tolerated) provides essential fatty acids and caloric density without overloading the gastroparetic stomach (DiBaise et al., 2019). On every plate, **salt** is added liberally to all components, and the meal is accompanied by a glass of electrolyte-enhanced water.

The Trifecta Plate is not about precise measurement. Nobody needs to weigh their broccoli. The visual division into quarters provides a rapid mental check at each eating occasion: Do I have protein? Do I have a complex carb? Do I have a vegetable? Did I add fat and salt? If the answer to all five is yes, the meal is likely contributing to all major trifecta targets simultaneously.

10.2 The Condition Decision Tree

Not all trifecta patients are affected equally by all three conditions. For some, MCAS dominates the clinical picture, producing frequent flares that overshadow POTS and EDS symptoms. For others, POTS is the primary driver of disability, with MCAS remaining relatively mild. Still others experience severe EDS-related GI dysfunction that creates the largest barrier to adequate nutrition. The **condition decision tree** helps patients prioritize which dietary strategies to implement in which order, rather than attempting to address everything simultaneously.

The decision tree works through three sequential questions.

Question 1: Which condition is currently causing the most dietary disruption? If MCAS flares are frequent and food-triggered, start with the low-histamine elimination protocol (Chapter 6.0) as the foundation. If POTS symptoms (presyncope, tachycardia, brain fog) dominate and are not well-controlled by hydration and medication, prioritize sodium and fluid targets (Chapter 7.0). If severe gastroparesis, nausea, or GI pain is the primary barrier to eating, begin with texture and volume modifications (Chapter 8.0).

Question 2: Is the first-priority strategy producing adequate improvement? After two to four weeks of focused implementation, evaluate the response. If symptoms have improved by 30% or more (using the symptom scoring system from section 6.11), maintain that foundation and add the next layer. If improvement is minimal, reassess with the medical team before adding additional dietary complexity.

Question 3: What is the next priority? Layer the second dietary strategy on top of the first, then the third. The anti-inflammatory overlay (Chapter 9.0) is typically added last because it builds on all three condition-specific foundations rather than replacing any of them.

This sequential approach prevents the overwhelm that comes from trying to implement four simultaneous dietary frameworks on day one. Research on health behavior change consistently demonstrates that staged implementation produces better adherence than all-at-once approaches (Prochaska & DiClemente, 1983). A patient who successfully establishes a low-histamine foundation over three weeks is better positioned to add sodium targets in week four than a patient who tries to simultaneously memorize histamine lists, count sodium milligrams, and modify meal textures from the first day.

10.3 Traffic Light Food Classification

The **traffic light system** provides a rapid decision-making tool for daily food choices. Every food that a trifecta patient encounters falls into one of three categories based on its compatibility with all three conditions.

Green foods are safe for all three conditions: low in histamine (when fresh), compatible with gastroparesis (when properly prepared), and easily incorporated into a high-sodium, protein-adequate eating pattern. Examples include fresh chicken breast, rice, oatmeal, zucchini, carrots, sweet potatoes, peeled pears, peeled apples, blueberries, olive oil, ghee, and fresh herbs. These are the foods that form the daily foundation. A patient who is having a bad symptom day and can't think clearly about food choices can default to green foods and know they are meeting basic trifecta requirements.

Yellow foods are conditionally safe, meaning they are compatible with one or two conditions but may be problematic for the third, depending on individual tolerance. Examples include eggs (tolerated by most but can be histamine liberators for some), bell peppers (tolerated by many but trigger nightshade sensitivity in a subset), fresh mozzarella (low histamine compared to aged cheese but may cause issues for lactose-sensitive individuals), and nuts (good protein and fat source but can worsen gastroparesis in some and trigger MCAS in others). Yellow foods are the testing zone. They expand the diet beyond the green foundation, and each patient's yellow list will differ based on individual tolerance established through the reintroduction protocol described in section 6.9.

Red foods are likely problematic for one or more trifecta conditions regardless of individual tolerance. These include aged cheeses, canned fish, smoked and cured meats, fermented foods (sauerkraut, kimchi, kombucha), alcohol, vinegar, soy sauce, leftover food stored more than 24 hours, and high-glycemic refined carbohydrates (white bread, candy, sugary drinks). Red foods are not absolutely forbidden (rigid prohibition creates its own psychological problems, as discussed in section 3.8 on ARFID), but they are foods that should be consumed rarely and with awareness that symptoms may follow.

The traffic light system is personal and dynamic. A food that is red during an MCAS flare may be yellow during a stable period. A food that is green for one patient may be yellow for another. The system's value lies not in creating a universal list but in giving each patient a framework for categorizing their own foods based on accumulated experience (Joneja, 2017).

10.4 Clotilde's Trifecta Plate in Action

Background

Clotilde, a 38-year-old occupational therapist, had been diagnosed with hEDS at 30, POTS at 33, and MCAS at 35. She had read extensively about each condition and had accumulated dietary advice from three different specialists, two online support groups, and numerous blog posts. She described her dietary situation as "paralyzed by information." She had lists of foods to avoid from each source, many of which contradicted each other, and no clear framework for making daily food decisions.

Presentation

Clotilde brought a binder to her dietitian appointment containing 14 pages of printed food lists from various sources. Her current diet consisted of approximately eight foods that she considered "safe" based on the intersection of all her lists: plain white rice, plain chicken breast, peeled cucumbers, boiled zucchini, peeled pears, olive oil, salt, and water. She was consuming approximately 1,100 calories daily, had lost 11 pounds over four months, and was experiencing worsening fatigue, hair thinning, and increased POTS symptoms. Her protein intake was approximately 40 grams daily (well below the 1.0 to 1.2 grams per kilogram target discussed in section 8.4).

Analysis

Clotilde's case illustrates what happens when dietary information is accumulated without a unifying framework. Each individual food list was partially correct, but the intersection of all lists produced a diet so restrictive that it was causing malnutrition, which in turn worsened all three trifecta conditions. Her situation resembled Dorothea's case from section 3.9, where layered restrictions led to caloric and nutritional crisis. The Trifecta Plate model and traffic light system were introduced as organizing frameworks to replace the contradictory lists.

Intervention

The dietitian helped Clotilde build a personal traffic light list starting from her eight confirmed green foods. Using the reintroduction protocol from section 6.9, they tested one new food every three to four days. The Trifecta Plate model provided structure for each meal: a quarter protein (chicken, then testing turkey and fresh fish), a quarter complex carbohydrate (rice, then testing sweet potato and oatmeal), a quarter cooked vegetable (zucchini, then testing carrots, broccoli, and cauliflower), and distributed fat (olive oil, then testing ghee). Salt was increased deliberately at each meal to target 5,000 milligrams daily.

Outcome

Over six weeks, Clotilde expanded her diet from 8 to 23 green-category foods and identified 7 yellow-category foods she could tolerate on most days. Her caloric intake rose to 1,650 calories. Her protein intake reached 72 grams daily. Her weight stabilized. She described the Trifecta Plate model as "the first time anyone gave me a framework instead of just another list." She discarded her 14-page binder.

Teaching Points

- Accumulating dietary advice from multiple sources without a unifying framework can produce restrictions so severe that the diet itself becomes harmful, worsening all three trifecta conditions through malnutrition

- The Trifecta Plate model provides a meal-level organizing structure that ensures multiple nutritional targets (protein, complex carbohydrates, vegetables, fats, sodium) are addressed at each eating occasion
- Structured food reintroduction with a traffic light classification system converts contradictory information into personalized, actionable categories

10.5 Building Your Safe Foods List

The **safe foods master list** is a living document that serves as the practical output of the traffic light system. Unlike the static lists printed from websites, the master list is built from personal experience, updated continuously, and reflects actual individual tolerance rather than theoretical risk.

The process of building the list begins with the elimination phase (section 6.9), during which the patient identifies a core group of 12 to 20 foods that are consistently tolerated. These become the initial green foods. As reintroduction progresses, each tested food is assigned a color based on the results: green if tolerated consistently (80% or more of attempts), yellow if tolerated under specific conditions (such as only when fresh, only in small amounts, or only when other histamine load is low), and red if it consistently triggers symptoms.

A useful format for the master list includes four columns: the food name, its traffic light color, any conditions for tolerance (such as "must be cooked within 24 hours" or "tolerated only in small amounts"), and the date it was last tested. The date column matters because tolerance can change over time. A food that was red during a period of active MCAS flaring may become yellow or even green once mast cell stabilizing medications take full effect (Afrin et al., 2016). Retesting red foods every three to six months prevents the list from becoming unnecessarily restrictive.

The safe foods list should span multiple food categories. A list that contains only proteins and grains but no vegetables or fruits signals a gap that needs attention. A list that contains only soft, cooked foods but no options for portable snacks signals a practical gap for eating outside the home. The goal is a list that can sustain varied, nutritionally adequate eating across all daily situations: home meals, work lunches, travel, social events, and low-energy days when cooking feels impossible.

10.6 Resolving Competing Dietary Needs

The most intellectually challenging aspect of trifecta nutrition is that the three conditions sometimes produce directly conflicting dietary recommendations. The most common conflicts, and their practical resolutions, deserve explicit attention.

Conflict 1: Fermented foods for gut health versus histamine avoidance. Conventional gut health advice emphasizes probiotics from fermented foods. MCAS management requires avoiding fermented foods. Resolution: as discussed in section 9.4, use capsule-form probiotic supplements containing strains that degrade rather than produce histamine (Schnedl & Enko, 2021). Support the microbiome through diverse tolerated plant fibers rather than fermented foods.

Conflict 2: High-fiber diets for IBS versus low-fiber for gastroparesis. IBS guidelines often recommend increased fiber. Gastroparesis guidelines often recommend reduced fiber. Resolution: distinguish between soluble and insoluble fiber. Soluble fiber (oatmeal, peeled cooked fruits, chia seeds when fully hydrated) is generally better tolerated in gastroparesis than insoluble fiber (raw vegetable skins, bran, whole grain husks). Adjust fiber type and quantity based on daily gastroparesis severity rather than following a single fixed rule (Thwaites et al., 2022).

Conflict 3: Salt restriction for MCAS flares versus salt loading for POTS. Some MCAS patients report that high sodium worsens certain mast cell symptoms, while their POTS requires aggressive sodium intake. Resolution: this conflict requires input from both the allergist/immunologist and the cardiologist or autonomic specialist. In most cases, the cardiovascular benefits of sodium for POTS outweigh the marginal effects on MCAS, but the hyperadrenergic POTS subtype (discussed in section 4.4) requires more cautious sodium dosing. Monitoring blood pressure responses to sodium changes helps identify the individual sweet spot.

Conflict 4: Nutrient-dense foods that are also high-histamine. Spinach, tomatoes, avocados, and citrus fruits are among the most nutrient-dense foods available, but all are high in histamine or are histamine liberators. Resolution: obtain those nutrients from alternative sources. Vitamin C from supplementation or peeled fruits (apples, pears, blueberries) rather than citrus. Iron from fresh meat, pumpkin seeds, and supplementation rather than spinach. Potassium from sweet potatoes and bananas rather than avocados and tomatoes (Maintz & Novak, 2007).

The overarching principle for resolving conflicts is that no dietary rule is more important than the patient's overall nutritional adequacy and clinical stability. A rule that produces malnutrition is a bad rule regardless of the evidence supporting it in isolation.

10.7 Erasmus's Conflicting Recommendations

Background

Erasmus, a 46-year-old civil engineer, had been managing the full trifecta for three years. He was seeing a cardiologist for POTS, an allergist for MCAS, and a gastroenterologist for EDS-related gastroparesis and GERD. Each specialist provided dietary advice specific to their condition, and none had reviewed the recommendations from the other two.

Presentation

Erasmus presented his three sets of instructions to his new integrative dietitian. His cardiologist had prescribed 8 to 10 grams of sodium daily with three liters of fluid. His allergist had recommended a strict low-histamine diet with no fermented foods, no leftovers, and no alcohol. His gastroenterologist had recommended a low-FODMAP, low-fat, low-fiber, small-meal plan for gastroparesis management. When Erasmus attempted to follow all three sets of instructions simultaneously, he found that many high-sodium foods were high in histamine (deli meats, aged cheese, canned soups, soy sauce), many of the foods his allergist approved were high in FODMAPs (apples, onions, garlic), and the low-fat restriction from his gastroenterologist conflicted with the calorie-dense diet he needed to prevent further weight loss.

Analysis

Erasmus's situation is common among trifecta patients receiving care from multiple specialists who do not communicate with each other. Each set of dietary recommendations was evidence-based for the individual condition but had not been integrated with the others. The result was a set of instructions that was internally contradictory and practically impossible to follow. The integrative dietitian's role was to identify the areas of genuine conflict, resolve them using the prioritization framework, and produce a single, coherent eating plan.

Intervention

The dietitian used the condition decision tree to identify Erasmus's primary dietary barrier: his gastroparesis was so severe that inadequate caloric intake was worsening both his POTS (through hypovolemia from malnutrition) and his MCAS (through immune dysregulation from nutritional deficiency). Gastroparesis-friendly texture modifications became the foundation. Low-histamine principles were layered on top (focusing on freshness rather than food elimination). Sodium targets were achieved through liberal salting and electrolyte drinks rather than through processed high-sodium foods. The low-FODMAP restriction was narrowed to the specific FODMAPs Erasmus had confirmed as personal triggers (fructans and polyols) rather than applied as a blanket elimination.

Outcome

The unified plan replaced three conflicting instruction sets with a single framework. Erasmus's caloric intake increased from 1,200 to 1,800 calories daily. His sodium reached 6,000 milligrams through cooking salt and electrolyte supplements. His MCAS symptoms remained stable because freshness principles were maintained. His gastroparesis symptoms improved modestly because the texture modifications were appropriate. He described the experience as "the first time my diet made sense as one plan instead of three impossible ones."

Teaching Points

- Trifecta patients receiving dietary advice from multiple specialists often encounter contradictory instructions that are each evidence-based in isolation but impossible to implement simultaneously
- An integrative dietitian or a single provider who understands all three conditions can reconcile conflicting recommendations by identifying which restrictions are essential, which are modifiable, and which can be replaced by alternative strategies
- The condition decision tree helps prioritize which dietary challenge to address as the foundation, with other modifications layered on top sequentially rather than simultaneously

10.8 Vegetarian and Vegan Adaptations

Trifecta dietary management becomes more complex for patients who follow vegetarian, vegan, or other restricted dietary patterns for ethical, cultural, or religious reasons. The additional constraints are manageable but require careful planning to prevent nutritional gaps.

Vegetarian adaptations primarily involve replacing animal proteins with plant-based options that are both low in histamine and gastroparesis-friendly. Eggs (if tolerated from a histamine perspective) are a versatile protein source. Fresh tofu (not fermented tempeh, which is high in histamine) provides approximately 10 grams of protein per half-cup serving and is soft enough for gastroparesis days (Comas-Basté et al., 2020). Legumes (lentils, chickpeas, black beans) offer protein and complex carbohydrates but may cause issues for FODMAP-sensitive patients and can worsen bloating in gastroparesis. Cooking legumes thoroughly and starting with small portions allows individual tolerance to be assessed.

Vegan adaptations remove eggs and dairy, creating a more substantial protein challenge. Without careful planning, vegan trifecta patients are at elevated risk for deficiencies in vitamin B12 (which has no reliable plant sources and is already commonly deficient in POTS patients, as discussed in section 5.4), iron (plant-based iron is less bioavailable than heme iron from animal sources), zinc, and omega-3 fatty acids (Melina et al., 2016). Supplementation is not optional for vegan trifecta patients; it is a clinical necessity. A vegan multivitamin plus individual B12 supplementation (1,000 micrograms daily of methylcobalamin), algae-based omega-3, and potentially iron bisglycinate (with serum ferritin monitoring) form the baseline supplement protocol.

Sodium targets can be met through the same cooking and electrolyte strategies described in Chapter 7.0, as sodium does not depend on animal products. Protein targets of 1.0 to 1.2 grams per kilogram require deliberate protein combining across multiple plant sources at each eating occasion. A vegan Trifecta Plate might include a quarter plate of well-cooked lentils, a quarter of rice, a quarter of cooked vegetables (carrots, zucchini), and olive oil drizzled throughout, with salt added liberally and a glass of electrolyte water alongside.

10.9 The 80/20 Consistency Principle

Perfectionism about dietary adherence is one of the most common psychological traps for trifecta patients. As discussed in section 3.8, the overlap between dietary restriction and ARFID (avoidant restrictive food intake disorder) is well-documented, with a positive ARFID screening independently associated with a 7.55 odds ratio for dietary alteration in hEDS patients (Topan et al., 2024). The pursuit of perfect dietary compliance can itself become a source of distress that worsens health outcomes.

The **80/20 consistency principle** provides a psychologically healthier framework. The goal is to follow trifecta dietary principles at approximately 80% of eating occasions while allowing 20% flexibility for imperfect meals, social eating, travel, and days when cooking from scratch is impossible. An 80% adherence rate to a sustainable dietary pattern produces better long-term health outcomes than 100% adherence to a pattern that causes burnout, social isolation, and eventual abandonment (Dansinger et al., 2005).

What the 20% looks like in practice: eating a restaurant meal without knowing the exact freshness of every ingredient. Having a piece of birthday cake at a family celebration. Eating a protein bar with imperfect ingredients because it was the only option available. Using day-old leftovers because the alternative was not eating at all. These are not failures. They are the normal fluctuations of real life that a sustainable dietary framework must accommodate.

The 80/20 principle also accounts for symptom variability. On good days (low symptoms, good energy, well-stocked kitchen), 95% adherence is easy. On bad days (flare, fatigue, pain, empty refrigerator), 60% adherence may be the best possible outcome. Averaging across weeks rather than judging each individual meal prevents the all-or-nothing thinking that drives restrictive eating spirals.

10.10 Nephele's Perfectionism Spiral

Background

Nephele, a 31-year-old graphic designer with hEDS and MCAS, had been following a strict low-histamine, high-sodium, gastroparesis-modified diet for 14 months. She tracked every gram of sodium, weighed her protein portions, timed her meals to the minute, and kept a detailed food journal that she reviewed nightly. She had not eaten at a restaurant or a friend's home since beginning the diet.

Presentation

Nephele described her dietary adherence as "basically perfect" but reported increasing anxiety around food, difficulty sleeping (she lay awake worrying about the next day's meal plan), and worsening social isolation. She had declined three dinner invitations, missed a friend's wedding reception, and eaten separately from her partner at home because she could not tolerate watching him eat foods she considered "red." Her MCAS symptoms were well-controlled, but her quality of life had deteriorated considerably. She described food preparation as "a second full-time job."

Analysis

Nephele's case demonstrates that dietary adherence exists on a spectrum where both extremes cause harm. At one end, complete disregard for trifecta dietary principles produces preventable symptoms and nutritional deficiencies. At the other end, rigid perfectionism produces anxiety, social isolation, and a relationship with food that resembles disordered eating (Topan et al., 2024). The goal is the functional middle ground where symptoms are adequately managed without sacrificing psychological wellbeing and social connection.

Intervention

Nephele's dietitian introduced the 80/20 principle and worked with her to identify specific flexibility opportunities. The first assignment was to eat one meal per week at her partner's table, eating the same base meal (she prepared her portion with modifications) but in a shared social context. The second was to identify three restaurants within driving distance that could accommodate a simple order (grilled chicken, plain rice, steamed vegetables, extra salt) and eat out once every two weeks. The third was to stop weighing food portions and instead use the visual Trifecta Plate model for meal composition.

Outcome

After two months, Nephele was eating with her partner daily, had eaten at two restaurants, and had attended a friend's dinner (bringing her own prepared meal, which the host warmed for her). Her MCAS symptoms did not worsen with the reduced rigidity. Her anxiety around food decreased noticeably. She described the shift as "realizing that an 85% diet that lets me have a life is better than a 100% diet that took my life away."

Teaching Points

- Dietary perfectionism in trifecta patients can produce psychological harm (anxiety, social isolation, disordered eating patterns) that offsets or exceeds the benefits of strict dietary adherence
- The 80/20 consistency principle provides a psychologically sustainable framework by explicitly permitting imperfect eating occasions without framing them as failures
- Gradual reintroduction of social eating (shared meals, restaurant visits) can occur without symptom worsening when the overall dietary pattern remains consistent

10.11 Daily Intake Target Summary

Translating the principles from Chapters 4.0 through 9.0 into concrete daily targets creates a practical reference for meal planning. These numbers represent evidence-based ranges for trifecta patients; individual targets should be established with a healthcare provider.

Fluid target: 2 to 3 liters daily, including water, electrolyte drinks, broth, and fluid-rich foods. The 2021 NIH Expert Consensus recommendation for POTS patients is 2 to 3 liters of water plus sodium supplementation (Vernino et al., 2021). Fluid should be distributed throughout the day, with the first 500 milliliters consumed before getting out of bed in the morning (as discussed in Marius's case, section 4.8).

Sodium target: 3,000 to 10,000 milligrams daily, individualized based on POTS subtype and blood pressure response. The 2015 Heart Rhythm Society consensus recommends up to 10 to 12 grams of salt daily (Sheldon et al., 2015). Patients with hyperadrenergic POTS may require lower targets. Sources include cooking salt, electrolyte drinks, salted foods, and salt tablets.

Protein target: 1.0 to 1.2 grams per kilogram of body weight daily, distributed across all eating occasions. For a 70-kilogram individual, this means 70 to 84 grams daily, or approximately 12 to 17 grams per eating occasion across five to six meals and snacks (DiBaise et al., 2019; Topan et al., 2024).

Fiber target: 20 to 30 grams daily for patients without active gastroparesis, adjusted downward (10 to 15 grams) during gastroparesis flares. Focus on soluble fiber sources (oatmeal, cooked vegetables, peeled fruits) rather than insoluble fiber sources (raw vegetable skins, bran). The general population recommendation of 25 to 38 grams may be unrealistic for patients with significant GI dysfunction (Steiner et al., 2023).

Micronutrient targets for supplementation (as established in Chapter 5.0): vitamin D at 5,000 IU D3 daily year-round, with monitoring of 25-hydroxyvitamin D levels (Gensemer et al., 2021); vitamin C at 750 to 1,000 milligrams daily for collagen support and mast cell stabilization (Hagel et al., 2013); vitamin B12 monitoring with supplementation as needed (particularly for patients on PPIs, with SIBO, or following vegan diets); magnesium glycinate at 200 to 400 milligrams daily (Steiner et al., 2023); and iron bisglycinate if ferritin is below 30 ng/mL, dosed on alternate days for improved absorption (Stoffel et al., 2017).

These targets are not all-or-nothing thresholds. Reaching 80% of a target most days is substantially better than reaching 100% some days and 30% on others. Consistency across weeks matters more than precision at individual meals.

10.12 Putting It All Together

The Trifecta Plate model, the condition decision tree, the traffic light food classification, the safe foods master list, the 80/20 principle, and the daily intake targets work together as an integrated system. No single tool is sufficient on its own. The plate provides meal-level structure. The decision tree provides sequence for implementation. The traffic light system provides rapid food-level decisions. The safe foods list provides accumulated personal data. The 80/20 principle provides psychological sustainability. And the daily targets provide measurable goals against which progress can be assessed.

The four preceding chapters (Chapters 6.0 through 9.0) provided the science. This chapter provides the translation. But translation without personalization is just another generic diet plan, and generic diet plans fail chronically ill patients because chronic illness is not generic. Each trifecta patient carries a unique combination of symptom severity, food tolerances, medication regimens, physical capabilities, financial constraints, and personal food preferences. The framework presented here accommodates that individuality by providing structure without rigidity, guidance without prescription, and targets without perfectionism.

In the chapters that follow (Part Three), we will move from framework to execution: specific meal plans, recipes adapted for trifecta compatibility, and practical cooking strategies for patients managing fatigue, pain, and limited kitchen energy. The framework you've built in this chapter will serve as the organizing structure for every meal plan and recipe that follows.

PART THREE: MEAL PLANS & PRACTICAL TOOLS

Chapter 11.0: Four Week Trifecta Meal Plan

Faustina spent three weeks reading about low-histamine eating, sodium targets, gastroparesis modifications, and anti-inflammatory strategies. She understood the science. She could explain why leftover chicken accumulates histamine and why sweet potatoes are preferable to white bread for POTS management. But at 6:30 on a Monday morning, standing in her kitchen with brain fog and aching joints, all that knowledge collapsed into a single, paralyzing question: what do I actually eat right now? The distance between understanding dietary principles and producing six trifecta-compatible eating occasions every single day, while managing fatigue, pain, and unpredictable symptoms, is where most patients abandon the entire effort. This chapter eliminates that distance.

The following four-week meal plan applies every principle established in Chapters 6.0 through 10.0. It is organized as a progressive framework:

- Week 1 establishes the baseline with simple, well-tolerated meals
- Week 2 expands ingredient variety while maintaining the trifecta framework
- Week 3 introduces greater flavor complexity through herbs, spices, and cooking methods
- Week 4 provides mix-and-match templates for independent meal planning
- Each day tracks sodium, histamine risk, fluid intake, prep time, and batch-cooking options

11.1 How to Use This Plan

This meal plan is a teaching tool, not a rigid prescription. The Trifecta Plate model from section 10.1 provides the structural foundation for every eating occasion: approximately one-quarter protein, one-quarter complex carbohydrate, one-quarter cooked vegetable, and distributed healthy fats, with liberal salt and electrolyte-enhanced fluid at every meal.

Each day includes six eating occasions: breakfast, mid-morning snack, lunch, afternoon snack, dinner, and evening snack. This frequency is based on the evidence discussed in section 7.4 showing that smaller, more frequent meals reduce postprandial hypotension and splanchnic blood pooling in POTS patients (Ganesh et al., 2020). Six smaller eating occasions also distribute protein intake across the day, supporting the 1.0 to 1.2 grams per kilogram target established in section 8.4 (Topan et al., 2024).

Every meal entry includes five tracking elements. The **sodium tally** shows the approximate milligrams of sodium in that eating occasion and a running daily total, targeting the 3,000 to 10,000 milligram range recommended by the 2021 NIH Expert Consensus (Vernino et al., 2021). The **histamine risk rating** uses a three-tier system: Low (all ingredients fresh or frozen, no known liberators), Moderate (contains one or two yellow-category foods from the traffic light system in section 10.3), or High (contains red-category foods, appropriate only for patients with confirmed tolerance). The **fluid target** tracks cumulative fluid intake toward the 2 to 3 liter daily goal. The **prep time estimate** gives realistic time ranges including cleanup. And the **batch-cooking indicator** marks meals that can be prepared in large quantities and frozen in individual portions for low-energy days.

Two cautions before proceeding. No meal plan can account for every individual's unique food tolerances, medication interactions, or symptom patterns. Use this plan as a starting point and modify it based on your personal safe foods master list (section 10.5). And if you are currently in an active MCAS elimination phase, begin with the specialized plan in Chapter 12.0 rather than this general four-week plan.

11.2 Foundation Week Structure

Week 1 uses the smallest, safest ingredient pool. Every food in this week falls into the green category of the traffic light system (section 10.3), meaning it is low-histamine when fresh, compatible with gastroparesis when properly cooked, and easily incorporated into high-sodium eating. The goal is not variety or excitement. The goal is establishing a reliable baseline from which symptoms can be assessed and future foods can be tested.

The foundation week rotates through a core ingredient list: fresh chicken breast, fresh turkey breast, fresh white fish (cod, tilapia, or sole), rice, oatmeal, sweet potatoes, zucchini, carrots, broccoli, peeled pears, peeled apples, blueberries, olive oil, ghee, fresh ginger, fresh garlic, turmeric, salt, and electrolyte drink mix. These 19 ingredients can produce dozens of different meals through variations in seasoning, cooking method, and combination.

A typical foundation day follows this pattern:

Breakfast (7:00 AM): Salted oatmeal cooked with water, topped with blueberries and a drizzle of ghee. One glass of electrolyte water (500 mL) consumed before getting out of bed (as recommended in section 4.7), plus 250 mL with breakfast. Sodium: approximately 800 mg from salted oatmeal and electrolyte drink. Histamine risk: Low. Prep time: 10 minutes. Batch-cook option: Prepare five servings of oatmeal base and refrigerate in individual containers; reheat within 24 hours only (to prevent histamine accumulation per section 6.2).

Mid-morning snack (9:30 AM): Salted rice cake with almond butter (if tolerated) or ghee, plus a peeled pear. Electrolyte water (250 mL). Sodium: approximately 400 mg. Histamine risk: Low. Prep time: 3 minutes.

Lunch (12:00 PM): Salted chicken breast (cooked fresh that morning or from frozen within 24 hours), rice, and steamed zucchini with olive oil and salt. Water (500 mL with meal). Sodium: approximately 1,200 mg. Histamine risk: Low. Prep time: 25 minutes. Batch-cook option: Cook four chicken breasts, portion individually, freeze three immediately.

Afternoon snack (3:00 PM): Blueberries with a small portion of salted rice. Electrolyte water (250 mL). Sodium: approximately 400 mg. Histamine risk: Low. Prep time: 5 minutes.

Dinner (6:00 PM): Salted white fish with roasted sweet potato wedges and steamed broccoli, all drizzled with olive oil and seasoned with fresh garlic, ginger, and turmeric. Water (500 mL). Sodium: approximately 1,400 mg. Histamine risk: Low. Prep time: 30 minutes.

Evening snack (8:30 PM): Small bowl of warm chicken broth (homemade, short-cooked per section 7.2 or low-histamine commercial brand) with a handful of plain rice. Sodium: approximately 800 mg from broth. Histamine risk: Low. Prep time: 5 minutes (reheating).

Daily totals for this sample day: Sodium approximately 5,000 mg. Fluid approximately 2.75 L. Protein approximately 85 g. Histamine risk: Low across all six occasions. Total active prep time: approximately 78 minutes (reducible to 30 minutes with batch cooking).

The foundation week repeats variations of this pattern, rotating between chicken, turkey, and fish as the protein source, alternating between rice, oatmeal, and sweet potato as the carbohydrate, and cycling through zucchini, carrots, and broccoli as the vegetable. The monotony is intentional. Research on elimination diets demonstrates that a brief period of dietary simplicity (two to four weeks) produces the clearest symptom baseline for subsequent food reintroduction (Joneja, 2017). Patients who start with too many variables cannot determine which foods they tolerate and which they don't.

11.3 Galatea's Foundation Week

Background

Galatea, a 29-year-old software developer with POTS, hEDS, and recently diagnosed MCAS, had been eating a standard American diet before her diagnoses. She consumed fast food three to four times weekly, drank minimal water (primarily coffee and soda), and had never cooked regularly. Her sodium intake was paradoxically adequate (processed food is high in sodium) but came packaged with histamine-rich ingredients, high-glycemic carbohydrates, and large infrequent meals that worsened her postprandial symptoms.

Presentation

Galatea described feeling overwhelmed by the dietary changes required: "I went from eating whatever I wanted to reading that practically everything I eat is wrong." She experienced daily presyncope, brain fog lasting two to four hours after meals, and MCAS flares (facial flushing, GI cramping) two to three times per week. She was eating two large meals daily, consuming less than one liter of water, and her sodium intake dropped from approximately 4,500 mg (from processed foods) to approximately 1,800 mg after she stopped eating fast food but didn't replace the sodium through cooking salt and electrolytes.

Analysis

Galatea's situation illustrates a common paradox in trifecta dietary transitions. Patients who eliminate processed foods (correctly, for histamine and glycemic reasons) often inadvertently reduce their sodium intake, worsening POTS symptoms (Vernino et al., 2021). The two-meal pattern was producing severe postprandial hemodynamic shifts (Mehr et al., 2018). Her minimal water intake compounded the hypovolemia. The foundation week plan addressed all three issues simultaneously: replacing processed-food sodium with cooking salt and electrolytes, distributing intake across six occasions, and increasing fluid to 2.5 liters daily.

Intervention

Galatea followed the foundation week plan with two modifications: she used a meal delivery service for pre-portioned fresh ingredients (reducing the shopping and planning burden during the transition) and set phone alarms for each eating occasion and fluid target. She batch-cooked chicken and rice on Sunday and Wednesday evenings, freezing portions immediately. Her partner helped with dinner preparation on weekdays.

Outcome

By day four, Galatea reported noticeable improvement in afternoon brain fog. By day seven, her standing heart rate had decreased from 135 to 118 (measured with a home pulse oximeter). Her MCAS facial flushing decreased from daily to twice that week. She described the foundation week as "boring but the first time in months I felt like my body was actually working." Sodium intake averaged 5,200 mg daily. Fluid averaged 2.4 liters. The structured framework eliminated decision fatigue around food, which she identified as a major unexpected benefit.

Teaching Points

- Patients transitioning from processed food diets to trifecta-compatible eating often experience a sodium deficit that worsens POTS symptoms, requiring deliberate replacement through cooking salt and electrolyte supplementation
- Phone alarms for eating occasions and fluid targets provide external structure that compensates for brain fog and executive dysfunction, common POTS symptoms that impair self-directed health behaviors
- Batch cooking with immediate freezing maintains freshness principles (section 6.2) while reducing the daily energy expenditure required for meal preparation

11.4 Building Variety in Week Two

Week 2 expands the ingredient pool from 19 to approximately 35 foods by introducing yellow-category items one at a time, following the reintroduction principles from section 6.9. The pace is one new food every one to two days, with at least 48 hours of monitoring between introductions to account for delayed reactions (Sánchez-Pérez et al., 2018).

New foods tested during Week 2 typically include: eggs (starting with yolks only, as egg whites are potential histamine liberators for some individuals, Reese et al., 2017), fresh mozzarella or cottage cheese (low-histamine dairy options), lamb, quinoa, asparagus, cauliflower, green beans, mango, watermelon, fresh basil, fresh cilantro, coconut oil, and almond or cashew butter.

The daily structure remains six eating occasions, but meals become more composed. Breakfast might include scrambled eggs (if tolerated from the Week 2 testing) with salt, sautéed zucchini in olive oil, and a side of rice, rather than the plain oatmeal of Week 1. Lunch might feature a chicken and vegetable bowl with quinoa, fresh basil, and olive oil dressing rather than the plain chicken-rice-steamed-vegetable combination. Dinner might include lamb chops (if tolerated) with roasted root vegetables and fresh herbs.

The sodium tracking continues, but by Week 2 most patients have internalized the habit of salting generously and drinking electrolyte-enhanced fluid. The tracking shifts from a teaching tool to a monitoring tool, used to verify that targets are being met rather than to learn how to meet them. Research on habit formation suggests that dietary behaviors require approximately 66 days to become automatic (Lally et al., 2010), so continued tracking through the full four weeks is appropriate even as the process becomes less effortful.

Batch-cooking expands in Week 2 to include component preparation rather than full-meal preparation. Cooking a large batch of quinoa, roasting a tray of mixed vegetables, and preparing two proteins on a single cooking day creates mix-and-match components that can be assembled into different meals with minimal additional effort. This approach reduces both cooking time and the food-decision burden that contributes to dietary fatigue (Dansinger et al., 2005).

11.5 Week Three Flavor Expansion

By Week 3, the patient has a confirmed safe foods list of 25 to 35 items and a stable symptom baseline. The focus shifts from safety to enjoyment. This shift matters because long-term dietary adherence correlates with food satisfaction more than it correlates with nutritional knowledge (Dansinger et al., 2005). Patients who eat food they enjoy maintain their dietary patterns. Patients who eat food they merely tolerate eventually abandon the effort.

Week 3 introduces greater **culinary complexity** through three avenues. The first is expanded seasoning. Fresh herbs (rosemary, thyme, oregano, dill, mint) and ground spices (cumin, coriander, paprika, cinnamon) are generally well-tolerated from a histamine perspective because they are not fermented and do not contain biogenic amines in meaningful quantities (Maintz & Novak, 2007). Each herb or spice should still be tested individually (small amount added to a known-safe meal, 48 hours monitoring), but the success rate is high. Garlic and ginger, already introduced in Week 1, can now be used more liberally.

The second avenue is **cooking method variety**. Week 1 relied primarily on boiling, steaming, and simple pan-cooking. Week 3 introduces roasting (which caramelizes natural sugars in vegetables, adding sweetness and depth), slow cooking (which allows morning prep with an evening meal ready, ideal for fatigue management), and sautéing with herbs and olive oil. These methods do not increase histamine content if the food is fresh and cooked promptly (Comas-Basté et al., 2020). They do increase flavor substantially.

The third avenue is **meal composition**. Instead of protein plus carbohydrate plus vegetable arranged separately on a plate, Week 3 introduces composed dishes:

chicken and vegetable stir-fry over rice with fresh ginger and garlic, lamb stew with root vegetables and fresh rosemary (slow cooker), fish packets with zucchini, lemon-safe herbs, and olive oil (baked in parchment). These composed dishes feel more like "real food" and less like a medical protocol, which is psychologically important for long-term adherence.

11.6 Ivo's Cooking Confidence

Background

Ivo, a 52-year-old retired firefighter with POTS and MCAS (no EDS), had been following a low-histamine diet for four months. His foundation was solid: he hit sodium targets consistently, maintained adequate fluid intake, and had a safe foods list of 28 items. But he described his meals as "survival food" and said he had stopped looking forward to eating. His wife cooked the same five meals in rotation because they were afraid that any change would trigger symptoms.

Presentation

Ivo's food journal showed adequate caloric intake (2,100 calories daily) and protein (95 grams), but he reported eating mechanically and with decreasing enjoyment. He had gained weight despite adequate caloric balance, which his physician attributed to decreased physical activity since his medical retirement. His mood had declined over the past two months, and he identified food monotony as a contributing factor: "Eating used to be one of my favorite things. Now it feels like taking medicine."

Analysis

Ivo's situation represents the psychological cost of dietary restriction discussed in section 3.8. While his nutritional status was adequate, the hedonic component of eating (the pleasure, social connection, and cultural meaning of food) had been eliminated. Research on dietary quality of life demonstrates that food enjoyment is an independent predictor of treatment adherence and overall wellbeing in patients with chronic conditions requiring dietary modification (Shepherd et al., 2019). Nutritional adequacy without food enjoyment is not a sustainable long-term outcome.

Intervention

Ivo and his wife followed the Week 3 flavor expansion protocol together. They tested fresh rosemary, thyme, cumin, and paprika individually over eight days, with no adverse reactions. They introduced roasting as a cooking method (roasted chicken thighs with rosemary, roasted sweet potato wedges with cumin and salt, roasted carrots with thyme). They prepared a slow-cooker lamb stew with root vegetables and herbs. Ivo's wife described the shift as "cooking again instead of just heating things."

Outcome

Within two weeks, Ivo reported that he looked forward to dinner again. His food journal showed the same caloric intake and macronutrient profile, but with 14 different meals across the two-week period instead of the previous five-meal rotation. His mood improved noticeably. He began inviting a neighbor couple for dinner (preparing the same trifecta-compatible meals, which the guests enjoyed without modifications). He described the herb and spice expansion as "getting my kitchen back."

Teaching Points

- Nutritional adequacy and food enjoyment are both necessary for sustainable long-term dietary adherence; addressing one without the other leads to eventual dietary abandonment or psychological decline
- Fresh herbs and ground spices are generally well-tolerated from a histamine perspective because they are not fermented, making them a low-risk avenue for expanding flavor in trifecta-compatible eating
- Social eating can be maintained with trifecta-compatible meals that do not require separate preparation for non-restricted guests, reducing the social isolation associated with dietary restrictions

11.7 Week Four Independence Templates

Week 4 transitions from following a prescribed plan to creating personalized meal plans using mix-and-match templates. This is the educational objective of the entire four-week program: building the patient's capacity for independent dietary decision-making within the trifecta framework.

The **mix-and-match template** uses the Trifecta Plate model (section 10.1) as a combinatorial framework. The patient selects one item from each of four categories for each eating occasion:

Protein options (from confirmed safe foods list): fresh chicken breast, fresh chicken thigh, fresh turkey, fresh white fish, fresh salmon (if tolerated), lamb, eggs, fresh tofu, cottage cheese, collagen peptides (for smoothies).

Complex carbohydrate options: rice, quinoa, oatmeal, sweet potato, millet, amaranth, gluten-free pasta (if tolerated).

Vegetable options: zucchini, carrots, broccoli, cauliflower, asparagus, green beans, sweet potato (counts as both carbohydrate and vegetable), butternut squash, cucumber (for raw options on good GI days).

Fat and flavor options: olive oil, ghee, coconut oil, almond butter, cashew butter, fresh herbs (rosemary, thyme, basil, cilantro, dill, mint), ground spices (cumin, coriander, paprika, turmeric, cinnamon), fresh garlic, fresh ginger, salt.

With 10 proteins, 7 carbohydrates, 9 vegetables, and 15 fat/flavor options, the combinatorial possibilities are in the thousands. The patient who felt trapped with eight safe foods in Week 1 now has the building blocks for months of varied eating without repeating the same meal twice.

Each combination is checked against the Trifecta Plate criteria: does it provide 15 to 20 grams of protein? Does it include a complex carbohydrate? Is there a vegetable component? Is fat distributed (not concentrated in one item)? Is it salted? Is it accompanied by fluid? If the answer to all six questions is yes, the meal is trifecta-compatible regardless of the specific combination chosen.

The Week 4 plan also introduces **meal planning as a weekly practice**. Setting aside 15 to 20 minutes each week to select combinations for the coming days, write a shopping list based on those selections, and identify one or two batch-cooking sessions reduces daily decision fatigue and ensures that the necessary fresh ingredients are available when needed. This weekly planning habit is the practical infrastructure that sustains trifecta eating beyond the structured four-week program.

11.8 Tracking and Adjustments

Throughout all four weeks, tracking sodium, fluid, protein, and symptoms provides the data needed to make informed adjustments. By Week 4, the tracking can be simplified. Rather than logging every milligram of sodium at every meal, patients can track three daily checkpoints: morning sodium (did I salt breakfast and have my first electrolyte drink?), afternoon sodium (have I had a second electrolyte serving and salted lunch and snack?), and evening sodium (did I salt dinner and have broth or an additional electrolyte serving?). If all three checkpoints are met, sodium targets are generally achieved without precise counting.

Fluid tracking follows a similar simplification. Rather than measuring every glass, patients can monitor urine color (pale yellow indicates adequate hydration, dark yellow indicates insufficient fluid, Ganesh et al., 2020) and track their large-volume fluid events: morning electrolyte drink before rising, water with each meal, and one to two additional glasses between meals.

The symptom journal, however, should continue beyond the four-week plan. Symptom patterns often become apparent only after several weeks of consistent data, and the journal remains the primary tool for identifying new triggers, confirming food tolerances during reintroduction, and tracking the effect of medication changes on dietary tolerability (Joneja, 2017). The food-symptom journal described in section 6.11 provides the format: time, all foods consumed, preparation method, portion size, and symptoms within 24 to 48 hours across skin, GI, neurological, cardiovascular, and respiratory categories.

11.9 Beyond the Four Weeks

The four-week meal plan is a training program, not a permanent protocol. Its purpose is to build three competencies: the practical skill of preparing trifecta-compatible meals efficiently, the personal knowledge of which foods you tolerate and which you don't, and the confidence to make independent dietary decisions using the Trifecta Plate model. Once these competencies are established, the meal plan becomes unnecessary. The patient eats using their safe foods list, their mix-and-match template, and their internalized understanding of trifecta principles.

Long-term dietary success in chronic illness requires flexibility, not rigidity. Research on dietary adherence in celiac disease (which shares the lifelong dietary restriction dimension with trifecta management) demonstrates that patients who develop flexible frameworks for food decisions maintain better adherence and higher quality of life over five or more years than patients who rely on rigid rules or prescribed meal plans (Hall et al., 2009). The 80/20 consistency principle from section 10.9 applies here: aiming for consistent application of trifecta principles across 80% of eating occasions, while allowing 20% flexibility for imperfect meals, social eating, and low-energy days when the best available option is not the textbook-ideal option.

Chapter 12.0 addresses the specialized situations that arise within this flexible framework: flare days, gastroparesis episodes, elimination phases, weight recovery, and eating away from home. Together, this chapter and the next provide the practical tools to sustain trifecta eating across the full spectrum of daily life.

Chapter 12.0: Specialized Situation Meal Plans

The four-week plan in Chapter 11.0 assumes a baseline level of stability: symptoms are partially managed, the patient can cook at least some of the time, kitchen access is consistent, and the primary challenge is establishing a sustainable daily eating pattern. But chronic illness does not stay at baseline. MCAS flares erupt. Gastroparesis worsens for weeks at a time. Weight drops. Travel disrupts routines. Teenagers need school-compatible options. Budgets tighten. Each of these situations demands a modified approach to trifecta eating, and the patient who has only one dietary mode (the standard plan) will abandon the framework entirely the first time circumstances change. This chapter provides eight specialized plans for the situations that arise most frequently.

This chapter covers the following situations:

- Flare day eating when symptoms are severe and energy is minimal
- Gastroparesis-specific modifications for periods of delayed gastric emptying
- Strict MCAS elimination phase eating during the initial diagnostic period
- Calorie-dense recovery eating for patients with unintentional weight loss
- Dietary transition plans for newly diagnosed post-COVID POTS patients
- Teen and young adult adaptations for the predominantly young female POTS population
- Budget-conscious trifecta eating when finances are limited
- Travel and restaurant strategies for maintaining dietary needs away from home

12.1 The Flare Day Plan

A **flare day** is any day when symptoms are so severe that normal functioning is substantially impaired. MCAS flares can produce widespread flushing, GI distress, cognitive dysfunction, and systemic inflammation that lasts hours to days (Afrin et al., 2016). POTS flares involve severe orthostatic intolerance that confines patients to bed or recline. EDS flares may involve acute joint instability, pain spikes, or GI crises. On these days, the standard meal plan is unrealistic. Standing in a kitchen for 30 minutes to prepare dinner is not possible when standing for 30 seconds triggers near-syncope.

The flare day plan has three requirements: zero to minimal cooking, maximum sodium and fluid delivery, and no histamine risk. Every item on the flare day plan can be prepared in under five minutes, consumed while lying down or reclined, and stored in a form that requires no advance preparation.

Flare day staples (stock these when you're feeling well, so they're available when you're not): commercial low-histamine chicken broth or bone broth (single-serve containers, read labels for additives), plain rice (cook a batch on a good day and freeze in single-serve portions), electrolyte drink mix or tablets, collagen peptide powder, peeled and frozen fruit (blueberries, mango chunks), plain rice cakes, almond butter or sunflower seed butter (single-serve packets if available), and applesauce (no sugar added).

A flare day eating pattern might look like this: warm broth with salt and collagen peptides (sipped in bed, 800 mg sodium, 18 g protein from collagen), electrolyte water throughout the morning, a rice cake with almond butter and salt for mid-morning, warm broth with a small amount of reheated frozen rice for lunch, a smoothie made with frozen blueberries, collagen peptides, and water in the afternoon (if a blender is manageable), warm broth for dinner, and applesauce with salt for an evening snack. This pattern delivers approximately 1,200 to 1,400 calories, 50 to 60 grams of protein, 4,000 to 5,000 milligrams of sodium, and 2 to 2.5 liters of fluid with virtually no preparation time and zero histamine risk.

The flare day plan is not nutritionally complete. It is designed for crisis management, not long-term sustenance. If flare days extend beyond three to four consecutive days, more substantial food intake becomes medically necessary, and the patient should communicate with their healthcare team about whether the flare requires clinical intervention (Tseng et al., 2021).

12.2 Faramond's Flare Day Protocol

Background

Faramond, a 43-year-old electrician with MCAS and POTS, experienced MCAS flares approximately twice monthly, lasting two to four days each. During flares, he experienced severe facial and trunk flushing, GI cramping with diarrhea, cognitive dysfunction ("can't think straight enough to follow a recipe"), and orthostatic intolerance that prevented standing for more than two to three minutes. Before developing his flare protocol, he ate nothing during flare days, then overate when the flare resolved, causing a secondary cycle of GI distress and postprandial hypotension.

Presentation

Faramond's pattern of fasting during flares followed by compensatory overeating was producing a boom-and-bust cycle that compounded his symptoms. The fasting periods worsened his POTS (hypovolemia from reduced fluid and sodium intake during the 48 to 96 hour flare period, Vernino et al., 2021), while the subsequent large meals overwhelmed his GI tract and triggered postprandial symptoms (Ganesh et al., 2020). His weight fluctuated by 5 to 8 pounds across each flare-recovery cycle. He described the situation as "I can't eat when I'm sick, and then I eat too much when I feel better."

Analysis

Faramond's fasting-then-overeating pattern reflects a lack of flare-specific dietary infrastructure rather than a lack of knowledge. He understood what he should eat; he simply didn't have the right foods available in the right forms when he was too symptomatic to shop or cook. The intervention focused on creating a permanent "flare shelf" in his pantry and a "flare drawer" in his freezer, stocked during well periods with items that required no preparation.

Intervention

Faramond built a flare kit containing 12 shelf-stable single-serve broth containers (low-histamine brand), electrolyte tablets, collagen peptide powder, rice cakes, single-serve almond butter packets, and applesauce cups. In his freezer, he maintained six individual-serve containers of plain cooked rice. He practiced the flare day eating pattern during a good day to confirm he could prepare everything while lying down or sitting (microwave for broth and rice, no standing required). His wife helped stock the flare kit after each use so it was always ready.

Outcome

Over his next three flare episodes, Faramond maintained oral intake throughout, consuming 1,200 to 1,500 calories, approximately 55 grams of protein, and 4,500 milligrams of sodium daily during flares. His POTS symptoms during and after flares improved noticeably because he was no longer compounding the flare with dehydration and sodium depletion. The post-flare overeating pattern disappeared because he wasn't arriving at recovery starved. His weight fluctuations decreased from 5 to 8 pounds per cycle to 1 to 2 pounds.

Teaching Points

- Flare day eating requires advance preparation during well periods, not real-time decision-making during acute symptoms, because cognitive dysfunction and physical limitation during flares prevent normal food preparation
- Maintaining even modest oral intake during flares (1,200 to 1,500 calories with adequate sodium and fluid) prevents the secondary dehydration and hypovolemia that compound POTS symptoms and prolong recovery

- The boom-and-bust pattern of fasting during flares followed by compensatory overeating creates its own cycle of GI distress that can be interrupted by consistent low-level intake throughout the flare period

12.3 The Gastroparesis Plan

When gastroparesis worsens (as it does episodically in many EDS patients, with 12.26 times higher odds ratio for gastroparesis compared to the general population, Thwaites et al., 2022), the standard meal plan requires specific modifications. The **gastroparesis plan** adjusts four variables: meal volume, texture, fiber type, and fat distribution.

Volume decreases from the standard 250 to 350 mL per meal to 150 to 200 mL per eating occasion, with corresponding increases in eating frequency from six to eight occasions daily. Smaller volumes reduce gastric distension and the sensation of fullness and nausea that accompany delayed emptying.

Texture shifts toward softer, more processed forms. Raw vegetables are replaced with pureed or very well-cooked vegetables. Chicken breast is replaced with ground chicken or chicken cooked until very tender and shredded. Rice is cooked slightly softer than usual. Smoothies replace whole-fruit snacks. Soups replace composed meals. Liquids and semi-liquids empty from the stomach faster than solid foods, with emptying rates following a hierarchy: clear liquids fastest, then thick liquids, then pureed foods, then soft solids, then firm solids (Thwaites et al., 2022).

Fiber is modified but not eliminated. Soluble fiber (oatmeal, peeled cooked fruits, well-cooked root vegetables) is generally tolerated because it dissolves in water and does not form the solid masses that insoluble fiber can create in a slowly-emptying stomach. Insoluble fiber (raw vegetable skins, seeds, husks, bran) is reduced because it can accumulate and form bezoars in patients with severe gastroparesis (DiBaise et al., 2019).

Fat is distributed across all eating occasions in small amounts rather than concentrated in one or two meals. Fat slows gastric emptying, so a meal containing 20 to 30 grams of fat may be tolerated poorly during a gastroparesis episode, while the same total fat distributed as 5 to 8 grams across four eating occasions is often manageable. Olive oil (1 teaspoon rather than 1 tablespoon per meal), small amounts of ghee, and almond butter (half a tablespoon rather than a full tablespoon) maintain caloric density without overwhelming the stomach.

Sodium and fluid targets remain the same during gastroparesis episodes, but delivery may shift toward broth, electrolyte drinks, and liquid-based meals rather than solid food with water alongside. Sipping fluid between meals rather than drinking large volumes with meals can also reduce gastric distension (Ganesh et al., 2020).

12.4 The MCAS Elimination Plan

The **MCAS elimination phase plan** is designed for the initial two to four week diagnostic period described in section 6.9, when the strictest possible low-histamine protocol is applied to establish a clear symptom baseline. This plan uses only foods from the lowest-risk tier: those with essentially no histamine content, no liberator activity, and no DAO-blocking properties.

The elimination phase food list is deliberately narrow: fresh chicken breast, fresh turkey breast, fresh cod or tilapia (cooked immediately from frozen), white rice, oatmeal, sweet potatoes, zucchini, carrots, peeled pears, peeled apples, blueberries, olive oil, ghee, salt, fresh ginger, and water. No dairy, no eggs, no nuts (potential liberators for some), no spices beyond salt and ginger, no reheated leftovers. Every protein is cooked fresh or from frozen within four hours of thawing.

This level of restriction is appropriate only for the initial diagnostic phase and should not extend beyond four weeks. As discussed in section 6.9, prolonged severe restriction reduces dietary diversity, impairs gut microbiome health (Staudacher et al., 2017), increases the risk of nutritional deficiency (Steiner et al., 2023), and can trigger or worsen ARFID-type food anxiety (Topan et al., 2024). The elimination phase is a diagnostic tool, not a lifestyle. Its purpose is to determine if dietary histamine is contributing to the patient's symptoms, after which systematic reintroduction begins.

Sodium targets during elimination must be met through cooking salt and electrolyte drinks because many traditional high-sodium foods (canned soups, processed meats, soy sauce) are histamine-rich and excluded during this phase. The homemade short-cooked broth described in section 7.2 is one of the few options that delivers substantial sodium (800 to 1,000 mg per cup) while remaining strictly low-histamine, provided it is cooked for two to four hours (not 24 hours), consumed immediately, or frozen in portions (Comas-Basté et al., 2020).

12.5 The Recovery and Weight Gain Plan

Unintentional weight loss is common in trifecta patients. The 2024 cross-sectional study of 680 hEDS patients found that 62.3% regularly skipped meals (Topan et al., 2024), and 10% of POTS patients at tertiary care centers required nutritional support at some point in their care (Tseng et al., 2021). The recovery plan is designed for patients who need to increase caloric intake substantially (by 400 to 800 calories daily) to halt weight loss and begin weight restoration.

The **calorie-dense trifecta strategy** adds calories through three mechanisms that do not increase meal volume (which would worsen gastroparesis) or histamine load (which would risk MCAS flares).

The first mechanism is **fat fortification**. Adding one tablespoon of olive oil or ghee to each of six eating occasions adds approximately 720 calories to the daily total without increasing volume or histamine risk. Drizzling oil on rice, stirring ghee into oatmeal, adding oil to smoothies, and cooking vegetables in oil rather than steaming them are simple additions that most patients can implement immediately.

The second mechanism is **collagen peptide supplementation**. Adding a scoop of hydrolyzed collagen peptides (typically 18 to 20 grams of protein and 70 to 80 calories per scoop) to one or two daily beverages (smoothies, broth, or warm water with electrolytes) increases both caloric and protein intake without adding volume, requiring cooking, or introducing histamine. Collagen peptides are pre-hydrolyzed, meaning they dissolve in liquids and do not require gastric digestion for absorption, making them well-tolerated even during gastroparesis episodes (DiBaise et al., 2019).

The third mechanism is **calorie-dense snack substitutions**. Replacing low-calorie snacks (plain fruit, rice cakes) with calorie-dense equivalents (fruit with almond butter, rice cakes with nut butter and ghee, oatmeal balls made with oats, almond butter, honey, and collagen peptides) increases daily intake by 200 to 400 calories without adding additional eating occasions.

The combined effect of these three mechanisms can increase daily intake by 900 to 1,200 calories, which is typically sufficient to halt weight loss and begin slow recovery (0.5 to 1 pound per week) for most trifecta patients (Tseng et al., 2021).

12.6 Melisande's Weight Recovery

Background

Melisande, a 24-year-old graduate student with hEDS, POTS, and MCAS, had experienced progressive weight loss over seven months, from 132 pounds (BMI 22.0) to 112 pounds (BMI 18.7). Her MCAS had been poorly controlled for several months, producing frequent GI symptoms that made eating aversive. She had developed significant food anxiety, eating only four foods (rice, plain chicken, zucchini, and pears) because she was afraid that any new food would trigger a flare. Her caloric intake averaged 900 to 1,000 calories daily.

Presentation

Melisande's laboratory results showed low prealbumin (indicating protein malnutrition), low ferritin (17 ng/mL, below the 30 ng/mL threshold recommended for POTS patients in section 5.6), and low vitamin D (18 ng/mL, well below the 40 to 60 ng/mL target discussed in section 5.3). Her POTS symptoms had worsened progressively as her nutritional status declined: resting heart rate had increased from 82 to 96, and standing heart rate from 120 to 145. Her hair was thinning, her bruising had increased, and she reported worsening fatigue even at baseline.

Analysis

Melisande's case illustrates the destructive cycle described in section 3.5: MCAS symptoms cause food restriction, which causes nutritional deficiency, which worsens POTS and EDS symptoms, which increases physiological stress, which may further activate mast cells, which worsens MCAS symptoms. Breaking this cycle requires simultaneous nutritional rehabilitation and MCAS management. Her gastroenterologist adjusted her mast cell stabilizing medications (adding cromolyn sodium before meals), which reduced her GI symptoms enough to tolerate dietary expansion.

Intervention

The recovery plan targeted 1,800 calories initially, increasing to 2,200 calories over four weeks. The three calorie-dense mechanisms were applied: one tablespoon of olive oil added to each of six eating occasions (+720 calories), collagen peptides added to two daily beverages (+150 calories), and nut butter added to two snacks (+200 calories). Her four safe foods remained the foundation, with gradual reintroduction of additional foods (sweet potato, carrots, oatmeal, ghee, blueberries) following the protocol in section 6.9. Iron bisglycinate supplementation (every other day for improved absorption, Stoffel et al., 2017), vitamin D3 at 5,000 IU daily, and vitamin C at 1,000 mg daily addressed her laboratory deficiencies.

Outcome

Over three months, Melisande's caloric intake stabilized at 1,900 to 2,100 calories daily. Her weight increased to 122 pounds. Her prealbumin normalized. Ferritin increased to 28 ng/mL (approaching target). Standing heart rate decreased from 145 to 125. Her food list expanded from four to 18 items. She described the olive oil fortification as "the easiest change that made the biggest difference" because it added substantial calories without adding volume, preparation time, or histamine risk.

Teaching Points

- Unintentional weight loss in trifecta patients often reflects a destructive cycle in which MCAS-driven food restriction leads to nutritional deficiency, which worsens POTS and EDS symptoms, which increases physiological stress and further activates mast cells
- Fat fortification (adding olive oil or ghee to existing meals) is the most efficient calorie-dense strategy for trifecta patients because it adds 120 calories per tablespoon without increasing volume, preparation time, or histamine risk
- Nutritional rehabilitation and MCAS medication management should proceed simultaneously rather than sequentially, because nutritional deficiency itself may perpetuate mast cell activation

12.7 The Post COVID Transition Plan

Post-COVID POTS now represents the largest subset of new POTS diagnoses, with estimates suggesting that 2 to 14% of COVID-19 survivors develop POTS symptoms (Blitshteyn & Whitelaw, 2021). These patients face a unique transition challenge: they were eating normally days or weeks before their diagnosis and must rapidly adopt a dietary pattern that differs substantially from the standard American diet.

The transition plan works through three two-week phases. **Phase one** (weeks 1 to 2) focuses on the two changes that produce the most immediate symptom improvement: increasing sodium to 5,000 milligrams daily and increasing fluid to 2.5 liters daily (Vernino et al., 2021). Patients add salt to every meal, begin drinking electrolyte-enhanced water, and consume one to two cups of broth daily. No other dietary changes are made in phase one. This limited scope prevents overwhelm and allows patients to experience the benefit of sodium and fluid before asking them to make additional modifications.

Phase two (weeks 3 to 4) introduces meal timing changes: shifting from two to three large meals to five to six smaller eating occasions, with protein at every occasion, to reduce postprandial hypotension (Ganesh et al., 2020). Patients also reduce high-glycemic carbohydrates (white bread, sugary drinks, candy) in favor of complex carbohydrates (rice, sweet potatoes, oats) to prevent the blood sugar spikes that worsen POTS tachycardia (Shibao et al., 2005).

Phase three (weeks 5 to 6) introduces low-histamine principles if MCAS symptoms are present, or focuses on anti-inflammatory dietary shifts (more vegetables, olive oil, fatty fish) if the primary presentation is POTS without MCAS features. Not all post-COVID POTS patients have MCAS, and low-histamine restrictions should not be applied universally without clinical indication (Afrin et al., 2016).

12.8 The Teen and Young Adult Plan

POTS disproportionately affects adolescent and young adult females, with typical onset during puberty and a female-to-male ratio of approximately 5:1 (Shaw et al., 2019). Dietary management in this population requires adaptations for school schedules, peer social dynamics, developmental nutritional needs, and the psychological risk of dietary restriction in a population already vulnerable to eating disorders.

School-compatible eating means packing portable trifecta meals and snacks that can be consumed during restricted lunch periods (typically 20 to 30 minutes) and between classes. Practical options include: salted rice with shredded chicken in a thermos container, nut butter and rice cakes in a bag, electrolyte water in a reusable bottle, and fruit with individual salt packets. Many schools allow students with medical conditions to carry water bottles and snacks if documentation is provided; a physician's letter specifying the need for frequent fluid, sodium, and food intake can facilitate this accommodation (Sheldon et al., 2015).

Peer dynamics present a genuine challenge. Teenagers eating differently from their friends face social pressure and potential stigma. Two strategies help: normalizing the diet by presenting trifecta-compatible foods that look similar to standard teen food (salted chicken rice bowls, smoothies, fruit and nut butter, plain burgers on compatible buns if gluten is tolerated), and developing a brief, matter-of-fact explanation for curious peers ("I have a condition that means I need extra salt and have to eat certain things"). Lengthy medical explanations are neither necessary nor socially advisable for most teens.

Nutritional needs during adolescence differ from adults. Calcium requirements are higher (1,300 mg daily for ages 9 to 18 versus 1,000 mg for adults, National Institutes of Health, 2021), and adequate nutrition supports ongoing bone mineralization, growth, and hormonal development. Iron requirements are elevated in menstruating adolescents (15 mg daily versus 8 mg for adult males). Caloric needs are often higher than adults assume, ranging from 1,800 to 2,400 calories daily depending on activity level and growth phase. Restricting a teenager's diet too aggressively can impair growth and development, so the clinical team must weigh symptom management against developmental nutritional needs (Shaw et al., 2019).

12.9 The Budget Friendly Approach

Trifecta eating does not require expensive specialty foods. The core trifecta-compatible ingredients (chicken, rice, oatmeal, root vegetables, cooking oil, salt) are among the least expensive items in any grocery store. Several strategies help patients manage trifecta nutrition on limited incomes.

Frozen vegetables and fruits are equally nutritious (and often more nutritious) than fresh produce, because flash-freezing preserves vitamins at the point of harvest while "fresh" produce loses nutrients during transportation and storage (Bouzari et al., 2015). Frozen vegetables are also lower in histamine than fresh produce that has been sitting in the grocery store for days, making them both cheaper and safer for MCAS patients. A bag of frozen broccoli, carrots, or green beans costs one to two dollars and provides four to six servings.

Whole chicken is substantially cheaper per pound than boneless skinless chicken breast, and yields both meat and bones for short-cooked broth (providing sodium and collagen-supporting amino acids). A whole chicken at standard grocery prices provides six to eight servings of protein plus two to three quarts of broth. The catch is that whole-chicken cooking requires more time and skill than prepackaged cuts, so this option works better for patients who have at least one higher-energy cooking day per week for batch preparation.

Dried grains and legumes (rice, oats, quinoa, lentils, chickpeas) are the least expensive complex carbohydrate and plant protein sources available. A one-pound bag of dried rice costs approximately one dollar and provides eight to ten servings. Oats cost even less. These staples form the carbohydrate backbone of trifecta eating at minimal cost.

Salt and electrolyte costs can be managed by using plain table salt for cooking (effectively free per serving) and making homemade electrolyte drinks from salt, water, and a small amount of fruit juice or citrus (if tolerated), rather than purchasing commercial electrolyte drink mixes, which can cost two to four dollars per serving. A simple recipe of 1/4 teaspoon salt, 1/4 teaspoon potassium-containing salt substitute, two tablespoons of honey, and 16 ounces of water provides a functional electrolyte drink for pennies.

12.10 Salome's Budget Trifecta Plan

Background

Salome, a 33-year-old single mother of two with POTS and hEDS, was living on disability benefits after leaving her nursing career due to worsening symptoms. Her monthly food budget was approximately $350 for the household. She had received dietary recommendations from her cardiologist that included expensive items:

specific brands of electrolyte drinks ($45 per month), grass-fed beef ($8 to $12 per pound), organic produce, and collagen peptide supplements ($35 per month). She calculated that following the recommended diet as specified would cost over $600 monthly for her alone, not including food for her children.

Presentation

Salome was eating approximately 1,500 calories daily, with sodium around 2,500 mg (well below her 5,000 mg target) because she couldn't afford commercial electrolyte drinks and didn't realize she could meet targets through cooking salt alone. She was buying conventional chicken breast (the cheapest fresh protein available) but not buying vegetables consistently because fresh produce was expensive and spoiled before she could use it during low-energy weeks. She described feeling that "this diet is for people with money."

Analysis

Salome's experience reflects a systemic barrier to dietary management of chronic illness: evidence-based dietary recommendations are often communicated through the lens of affluent patient populations, using brand-name products and specialty ingredients that are unnecessary for achieving the nutritional targets. The actual trifecta requirements (adequate sodium, fluid, protein, low-histamine fresh or frozen foods, and basic micronutrient supplementation) can be met with standard grocery items at standard prices.

Intervention

A dietitian restructured Salome's approach around budget staples. Whole chickens ($1.29 per pound) replaced boneless breasts ($3.99 per pound), yielding meat plus broth. Frozen vegetables ($1.00 to $1.50 per bag) replaced fresh. Rice and oats became the primary carbohydrates. Homemade electrolyte drinks (salt, potassium substitute, water, small amount of juice) replaced commercial mixes. A store-brand multivitamin ($8 per month) replaced multiple specialty supplements. Vitamin D3 as a standalone supplement ($5 for three months' supply) and vitamin C ($6 for two months' supply) were the only individual supplements added.

Outcome

Salome's monthly food budget for herself came to approximately $180, well within her household budget constraints. Her sodium intake increased to 4,800 mg daily through aggressive cooking salt use and homemade electrolyte drinks. Her protein intake increased to 75 grams daily (from approximately 50 grams) through whole-chicken meal prep. Frozen vegetables provided consistent produce access regardless of energy levels. She described the experience as "finding out the diet was actually accessible once someone stripped away the fancy stuff."

Teaching Points

- Evidence-based trifecta dietary recommendations can be met with standard grocery items at standard prices, and the perception that trifecta eating requires specialty or expensive products reflects communication bias rather than nutritional reality
- Frozen vegetables and fruits are equivalent to or better than fresh produce for trifecta patients because flash-freezing both preserves nutrients and prevents histamine accumulation, while costing substantially less
- Homemade electrolyte drinks using salt, potassium substitute, and water provide comparable electrolyte delivery to commercial products at a fraction of the cost

12.11 Travel and Eating Out

Maintaining trifecta dietary principles away from home requires advance planning rather than real-time improvisation. Travel and restaurant eating cannot perfectly replicate home cooking, but the 80/20 principle from section 10.9 provides the framework: aim for trifecta compatibility at most meals while accepting that some travel meals will be imperfect.

Restaurant strategies begin with menu selection. Most restaurants can prepare simply seasoned grilled chicken, plain rice, and steamed vegetables, which constitutes a green-category Trifecta Plate meal. Adding extra salt at the table and ordering plain water with an electrolyte tablet or packet maintains sodium and fluid targets. Restaurants where this approach works well include American grill restaurants, Asian restaurants (where plain rice is always available), and Mediterranean restaurants (where olive oil, grilled proteins, and vegetables are standard offerings). Fast food can work in emergencies: a plain grilled chicken sandwich without the bun plus a side salad provides protein and vegetables, and salt packets are free.

The primary restaurant risks are freshness uncertainty (you can't verify when the chicken was defrosted or how long the food sat before serving), hidden ingredients (sauces and dressings may contain histamine-rich ingredients like soy sauce, vinegar, or fermented compounds), and portion size (restaurant portions are typically larger than trifecta-friendly meal volumes). Managing these risks involves asking for simply prepared food with sauce on the side, requesting freshly cooked rather than pre-prepared items, and eating a trifecta-appropriate portion while taking the rest home or leaving it.

Travel preparation means packing a travel kit with non-perishable trifecta staples: electrolyte tablets or powder (enough for the entire trip plus two buffer days), salt packets, rice cakes, individual nut butter packets, collagen peptide powder (single-serve packets), and a refillable water bottle. For air travel, these items all pass through security without issue. For road trips, a cooler with ice packs can maintain fresh cooked chicken, rice portions, and peeled fruit for six to eight hours. For longer trips, booking accommodation with kitchen access (apartment rental or hotel with kitchenette) provides the option to cook trifecta meals with locally purchased fresh ingredients.

12.12 Summary

The specialized plans in this chapter share a common principle with the four-week plan in Chapter 11.0: structure enables flexibility. The patient who has a flare day protocol stocked and ready is more flexible during a flare than the patient who has no plan. The patient who knows how to order a trifecta-compatible restaurant meal is more flexible while traveling than the patient who avoids restaurants entirely. The teen who can pack a school-compatible trifecta lunch is more flexible in their social life than the teen who skips eating until they get home.

Each specialized plan modifies the trifecta framework for its specific context without abandoning the framework's core principles. Sodium targets remain consistent across all plans because POTS physiology doesn't change during a gastroparesis flare or a family vacation. Low-histamine freshness principles remain consistent because MCAS biology doesn't take days off. Protein distribution across multiple eating occasions remains consistent because connective tissue needs don't decrease during budget constraints. What changes is the practical implementation: the specific foods, the preparation methods, the eating schedule, and the level of strictness applied to each trifecta dimension.

The chapters that follow in Part Four will address the psychosocial dimensions of trifecta eating: the emotional relationship with food, managing dietary restrictions in relationships and families, communicating dietary needs to healthcare providers, and building a sustainable long-term relationship with eating that serves health without consuming identity. The practical foundation built in these two chapters, together with the scientific foundation from Part Two, provides the knowledge and the tools. What remains is the human experience of living with dietary restrictions in a world that doesn't always accommodate them.

Chapter 13.0: Shopping, Pantry and Kitchen Setup

Berenice stood in the grocery store holding two cans of chicken broth, squinting at ingredient lists through brain fog so thick that the words blurred together. One brand listed "natural flavors" without specifying what those flavors contained. The other included tomato paste, a histamine liberator she had learned about in Chapter 6.0. Her cart already held a bag of frozen chicken breasts that had been sitting in the store's open freezer case for an unknown duration, a package of pre-cut vegetables whose "packaged on" date was four days earlier, and a bottle of electrolyte drink containing citric acid. She had spent 40 minutes in the store. Her standing heart rate was climbing past 110. Her ankles were beginning to swell. And she still didn't have enough food for two days. This is where trifecta eating fails for most people. Not in the meal plan. Not in the science. In the grocery store, in the pantry, and in the kitchen itself.

This chapter provides the practical infrastructure that turns dietary knowledge into daily eating:

- Shelf-stable, refrigerator, and freezer staple lists organized for trifecta compatibility
- Freshness management strategies that minimize histamine accumulation in stored foods
- Week-by-week shopping lists aligned with the four-week meal plan from Chapter 11.0
- Budget strategies for affordable trifecta eating on any income
- Adaptive kitchen setup for patients managing joint hypermobility, fatigue, and chronic pain
- The "cook once, eat three times" batch preparation approach for low-energy days
- Label reading skills for identifying hidden histamine, hidden sodium, and problematic additives

13.1 The Trifecta Pantry

A well-stocked **trifecta pantry** contains shelf-stable items that form the backbone of daily eating. These foods do not accumulate histamine because they are dry, sealed, or otherwise preserved in forms that prevent the bacterial conversion of histidine to histamine that occurs in protein-rich perishable foods (Comas-Basté et al., 2020). A pantry organized by trifecta category means that even on a zero-energy day, the raw materials for a compatible meal sit within arm's reach.

Grains and starches serve as the carbohydrate foundation of the Trifecta Plate described in section 10.1. White rice (long-grain, basmati, or jasmine) is the single most reliable grain because it is naturally low-histamine, well-tolerated during gastroparesis flares due to rapid gastric emptying (Thwaites et al., 2022), and inexpensive. Rolled oats provide soluble fiber and can be prepared as overnight oats or quick stovetop porridge. Quinoa and millet offer higher protein content than rice and diversify the carbohydrate rotation. Rice pasta and gluten-free corn pasta (if individually tolerated) provide variety without wheat exposure. All grains should be stored in airtight containers after opening to prevent moisture absorption and contamination.

Cooking fats include extra virgin olive oil (whose oleocanthal compound provides anti-inflammatory activity comparable to low-dose ibuprofen, as discussed in section 9.2; Beauchamp et al., 2005), coconut oil for higher-heat cooking, and ghee for both cooking and flavor. Ghee is shelf-stable when unopened and typically well-tolerated even by patients who react to butter, because the clarification process removes most milk proteins (Reese et al., 2017).

Flavor builders are where pantry organization directly impacts dietary adherence. Salt is the most therapeutically important pantry item for POTS patients, with the 2021 NIH Expert Consensus recommending up to 10 to 12 grams of salt daily (Vernino et al., 2021). Fresh garlic lasts weeks at room temperature and adds flavor without histamine concerns. Dried herbs (rosemary, thyme, oregano, basil, dill) and ground spices (turmeric, cumin, coriander, ginger, black pepper) are generally well-tolerated because they are not fermented (Maintz & Novak, 2007). Turmeric deserves special mention for its anti-inflammatory curcumin content discussed in section 9.3.

Emergency flare supplies (complementing the flare day protocol from section 12.1) should occupy a single, dedicated, visible shelf: shelf-stable single-serve broth containers, rice cakes, single-serve nut butter packets, no-sugar-added applesauce cups, electrolyte drink tablets, and collagen peptide powder for adding protein to beverages without cooking.

Supplements complete the pantry: vitamin D3 (5,000 IU daily as discussed in section 5.3; Gensemer et al., 2021), vitamin C (750 to 1,000 mg daily for collagen support and mast cell stabilization; Hagel et al., 2013), and magnesium glycinate (200 to 400 mg daily; Steiner et al., 2023).

13.2 Freshness and the Fridge

The refrigerator is where freshness management matters most, because refrigerated protein-rich foods are the primary site of histamine accumulation in trifecta eating.

The foundational principle from section 6.2 bears repeating here in practical terms: **histamine content is a function of time and temperature**, not a fixed property of the food itself (Maintz & Novak, 2007). A chicken breast purchased today and cooked tonight is low-histamine. That same chicken breast sitting in the refrigerator until Thursday is not.

Histamine accumulation occurs through bacterial decarboxylation, a process in which bacteria naturally present on food convert the amino acid histidine into histamine as the food ages (Comas-Basté et al., 2020). This conversion accelerates at refrigerator temperatures (4°C/40°F) compared to freezing, which halts bacterial activity entirely. The practical consequence is straightforward: the longer a protein-rich food sits in the refrigerator, the more histamine it contains, regardless of how it smells, looks, or tastes. Food can pass every conventional freshness test and still contain enough histamine to trigger an MCAS flare in a sensitive patient (Sánchez-Pérez et al., 2018).

The **buy small, cook quickly, freeze portions** approach operationalizes this biochemistry into purchasing habits. Buy fresh proteins in quantities you can cook within 24 hours of purchase. For a single person eating protein at five to six occasions daily, this means purchasing approximately one to two pounds of fresh meat or fish every two to three days rather than buying a week's supply at once. The inconvenience of more frequent shopping trips is offset by dramatically reduced histamine exposure.

Fish requires even greater urgency. Seafood accumulates histamine faster than poultry or red meat due to higher histidine content in fish muscle tissue (Sánchez-Pérez et al., 2018). Fresh fish should ideally be cooked the same day it is purchased. If same-day cooking isn't possible, freeze the fish immediately upon arriving home and thaw it the day you plan to cook it.

Leftovers are the most counterintuitive aspect of trifecta refrigerator management, and the single most common source of "mystery" MCAS flares. Cooked food begins accumulating histamine immediately upon cooling. Reheating does not destroy histamine because histamine is heat-stable (Kovacova-Hanuskova et al., 2015). A meal reheated to steaming contains the same histamine as the cold leftover. The trifecta rule for leftovers: portion cooked food into individual serving containers within 30 minutes of cooking, refrigerate what you will eat within 24 hours, and freeze everything else immediately. Food that has sat in the refrigerator for 48 hours or longer should not be consumed by histamine-sensitive patients.

Refrigerator staples that tolerate longer storage include fresh vegetables (which accumulate histamine far more slowly than proteins; intact, uncut vegetables remain safe for approximately a week), peeled and cut fruit (in airtight containers, consumed within 48 hours), fresh herbs (wrapped in damp paper towel inside a bag), fresh ginger root, and eggs (if individually tolerated).

13.3 The Freezer as Safety Net

The freezer is the trifecta patient's most underutilized and most powerful tool. **Flash-freezing halts bacterial activity**, which means it halts histamine production entirely (Comas-Basté et al., 2020). A properly organized freezer transforms a zero-energy day from a dietary crisis into a five-minute meal assembly.

Commercially frozen foods often contain less histamine than their "fresh" counterparts at the grocery store. This surprises many patients. A frozen salmon fillet that was flash-frozen within hours of harvest at a processing plant contains less histamine than a "fresh" salmon fillet that traveled two to three days in refrigerated transit before reaching the store's display case (Maintz & Novak, 2007). The same principle applies to vegetables: frozen broccoli, green beans, cauliflower, and mixed vegetable blends that were flash-frozen at harvest retain nutritional content equivalent to or better than "fresh" produce that has traveled long distances and sat in warehouse and store refrigeration (Bouzari et al., 2015).

Stock the freezer with individually quick-frozen (IQF) chicken breasts or thighs (so individual pieces can be removed without thawing the entire package), frozen white fish fillets (cod, tilapia, sole), frozen vegetable blends without sauce, and frozen fruit (blueberries, mango chunks, peach slices for smoothies).

Home-frozen batch-cooked items are the second freezer category. Cooked rice portioned into individual servings in freezer-safe containers reheats in the microwave in two to three minutes. Shredded or sliced cooked chicken, portioned individually and frozen within 30 minutes of cooking, maintains quality for two to three months. Homemade short-cooked broth (two to four hours of simmering, not the 24-hour bone broth that accumulates histamine during extended cooking) frozen in ice cube trays and then transferred to freezer bags provides single-serve sodium delivery. Blended smoothie packs (pre-measured frozen fruit and collagen peptides in individual bags, ready to blend with water) eliminate all preparation on exhausted mornings.

Freezer organization matters for accessibility. Group items by category: proteins together, vegetables together, grains and starches together, broths and liquids together. Label everything with the contents and the date frozen. Use the **first-in, first-out** principle: move older items to the front when adding new ones. Most properly stored frozen foods maintain quality for three to six months and remain safe indefinitely, though texture and nutrient content may decline over longer periods (U.S. Department of Agriculture, 2023).

13.4 Berenice's Kitchen Overhaul

Background

Berenice, a 52-year-old retired pharmacist with hEDS, POTS, and MCAS, had been managing trifecta eating for two years. She understood the dietary principles thoroughly and maintained a confirmed safe foods list of 28 items. But her kitchen was working against her. Her pantry mixed trifecta-compatible items among old processed foods. Her freezer contained unmarked containers frozen at unknown dates. Her refrigerator held fresh chicken purchased five days earlier that she hadn't had the energy to cook.

Presentation

Berenice described a repeating cycle: she felt well on shopping day, bought fresh produce and proteins with ambitious meal plans, then experienced a fatigue crash or POTS flare that prevented cooking for two to three days. By the time she recovered, the fresh food had passed its histamine-safe window. She threw it away, felt guilty, and ate from her freezer stash of old, unlabeled containers whose freshness she could not verify. She estimated food waste of $50 to $70 monthly. Her histamine exposure was unpredictable because she could not assess the freshness of unmarked frozen items, and she experienced approximately three MCAS flares monthly that she described as "coming from nowhere."

Analysis

Berenice's problem was not knowledge or motivation. It was **kitchen infrastructure**. Her purchasing pattern assumed consistent daily energy, which POTS and EDS simply do not provide (Hakim et al., 2017). Her storage systems did not account for the gap between purchasing and cooking. And her freezer, which should have been her primary safety mechanism, was unreliable because of poor labeling and organization. The "mystery" flares likely traced to consuming foods with unverifiable histamine histories.

Intervention

A dietitian helped Berenice restructure her kitchen in three steps. She cleared the pantry and reorganized it by trifecta category (grains, fats, seasonings, electrolyte supplies, flare kit on a single visible shelf). She emptied the freezer completely, discarding anything unlabeled or older than three months, and reorganized by food type with dated labels. She shifted her shopping pattern from one large weekly trip to two smaller trips, purchasing only the fresh protein and vegetables she could cook within 48 hours. On shopping day, she immediately cooked all purchased protein, portioned it, and froze everything she wouldn't eat within 24 hours.

Outcome

Over two months, Berenice's food waste decreased from $50 to $70 monthly to less than $10. Her histamine exposure became more predictable because every protein she consumed was either freshly cooked or frozen within 30 minutes of cooking. Her MCAS flares decreased from approximately three per month to one or none, which she attributed to reduced histamine variability. She described the labeled, organized freezer as "my insurance policy for bad days."

Teaching Points

- Kitchen infrastructure (pantry organization, freezer labeling, purchasing frequency) directly affects histamine exposure and dietary consistency, independent of the patient's dietary knowledge or motivation
- Purchasing patterns should match the patient's realistic energy availability rather than assuming consistent daily cooking capacity
- The freezer functions as the primary safety mechanism for histamine-sensitive eating, but only when properly organized, labeled with dates, and maintained with regular rotation

13.5 Weekly Shopping Lists

The four-week progressive meal plan from Chapter 11.0 requires different ingredients at each stage. Rather than presenting a single large shopping list that overwhelms, the week-by-week approach ensures patients buy only what each phase demands, reducing waste, cost, and decision burden.

Week 1 (Foundation) centers on the safest green-category foods from the traffic light system (section 10.3): fresh chicken breast (two pounds, cooked day of purchase and frozen in portions), fresh turkey breast or ground turkey (one pound), fresh white fish fillets (one pound, cooked same day), white rice (two-pound bag), rolled oats (one-pound canister), sweet potatoes (three to four medium), zucchini (three to four medium), carrots (one-pound bag), broccoli (one large head or one bag frozen), peeled pears (three to four), apples (three to four), blueberries (one pint fresh or one bag frozen), olive oil, ghee, fresh ginger root, fresh garlic, ground turmeric, salt, electrolyte drink mix, rice cakes, and almond butter. Approximate cost at standard grocery prices: $35 to $50 depending on region. This list covers approximately four to five days; a second smaller trip mid-week replenishes fresh proteins and perishable vegetables.

Weeks 2 through 4 expand progressively as tested foods are added through the reintroduction protocol from section 6.9. The shopping list grows to include eggs (if tolerated), fresh mozzarella or cottage cheese (if tolerated), lamb, quinoa, asparagus, cauliflower, green beans, mango, watermelon, fresh herbs (basil, cilantro, rosemary), and coconut oil. Each new food appears on the shopping list only after successful tolerance testing.

13.6 Budget Shopping Strategies

Trifecta eating need not be expensive. The perception that eating for chronic illness requires premium products is a barrier that discourages patients before they begin.

Store brands versus name brands are nutritionally identical for basic ingredients. Store-brand rice, oats, frozen vegetables, olive oil, and salt cost 20 to 40% less than name-brand equivalents with no difference in quality, nutritional content, or safety (Volpe et al., 2013). The exception is products where specific formulations matter (such as electrolyte mixes where ingredient ratios affect absorption), but even here, homemade electrolyte drinks using salt, potassium-containing salt substitute, honey, and water provide equivalent function at a fraction of the cost.

Seasonal produce is both cheaper and fresher than out-of-season produce, which has typically traveled longer distances and been stored longer, increasing both cost and histamine accumulation time. The practical approach: buy whatever local, in-season vegetables and fruits are cheapest each week (checking against your safe foods list from section 10.5), supplement with frozen produce for consistency, and accept that vegetable rotation will shift across the year.

Buying proteins strategically produces the largest savings. Whole chickens yield meat plus bones for broth at the lowest per-pound cost ($1 to $2 per pound versus $4 to $5 for boneless breasts). Frozen fish is both cheaper and lower in histamine than fresh fish counter options. Watching for sales on fresh turkey, lamb, and chicken provides opportunities to purchase, portion, and freeze immediately. Over a month of daily protein consumption at five to six eating occasions, the cost difference between boneless skinless chicken breast and whole chicken amounts to $60 to $100 in savings (Volpe et al., 2013).

Grains in bulk represent the least expensive calories available in trifecta-compatible eating. A 10-pound bag of rice costs $8 to $12 and provides approximately 50 servings. Rolled oats in large canisters cost $3 to $5 for approximately 30 servings. At less than $0.20 per serving, these grains make the carbohydrate quarter of the Trifecta Plate nearly free.

13.7 Adaptive Kitchen Setup

The physical demands of cooking create a distinct barrier for EDS patients. Joint hypermobility causes pain and instability during gripping, chopping, stirring, and lifting. POTS causes tachycardia, lightheadedness, and presyncope during prolonged standing. Fatigue from all three conditions limits the total time and energy available for food preparation. Occupational therapy research for EDS emphasizes environmental modification and adaptive equipment as primary interventions for maintaining functional independence (Chopra et al., 2017).

A **perching stool** (a tall stool that allows sitting at counter height while maintaining a semi-standing posture) is the single most impactful kitchen adaptation for POTS patients. It eliminates the need to stand fully upright while cooking, reducing orthostatic stress, decreasing tachycardia, and extending cooking tolerance from 10 to 15 minutes (while standing) to 30 to 45 minutes (while perching). Perching stools cost $50 to $150 and are available at medical supply stores or online retailers. For patients who cannot tolerate any standing, a standard chair at a lower work surface (kitchen table rather than counter) serves the same purpose.

Lightweight cookware reduces the injury risk associated with heavy pots and pans. Cast-iron skillets weigh five to eight pounds empty and 10 or more pounds with food, creating subluxation risk for hypermobile wrists and shoulders (Castori et al., 2012). Ceramic-coated aluminum pans weigh one to two pounds and perform adequately for all trifecta cooking methods. Smaller pot sizes (1.5 to 2 quarts rather than 4 to 6 quarts) further reduce both weight and the lifting force required.

Ergonomic cutting tools address the gripping and wrist instability common in EDS. Knives with large padded handles reduce the grip force needed for chopping. Rocker knives cut with a downward rocking motion rather than a forward sawing motion, reducing wrist strain. Electric food choppers ($20 to $40) replace manual chopping entirely for patients with severe hand involvement. Jar openers mounted under the cabinet provide mechanical advantage without requiring grip strength.

Workflow organization arranges the kitchen so that the most frequently used items (salt, oil, primary spices, daily cookware) sit at waist to chest height. Overhead reaching above shoulder level risks subluxation. Bending to floor-level cabinets worsens POTS symptoms by rapidly changing the body's position relative to gravity (Vernino et al., 2021). A kitchen cart on wheels can transport multiple items from refrigerator to stove to table in a single trip, reducing total standing and walking steps.

Energy-conserving appliances shift cooking labor from continuous standing and active monitoring to brief setup and passive operation. Slow cookers allow 10 to 15 minutes of morning preparation with a ready meal by evening. Rice cookers produce perfectly cooked rice without monitoring. Instant Pots combine pressure cooking and slow cooking functions, cooking frozen chicken breasts to safe internal temperature in 15 to 20 minutes. Each of these appliances converts an active cooking task into a passive one, preserving limited daily energy for activities beyond food preparation (Simmonds et al., 2017).

13.8 Faramond's Energy Budget

Background

Faramond, a 39-year-old freelance illustrator with POTS and hEDS, worked from home. His POTS was moderately controlled with midodrine and fludrocortisone, but he experienced two to three low-energy days per week when standing for more than 10 minutes triggered presyncope and heart rates above 130. He lived alone with no one to prepare meals for him.

Presentation

On good-energy days, Faramond prepared meals following the trifecta framework with reasonable success. On low-energy days, he defaulted to processed convenience foods (frozen pizza, instant ramen, crackers with aged cheese) because they required minimal standing and preparation. These foods were high in histamine (aged cheese, processed meats in pizza), high in refined carbohydrates, and ironically adequate in sodium but from sources that worsened his MCAS. He estimated that 35 to 40% of his eating occasions involved processed convenience foods, undermining the trifecta framework he followed the other 60 to 65% of the time.

Analysis

Faramond's situation illustrates the concept of **energy budgeting** in chronic illness. Each day provides a limited pool of physical energy, and cooking competes with work, hygiene, household tasks, and social activities for shares of that pool (Jason et al., 2010). On low-energy days, the cooking share drops to near zero. The solution is not motivation or willpower. It is reducing the energy cost of meal preparation below the threshold that low-energy days can accommodate. This requires both adaptive equipment (section 13.7) and the **cook once, eat three times** batch strategy described in section 13.9.

Intervention

Faramond implemented three changes. He purchased a perching stool, which he estimated reduced his standing energy expenditure during cooking by approximately 40% based on heart rate monitoring while cooking seated versus standing. He adopted the cook-once batch approach: on his two highest-energy days each week, he spent 45 to 60 minutes batch-cooking three base components (a protein, a grain, and roasted vegetables), portioning into individual containers, and freezing everything not intended for consumption within 24 hours. He also prepared five frozen smoothie packs per batch session. On low-energy days, his meals consisted entirely of reheated frozen home-cooked portions and blended smoothies, each requiring less than five minutes of preparation.

Outcome

Over four weeks, Faramond's processed food consumption dropped from 35 to 40% of eating occasions to less than 10%. His POTS symptoms improved modestly, which he attributed to more consistent sodium intake (home-cooked meals were salted to target, while convenience foods had unpredictable sodium levels) and reduced histamine exposure. He described the perching stool and batch cooking as "the two things that actually made this diet livable for someone who lives alone."

Teaching Points

- Low-energy days in chronic illness require dietary solutions designed around reduced physical capacity rather than motivational approaches that assume full capacity
- The cook-once batch-cooking approach concentrates cooking labor on high-energy days and distributes the results across low-energy days via frozen individual portions
- A perching stool functions as a medical accommodation that extends cooking tolerance, not merely a convenience item, and should be considered a primary intervention for POTS patients who cook

13.9 Batch Cooking Strategies

The **cook once, eat three times** approach deserves detailed explanation because it addresses the most common practical barrier to sustained trifecta eating. Research on dietary adherence in chronic illness consistently identifies meal preparation burden as a primary predictor of non-adherence, more predictive than knowledge, motivation, or even symptom severity (Dansinger et al., 2005).

The approach works through three principles. The first is **concentrating labor**. Rather than cooking from scratch at each of six daily eating occasions (which would require approximately two to three hours of total kitchen time per day, or 14 to 21 hours weekly), concentrate all cooking into one or two sessions per week. A single 60 to 90 minute session on a high-energy day can produce enough cooked protein, grains, and vegetables for 15 to 18 individual portions, covering approximately three days of eating across six occasions daily. If a second shorter session occurs mid-week (30 to 45 minutes), the full week is covered. Total weekly kitchen time: approximately three hours versus 14 or more hours without batching.

The second principle is **immediate portioning and freezing**. As discussed in section 13.2, cooked food begins accumulating histamine as soon as it cools to room temperature. Portioning into individual containers and moving them to the freezer within 30 minutes of cooking arrests this process completely. Each container should hold one eating occasion's worth of food (approximately 250 to 350 mL for a meal, 150 to 200 mL for a snack). Label each container with contents and date.

The third principle is **component cooking** rather than full-meal cooking. Cook proteins, grains, and vegetables separately rather than as combined dishes. This creates maximum flexibility: a container of shredded chicken can become chicken over rice with broccoli for lunch, chicken stirred into oatmeal with salt for a savory breakfast, or chicken added to broth for an evening soup. Component cooking also simplifies reintroduction testing from section 6.9 because each ingredient remains separate and identifiable (Joneja, 2017).

A typical batch session might include four chicken breasts (seasoned with salt, garlic, and olive oil, baked at 400°F for 22 to 25 minutes, then shredded), two cups of dry rice (cooked in a rice cooker with salt), one head of broccoli and four zucchini (roasted with olive oil and salt at 400°F for 20 minutes), and four sweet potatoes (baked whole at 400°F for 45 minutes). Total active preparation: approximately 20 minutes. Passive oven time: 45 minutes (during which the patient can sit or rest). Portioning and freezing: 15 minutes. Yield: approximately 16 to 20 individual portions.

13.10 Reading Food Labels

Label reading is a necessary skill because processed and packaged foods frequently contain hidden histamine sources, unpredictable sodium levels, and additives that can trigger MCAS reactions. The ingredient list on packaged food provides more useful information for trifecta patients than the nutrition facts panel, because the specific ingredients matter more than the macronutrient totals.

Hidden histamine sources on ingredient labels include: "natural flavors" (a regulatory category that can include fermented or aged flavor compounds without specifying which ones; Reese et al., 2017), yeast extract (a flavor enhancer produced by autolysis of yeast cells, which generates histamine and free glutamate), soy sauce or soy protein (fermented soy is high-histamine), vinegar (all vinegar is produced through fermentation, including white vinegar and apple cider vinegar), citric acid (which may be derived from mold fermentation and can trigger reactions in sensitive MCAS patients), and "spices" without specification (which may contain individual trigger spices).

Hidden sodium works in two directions for trifecta patients. For POTS patients, sodium is therapeutic rather than harmful, so foods with higher sodium content can be allies. But the sodium must come from compatible sources. A can of soup providing 800 mg of sodium is only useful if the other ingredients are low-histamine and well-tolerated. "Low sodium" versions of products contain 40 to 50% less sodium than regular versions, which actually works against POTS targets (Sheldon et al., 2015). Pure salt added during cooking remains the most controllable and cleanest sodium source.

Problematic additives for MCAS patients include: sulfites (preservatives used in dried fruits, wine, and some medications; can trigger mast cell degranulation in sensitive individuals; Vally & Misso, 2012), artificial colors (particularly tartrazine and other azo dyes, which have been associated with mast cell activation; Vojdani & Vojdani, 2015), benzoates (preservatives in beverages and condiments), and carrageenan (a thickener derived from seaweed that can trigger GI inflammation in some individuals).

The practical approach is the **three-scan method**: scan the ingredient list for any known personal triggers from your traffic light list (section 10.3), scan for hidden histamine categories listed above, and scan the nutrition facts for sodium content (to add to your daily tally). If all three scans are clear, the product is likely compatible. If any scan raises a flag, choose an alternative or test the product cautiously through the reintroduction protocol from section 6.9.

13.11 Galatea's Label Lessons

Background

Galatea, a 29-year-old veterinary assistant with MCAS and POTS, had been following a low-histamine diet for four months with moderate symptom improvement. She had successfully identified and removed obvious high-histamine foods (aged cheese, canned fish, fermented foods) but continued to experience two to three unexplained MCAS flares weekly. She described these flares as "random" because they did not correlate with any food she recognized as problematic.

Presentation

When Galatea's dietitian reviewed her food diary, the recorded foods appeared compatible with trifecta principles: chicken, rice, vegetables, olive oil. But closer examination revealed that she was using a commercial chicken broth listed as "organic" (which she assumed meant safe), a store-bought salad dressing labeled "all natural," and a protein bar she consumed daily as an afternoon snack. She had not examined the ingredient lists of any of these products because the front-of-package marketing language ("organic," "natural," "clean ingredients") had seemed reassuring.

Analysis

The dietitian examined the ingredient lists of Galatea's three suspect products. The organic chicken broth contained yeast extract and "natural flavors," both potential histamine sources. The salad dressing contained apple cider vinegar and lemon juice (both histamine liberators for some MCAS patients; Kovacova-Hanuskova et al., 2015). The protein bar contained soy protein isolate (derived from soy, a fermented legume product in many processing methods), citric acid, and "natural flavors." Between these three products, Galatea was consuming histamine-triggering ingredients at one to two eating occasions daily without realizing it. Front-of-package claims like "organic" and "natural" carry no meaning for histamine content and do not substitute for reading the full ingredient list (Reese et al., 2017).

Intervention

The dietitian taught Galatea the three-scan label reading method. She replaced the commercial broth with homemade short-cooked broth (frozen in individual portions), replaced the salad dressing with olive oil and salt, and replaced the protein bar with a homemade smoothie pack containing frozen blueberries, collagen peptides, and a pinch of salt. No other dietary changes were made.

Outcome

Over the following three weeks, Galatea's unexplained MCAS flares decreased from two to three weekly to approximately one every 10 days. She had not eliminated any food. She had eliminated three packaged products whose ingredient lists contained hidden histamine sources. She described the experience as "realizing that 'natural flavors' is the most suspicious phrase on any food label."

Teaching Points

- Front-of-package marketing claims ("organic," "natural," "clean") carry no information about histamine content and should never substitute for reading the full ingredient list

- Hidden histamine sources in packaged foods (yeast extract, natural flavors, vinegar, soy protein, citric acid) can produce MCAS flares that appear "random" because the patient does not recognize these ingredients as histamine-related
- Replacing packaged products with simple homemade alternatives (homemade broth, oil-and-salt dressing, smoothie packs) often resolves unexplained flares without requiring additional food elimination

13.12 Practical Foundations Review

The kitchen infrastructure described in this chapter is not supplementary to the dietary framework from Chapters 6.0 through 12.0. It is foundational. The most evidence-based meal plan produces no benefit if the patient can't execute it in their actual kitchen, with their actual energy levels, using their actual grocery budget.

The trifecta pantry, refrigerator, and freezer systems ensure that compatible ingredients are always available. Freshness management rules (buy small, cook quickly, freeze immediately) operationalize the histamine biochemistry from Chapter 6.0 into daily purchasing and storage habits. Adaptive kitchen setup translates occupational therapy research into specific equipment and organizational choices that reduce pain, conserve energy, and prevent injury. The cook-once batch approach distributes cooking labor across the patient's variable daily energy, concentrating effort on good days and distributing results across difficult ones. Label reading skills protect against the hidden histamine, unexpected additives, and sodium ambiguity that packaged foods introduce.

The meal plans from Chapters 11.0 and 12.0 describe what to eat. This chapter describes how to make that eating possible, consistently, across the full range of good days and bad days that define life with these conditions. Chapter 14.0 addresses the next practical skill: tracking what you eat, monitoring how your body responds, and using that data to refine your individual dietary approach over time.

Chapter 14.0: Tracking and Troubleshooting

A trifecta patient follows her low-histamine, high-sodium, gastroparesis-friendly meal plan for three weeks and feels noticeably better. Then, on a Tuesday, she eats the same chicken-rice-broccoli combination she has eaten 15 times before and experiences a severe MCAS flare: flushing, GI cramping, brain fog, and tachycardia lasting four hours. She is baffled. She ate the same food, prepared the same way, in the same kitchen. What went wrong? Without a detailed tracking diary, she will never know. With one, she might discover that Tuesday was also the day her menstrual period started (hormonal mast cell activation), or that she slept only four hours the previous night (stress-mediated immune activation), or that she used chicken purchased three days earlier instead of her usual 24-hour window (histamine accumulation). The answer is almost always in the data. But only if the data is being collected.

This chapter teaches the systematic approach to dietary tracking and troubleshooting for trifecta patients:

- The Trifecta Food and Symptom Diary template and how to use each tracking category
- Pattern recognition techniques for identifying genuine triggers versus coincidental associations
- Common pitfalls that undermine trifecta eating, from over-restriction to supplement over-reliance
- How to distinguish food triggers from non-food triggers like stress, sleep, heat, and hormones
- Red flags that indicate professional help from an RDN, allergist, or GI specialist is needed
- How to find registered dietitians and specialists who understand trifecta conditions

14.1 The Trifecta Diary Template

The **Trifecta Food and Symptom Diary** extends well beyond the basic food journal discussed in section 6.11. A simple food log records what was eaten and what symptoms followed. The trifecta diary tracks multiple dimensions simultaneously because symptoms in these conditions arise from the interaction of dietary, hormonal, environmental, and behavioral factors (Afrin et al., 2016). A diary that tracks only food and symptoms will generate false associations because it cannot distinguish dietary triggers from non-dietary triggers that happened to coincide with specific meals.

The trifecta diary captures eight categories of information at each eating occasion and four categories of daily context.

Eating-occasion categories include: the time of eating, all foods consumed (including brands for packaged items), the preparation method for each food (fresh, frozen then cooked, leftover with number of hours since cooking), estimated portion sizes, estimated sodium for the eating occasion, fluids consumed with the meal, and any medications or supplements taken at that time. The preparation method column matters more than any other single category, because the same food prepared differently produces different histamine outcomes. Chicken cooked fresh this morning is a different exposure than chicken from a container cooked 48 hours ago, even though both appear as "chicken" in a basic food log (Maintz & Novak, 2007).

Daily context categories capture the non-food variables that influence trifecta symptoms: sleep quality and duration the previous night (rated on a 1 to 5 scale), overall activity level and specific physical exertions (including type, duration, and intensity), stress level (rated on a 1 to 5 scale), and for menstruating patients, current phase of the menstrual cycle.

Why track sleep? Because sleep deprivation increases systemic inflammation through elevation of pro-inflammatory cytokines and increases mast cell activation (Irwin et al., 2016). Why track physical activity? Because exertion can trigger both POTS symptoms and mast cell degranulation (Vernino et al., 2021). Why track stress? Because psychological stress activates mast cells directly through corticotropin-releasing hormone (CRH) receptors on the mast cell surface (Theoharides & Cochrane, 2004). Why track menstrual phase? Because estrogen directly influences histamine release, with rising estrogen increasing mast cell activation, and the estrogen drop before menstruation triggering degranulation in many patients (Zierau et al., 2012). Many trifecta patients report predictable symptom worsening during the late luteal phase and during menstruation itself (Raj et al., 2020).

Symptom tracking uses a 0 to 3 severity rating across five organ-system categories: skin (flushing, hives, itching), gastrointestinal (nausea, cramping, diarrhea, bloating), neurological (headache, brain fog, dizziness), cardiovascular (tachycardia, palpitations, presyncope), and respiratory (nasal congestion, throat tightness, shortness of breath). Recording time of symptom onset matters because some food reactions occur within minutes (suggesting IgE-mediated allergy or direct histamine effect) while others are delayed 6 to 48 hours (suggesting histamine accumulation, DAO pathway overload, or immune-mediated responses; Joneja, 2017). This multi-category scoring captures the diverse symptom presentation of MCAS, which can affect multiple organ systems simultaneously (Molderings et al., 2011).

14.2 Pattern Recognition Techniques

A single diary entry tells you almost nothing. A week of entries tells you a little. A month of consistent entries begins revealing patterns that would be invisible without systematic tracking. **Pattern recognition** in trifecta diaries operates across three dimensions: frequency, confounders, and time delay.

Frequency counting is the most straightforward technique. After two to four weeks of diary data, count how many times a specific food was consumed and how many of those occasions were followed by symptoms within the relevant time window (0 to 48 hours for most reactions). A food consumed 10 times with symptoms following 8 to 10 times is a probable trigger. A food consumed 10 times with symptoms following 2 to 3 times requires further analysis, because the symptomatic occasions may reflect confounding variables rather than the food itself. The minimum number of consistent exposures needed to identify a trigger with reasonable confidence is typically three to five positive associations across different days and contexts (Joneja, 2017).

Confounding variable analysis examines what else was happening on symptomatic days versus non-symptomatic days when the same food was consumed. If blueberries were consumed 10 times and the three symptomatic occasions all fell on days with poor sleep, high stress, or heat exposure, blueberries are not the trigger. The non-dietary variables are. This analysis is precisely why the trifecta diary captures context data (sleep, activity, stress, menstrual phase) that a simple food log does not.

Elimination-rechallenge confirmation remains the gold standard for confirming a suspected trigger identified through diary patterns. Remove the suspected food for two to four weeks while keeping all other variables as constant as possible. If symptoms decrease during removal, reintroduce the food in a controlled single-variable test: one moderate serving, on a day with good sleep, low stress, no unusual activity, and a stable menstrual phase. Monitor for 48 hours. If symptoms return, the association is confirmed. If they do not, the food is cleared and the original association was coincidental or confounded (Joneja, 2017).

Time-delay analysis tracks the interval between food consumption and symptom onset. Consistent patterns (symptoms always appearing four to six hours after consuming a particular food) strengthen the case for a genuine trigger. Variable patterns (symptoms sometimes appearing two hours after consumption and sometimes 36 hours after) suggest confounding or coincidence rather than causation. The consistency of the delay is often more informative than the delay length itself.

14.3 Simeon's Diary Discovery

Background

Simeon, a 35-year-old high school teacher with POTS and MCAS, had been tracking food and symptoms in a simple journal (food items and symptoms only, without preparation method, sleep, stress, or cycle data) for three months. He had identified 11 foods he believed triggered his MCAS, including sweet potatoes, blueberries, oatmeal, and fresh chicken breast. All four are green-category foods on the traffic light system from section 10.3. Their elimination had left him with a dangerously narrow diet of 10 foods providing approximately 1,250 calories daily.

Presentation

Simeon's dietitian was skeptical that four low-histamine, non-liberator foods were genuine MCAS triggers. She asked him to switch from his simple food-symptom journal to the full trifecta diary template for four weeks, adding sleep quality, activity level, stress rating, and preparation method to each entry. She also asked him to note the day of the week for each entry.

Analysis

After four weeks, a pattern emerged immediately. All 11 "trigger" foods had been tested during the school week (Monday through Friday). Most reactions occurred on Monday or Tuesday. Weekend eating (Saturday and Sunday) produced almost no reactions, even when Simeon consumed the same foods prepared the same way. The confounding variable was obvious once the contextual data was present: school days involved six hours of standing and walking in a warm building (a double trigger of prolonged upright posture plus heat for a POTS/MCAS patient), while weekends were spent at home in climate-controlled conditions with minimal standing. His symptoms were being triggered by his work environment, not by his food. The temporal association with specific foods was coincidental, created by the fact that he tested new foods on weekdays when he was already symptomatic from environmental triggers (Theoharides et al., 2019).

Intervention

The dietitian supervised reintroduction of all 11 "trigger" foods on weekends, one at a time, while Simeon rested in his air-conditioned home with adequate hydration and sodium loading. She also recommended discussing workplace accommodations with his employer: access to a perching stool for his classroom, permission to carry and drink electrolyte water during class, and a portable fan for his desk.

Outcome

Nine of 11 foods produced no symptoms when tested under controlled weekend conditions. Sweet potatoes and blueberries, the two Simeon had been most certain about, were completely tolerated. Two foods (canned black beans and store-bought hummus) did produce mild GI symptoms that the dietitian attributed to the canned and processed preparation methods, consistent with histamine concerns about processed foods (Reese et al., 2017), rather than the foods themselves. His diet expanded from 10 to 22 foods. His caloric intake increased to 1,900 calories daily. He described the experience as "the diary showed me I was blaming food for what the building was doing to me."

Teaching Points

- Non-food triggers (heat, prolonged standing, environmental stress) can produce MCAS symptoms that patients incorrectly attribute to food because the food and the environmental trigger co-occur in predictable patterns, particularly on work days
- The trifecta diary's contextual tracking (sleep, stress, activity, temperature exposure) distinguishes dietary triggers from environmental ones by revealing which variables most consistently predict symptoms
- Controlled reintroduction testing on rest days with managed environmental conditions prevents unnecessary food elimination and protects against the progressive dietary restriction that leads to malnutrition

14.4 Common Dietary Pitfalls

Five pitfalls undermine trifecta eating more frequently than all others combined. Each represents a predictable failure mode that the diary can help detect and correct.

Pitfall 1: Over-restriction leading to malnutrition. This is the most dangerous pitfall, addressed repeatedly throughout this book (sections 3.5, 6.9, 8.7, 10.9, 12.5) because the consequences are severe. A 2024 cross-sectional study of 680 hEDS patients found that 62.3% regularly skipped meals, and a positive ARFID screening was independently associated with 7.55 times higher odds of dietary alteration (Topan et al., 2024). Each food eliminated from the diet reduces the pool of available nutrition. Patients who eliminate 15 to 20 foods based on uncontrolled observations risk caloric and nutritional deficiency that worsens all three trifecta conditions simultaneously. The rule: never eliminate a food permanently without confirmation through the elimination-rechallenge protocol under controlled conditions (section 6.9).

Pitfall 2: Ignoring histamine variability. The same food has different histamine levels depending on freshness, preparation method, and source, as established in Chapter 6.0 (Comas-Basté et al., 2020). A patient who tolerates fresh chicken cooked within 24 hours but reacts to chicken from the same package stored for three days is not "developing a chicken sensitivity." She is experiencing histamine accumulation in the stored chicken. The diary detects this pitfall when the preparation method column reveals that symptomatic meals used older ingredients while asymptomatic meals used fresher ones.

Pitfall 3: Supplement over-reliance. Supplements support dietary intake; they do not replace it. A patient taking quercetin, vitamin C, omega-3 fish oil, collagen peptides, magnesium, vitamin D, and a multivitamin while consuming 1,000 calories of food is not achieving adequate nutrition. The micronutrients in supplements cannot compensate for insufficient macronutrient intake (calories, protein, fat, carbohydrates) or for the fiber, phytonutrients, and prebiotic compounds that come only from whole foods (Steiner et al., 2023). Darian's case in section 9.7 illustrated this pattern clearly. The diary detects it when supplement entries are extensive but food entries are sparse.

Pitfall 4: Not accounting for non-food triggers. As Simeon's case (section 14.3) demonstrated, attributing all symptoms to food when heat, stress, sleep deprivation, or hormonal fluctuations are contributing leads to unnecessary dietary restriction and progressive malnutrition. Research on MCAS demonstrates that mast cell activation is triggered by heat, cold, psychological stress, hormonal shifts, infections, exercise, medications, and environmental chemicals in addition to dietary histamine (Afrin et al., 2016). A food diary that does not track these variables will misattribute environmentally triggered symptoms to whatever food was consumed in the relevant time window.

Pitfall 5: Abandoning the framework during setbacks. A severe MCAS flare, a week of travel, or a period of emotional distress can disrupt trifecta eating. If the patient interprets this disruption as failure ("I can't maintain this diet") rather than as a temporary deviation requiring recovery, she may abandon the framework entirely. The 80/20 principle from section 10.9 provides the psychological architecture for absorbing setbacks without abandoning the overall approach (Dansinger et al., 2005). The diary helps by providing visual evidence of consistency across weeks, even when individual days are imperfect.

14.5 Leocadia's Shrinking Diet

Background

Leocadia, a 28-year-old veterinary technician with hEDS and MCAS, began a low-histamine elimination diet seven months earlier after her MCAS diagnosis. Her initial elimination phase had been successful, reducing symptom frequency from daily to weekly. But the reintroduction phase had stalled. She tested one food every two weeks (far slower than the recommended three to four days between tests described in section 6.9) and declared any food that produced even a mild or ambiguous symptom as "failed." She had not successfully reintroduced any food in four months.

Presentation

Leocadia's safe foods list had actually shrunk from the 16 foods in her initial elimination phase to 11. She had removed eggs, bell peppers, blueberries, ghee, and oatmeal after experiencing what she described as "slight nausea" or "a little foggy" after eating them. On review, these symptoms were rated 1 out of 3 (mild) and lasted less than 30 minutes each. Her caloric intake averaged 1,050 calories daily. She had lost 14 pounds over five months. Her hair was thinning. Her ferritin was 12 ng/mL (well below the 30 ng/mL threshold for POTS patients discussed in section 5.6). She was experiencing frequent joint subluxations that her physical therapist attributed to muscle wasting from inadequate protein intake.

Analysis

Leocadia's diary revealed the over-restriction pattern described in pitfall 1 above. Her reintroduction protocol had become dysfunctional rather than diagnostic: the threshold for "failure" was set so low (any symptom, regardless of severity, duration, or reproducibility) that normal physiological variation was being interpreted as food intolerance. Mild, transient symptoms after eating (slight nausea, brief brain fog) are common in patients with gastroparesis and POTS regardless of the specific food consumed, because eating itself triggers postprandial hemodynamic changes that can produce these sensations (Mehr et al., 2018). Using these nonspecific post-meal symptoms as evidence of food intolerance leads to progressive food elimination with no logical stopping point.

Intervention

Leocadia's dietitian recalibrated her reintroduction criteria. A food would be classified as "failed" only if it produced symptoms rated 2 or higher (moderate to severe) or if it produced consistent mild symptoms across three separate exposures on different days under controlled conditions. Ambiguous single-test results would be repeated twice more before classification. The five "failed" foods were reclassified as "needs retesting." A psychologist specializing in chronic illness was consulted to address the food anxiety component, which met screening criteria for ARFID (avoidant restrictive food intake disorder, as discussed in section 3.8). Iron supplementation with bisglycinate was initiated on alternate days to address the ferritin deficiency (Stoffel et al., 2017).

Outcome

Over six weeks of recalibrated reintroduction, Leocadia successfully reintroduced four of the five removed foods (eggs, blueberries, ghee, and oatmeal). Bell peppers remained a genuine trigger, producing moderate GI symptoms across three separate tests. Her safe foods list expanded to 21 items. Caloric intake increased to 1,550 calories. Weight loss halted. The psychological intervention reduced her food anxiety, and she described the recalibrated criteria as "giving me permission to eat again without being terrified."

Teaching Points

- Reintroduction failure criteria must distinguish between genuine food-triggered symptoms (moderate to severe, reproducible across multiple controlled exposures) and normal postprandial physiological variation (mild, transient, inconsistent), because conflating the two leads to progressive unnecessary restriction
- ARFID can develop as a secondary condition following medically necessary dietary restriction when food anxiety accumulates over months of elimination dieting, and early identification plus psychological intervention prevents further deterioration
- Over-restriction produces its own medical consequences (weight loss, micronutrient deficiency, muscle wasting, worsening POTS) that can be more harmful than the symptoms the elimination diet was intended to manage

14.6 Beyond Food Triggers

For menstruating trifecta patients (the majority of POTS patients are young women, with a female-to-male ratio of approximately 5:1; Shaw et al., 2019), the **menstrual cycle** represents a systematic, predictable source of symptom variability that must be tracked alongside dietary data to prevent false trigger identification.

Estrogen directly influences mast cell activity. Mast cells carry estrogen receptors, and fluctuations in estrogen levels (particularly the drop that occurs just before menstruation) can trigger degranulation independent of any dietary histamine exposure (Zierau et al., 2012). Progesterone exerts partially counterbalancing anti-inflammatory effects. The practical result: many trifecta patients experience predictable symptom worsening during the late luteal phase (the premenstrual week) and during menstruation itself, with relative improvement during the follicular phase (Shibao et al., 2005).

A patient who tests a new food during her premenstrual week and experiences a flare may be experiencing hormonally mediated mast cell reactivity rather than a food reaction. Tracking cycle phase in the trifecta diary allows this distinction. If symptoms consistently worsen during cycle days 21 to 28 regardless of dietary composition, the pattern is hormonal. If symptoms worsen only when specific foods are consumed regardless of cycle phase, the pattern is dietary. If symptoms worsen when specific foods are consumed during specific cycle phases but not during others, the interaction between dietary and hormonal triggers provides actionable planning information: avoid yellow-category foods during the premenstrual week while tolerating them during the follicular phase.

Heat and temperature deserve similar attention. Heat is one of the most common non-food mast cell triggers. Temperatures above 80°F, hot showers, and humid weather can trigger widespread mast cell degranulation independently of dietary intake (Theoharides et al., 2019). A patient who experiences MCAS symptoms every time she eats lunch on her outdoor patio in July may be reacting to the heat, not the food.

Psychological stress activates mast cells directly. CRH, released during the stress response, binds to CRH receptors on mast cells and triggers degranulation (Theoharides & Cochrane, 2004). A patient who flares after every Monday lunch may be reacting to the accumulated stress of the work week, not to her lunch ingredients. The diary distinguishes these patterns by tracking stress alongside food, making the correlation visible.

14.7 Professional Referral Criteria

Self-directed trifecta dietary management is appropriate for patients with mild to moderate symptoms whose conditions are medically managed and whose nutritional status is stable. Several situations indicate that professional support is needed.

Red flags for registered dietitian referral: unintentional weight loss exceeding 5% of body weight over three months, caloric intake consistently below 1,200 calories daily despite attempts to increase it, a safe foods list that is shrinking rather than growing over time, laboratory evidence of nutritional deficiency (low ferritin, low vitamin D below 20 ng/mL despite supplementation, low prealbumin, low albumin), persistent food anxiety or eating behaviors that meet ARFID screening criteria, and inability to meet sodium or protein targets despite following the trifecta framework.

Red flags for allergist or immunologist referral: MCAS symptoms that do not improve after four to six weeks of strict low-histamine eating (suggesting dietary histamine is not the primary trigger), symptoms triggered by most or all foods regardless of histamine content, anaphylaxis or severe allergic-type reactions including throat tightness or anaphylaxis (Vlieg-Boerstra et al., 2005), and symptoms worsening despite adequate dietary management (suggesting the need for mast cell stabilizing medications such as H1 and H2 antihistamines or cromolyn sodium; Afrin et al., 2016).

Red flags for gastroenterologist referral: progressive weight loss with severe nausea and vomiting suggesting severe gastroparesis requiring prokinetic medications or nutritional support (Thwaites et al., 2022), blood in stool (which requires endoscopic evaluation to rule out inflammatory bowel disease or structural pathology), persistent diarrhea or constipation not responding to dietary modification, and symptoms consistent with small intestinal bacterial overgrowth (SIBO) that may be complicating both MCAS and nutritional absorption.

14.8 Finding Qualified Providers

Finding healthcare providers who understand the intersection of POTS, EDS, and MCAS remains a genuine challenge. A survey of 4,835 individuals with POTS found that 73% felt their healthcare providers had inadequate knowledge of their condition, and the average time to diagnosis was 4.1 years (Shaw et al., 2019).

For **registered dietitians**, the Academy of Nutrition and Dietetics maintains a searchable database of RDNs by specialty. Filtering for "food allergies and intolerances," "gastrointestinal disorders," or "eating disorders" (relevant for ARFID management) identifies practitioners with adjacent training. Patients should ask prospective RDNs directly if they have experience with MCAS, low-histamine diets, and POTS. A productive screening question is "How do you balance dietary restriction with nutritional adequacy in patients managing food sensitivities?" The answer reveals the provider's awareness of the over-restriction risk more effectively than any credential alone (Ganesh et al., 2020).

For **allergists and immunologists**, academic medical centers with mast cell disease programs offer the highest concentration of MCAS expertise. The Mastocytosis Society and Mast Cell Disease Society maintain provider directories. Community allergists may be less familiar with MCAS as a distinct entity from traditional allergy and mastocytosis, so patients should verify that the provider has experience with **mast cell activation syndrome** specifically rather than only mast cell neoplastic diseases.

For **POTS specialists**, Dysautonomia International maintains a provider directory listing clinicians experienced in autonomic disorders. Cardiology, neurology, and internal medicine divisions at academic centers are the most common settings for POTS expertise (Vernino et al., 2021).

For **EDS evaluation**, the Ehlers-Danlos Society maintains a provider directory. Genetics, rheumatology, and physical medicine departments at academic centers are typical referral targets for formal EDS diagnosis and management (Malfait et al., 2017).

Telehealth has expanded access considerably. Many dietitians who specialize in POTS, EDS, or MCAS conditions offer virtual consultations across state lines (where licensure permits). When a trifecta-specialized dietitian is not available locally, telehealth may be the most practical option.

The trifecta diary (section 14.1) serves double duty as both a self-management tool and a clinical communication document. Bringing a completed month of diary data to any healthcare appointment provides the provider with immediate insight into the patient's dietary patterns, symptom trends, and treatment responses, reducing the need to reconstruct this information from memory during a brief office visit.

14.9 Apollonia's Care Team

Background

Apollonia, a 25-year-old graduate student with hEDS and self-suspected MCAS, had been self-managing her diet for 11 months using online resources and patient community forums. She had not been formally evaluated for MCAS but had self-diagnosed based on her symptom pattern and had implemented a strict low-histamine diet. She had progressively eliminated foods based on self-reported reactions until her diet consisted of eight foods providing approximately 1,000 calories daily.

Presentation

Apollonia's primary care physician referred her to a registered dietitian after laboratory work revealed low albumin (2.9 g/dL; normal 3.5 to 5.0), ferritin of 9 ng/mL (iron deficiency), vitamin D of 14 ng/mL (severe deficiency), and BMI of 17.1 (underweight). She reported hair loss, easy bruising, frequent infections, and worsening orthostatic symptoms (resting heart rate 100, standing heart rate 148).

She had not seen an allergist, immunologist, or gastroenterologist at any point during her 11 months of self-management.

Analysis

Apollonia's case illustrates the danger of self-directed MCAS management without professional oversight. While her symptom pattern was consistent with possible MCAS, she had never undergone the laboratory testing needed for formal diagnosis (serum tryptase, 24-hour urine prostaglandin D2 metabolites, or urinary N-methylhistamine; Afrin et al., 2016). Her progressive dietary restriction had produced severe malnutrition that was now independently worsening her orthostatic symptoms (through hypovolemia from inadequate intake; Vernino et al., 2021) and potentially causing symptoms she was misattributing to food reactions. Nutritional deficiency itself produces fatigue, brain fog, muscle weakness, and immune dysfunction that can mimic MCAS symptoms, creating a feedback loop in which restriction produces symptoms that motivate further restriction.

Intervention

The RDN initiated nutritional rehabilitation targeting 1,600 calories initially with gradual increase to 2,000, while simultaneously referring to an allergist for formal MCAS evaluation and a gastroenterologist for assessment of upper GI symptoms. The allergist ordered appropriate laboratory testing. The gastroenterologist performed endoscopy to evaluate persistent nausea and early satiety. Meanwhile, the RDN supervised controlled food reintroduction using the protocol from section 6.9, beginning with the safest green-category foods and expanding from there.

Outcome

MCAS was confirmed through elevated urinary prostaglandin D2 metabolites. The allergist initiated H1 and H2 antihistamines plus cromolyn sodium as mast cell stabilizing medications. With medication managing baseline mast cell activity, Apollonia tolerated food reintroduction far more successfully than she had during unmedicated self-management. Her diet expanded from 8 to 22 foods over eight weeks. Caloric intake stabilized at 1,750 calories. Albumin, ferritin, and vitamin D began improving with targeted supplementation and increased dietary intake. The RDN described the case as a reminder that "MCAS medication and dietary management work together as partners, not as alternatives to each other."

Teaching Points

- Self-directed MCAS dietary management without formal diagnosis and medical oversight risks progressive restriction, malnutrition, and the development of nutritional deficiency symptoms that mimic and compound the condition being managed

- Formal MCAS diagnosis through appropriate laboratory testing enables medication interventions (H1/H2 antihistamines, mast cell stabilizers) that reduce baseline mast cell reactivity and make dietary reintroduction more successful
- A multidisciplinary care team (RDN, allergist, gastroenterologist) addresses the trifecta more effectively than any single provider or any amount of self-directed management, because each specialist contributes diagnostic and therapeutic expertise that the others lack

14.10 Core Concepts Recap

Tracking and troubleshooting are the skills that convert trifecta eating from a static set of rules into a dynamic, personalized system that improves over time. The trifecta diary captures data across food, preparation method, sodium, fluid, medications, symptoms, sleep, stress, activity, and menstrual cycle. Pattern recognition extracts meaning from that data through frequency counting, confounding variable analysis, elimination-rechallenge confirmation, and time-delay analysis. Awareness of common pitfalls (over-restriction, ignoring histamine variability, supplement over-reliance, neglecting non-food triggers, and abandoning the framework during setbacks) prevents the predictable errors that undermine long-term dietary management.

The most important lesson from this chapter may be the most counterintuitive: not everything is about food. Trifecta patients, understandably, focus intensely on their diets because food is the variable they can most directly control. But hormonal fluctuations, sleep quality, emotional stress, physical exertion, temperature exposure, and medication timing all influence symptoms as much as dietary choices in many patients (Theoharides et al., 2019). The trifecta diary captures all of these variables precisely because symptoms arise from the interaction of multiple systems, not from any single trigger acting in isolation.

Part Three of this book has now provided the complete practical toolkit for trifecta eating: personalized frameworks (Chapter 10.0), structured meal plans (Chapter 11.0), specialized situation plans (Chapter 12.0), kitchen infrastructure (Chapter 13.0), and tracking and troubleshooting systems (this chapter). Part Four addresses the dimension of trifecta eating that no meal plan or tracking diary can fully resolve: the emotional, social, and psychological experience of living with permanent dietary modifications in a world that does not always understand or accommodate them.

PART FOUR: RECIPES

Chapter 15.0: Breakfast and Morning Fuel

Dorothea woke at 7:15 a.m. with a resting heart rate of 92 and the familiar heaviness behind her eyes that signaled a moderate symptom day. She had 40 minutes before she needed to leave for work. Standing up from bed produced an immediate spike to 118 beats per minute, a 26-point orthostatic increase that made the room tilt slightly before her cardiovascular reflexes caught up. She needed to eat. She needed sodium. She needed fluids. She needed something that wouldn't trigger her MCAS. And she needed all of it assembled and consumed before her body's morning cortisol surge faded and the fatigue deepened. She opened the refrigerator to three containers of overnight chia pudding she had prepared on Sunday, grabbed one, sprinkled salt on top, and sat down. Within 10 minutes she had consumed 350 calories, 1,200 mg of sodium, 16 ounces of fluid (embedded in the pudding and her electrolyte tonic), and zero histamine triggers. Her heart rate settled to 96. The day was manageable.

This chapter provides 15 trifecta-compatible breakfast recipes designed around the physiological realities of morning eating with POTS, EDS, and MCAS:

- Make-ahead options that require zero morning preparation energy
- High-sodium recipes that address the orthostatic demands of the first upright hour
- Low-histamine formulations using only green and tested yellow-category ingredients
- Batch-friendly preparations aligned with the cook-once approach from section 13.9
- Scalable recipes that accommodate both high-energy and crash days

15.1 Morning Physiology Explained

Breakfast matters more for trifecta patients than for the general population, and it matters for different reasons. The standard nutritional argument for breakfast centers on metabolic activation and cognitive performance (Adolphus et al., 2013). For POTS patients, the argument is hemodynamic. Overnight fasting depletes intravascular volume through insensible fluid loss (respiration and perspiration during sleep), and the transition from supine to upright posture upon waking demands immediate cardiovascular compensation (Vernino et al., 2021). Without sodium, fluid, and calories in the first 30 to 60 minutes after rising, the compensatory mechanisms that maintain blood pressure and cerebral perfusion during upright posture operate at a deficit.

Orthostatic intolerance peaks in the morning for most POTS patients. A 2019 cross-sectional survey of 4,835 POTS patients found that morning symptoms (dizziness, tachycardia, brain fog, nausea) were reported as the most disabling time-of-day symptom by 67% of respondents (Shaw et al., 2019). The physiological explanation involves the convergence of overnight volume depletion, the natural morning surge in cortisol and catecholamines that raises heart rate, and the abrupt gravitational challenge of standing from a supine position (Raj et al., 2020). Eating breakfast, particularly a breakfast rich in sodium and fluid, partially offsets the volume deficit and supports the hemodynamic response to upright posture.

Postprandial hemodynamic shifts create a second consideration. Eating diverts blood flow to the splanchnic (gut) circulation for digestion, which can worsen orthostatic symptoms in some POTS patients, particularly after large meals (Mehr et al., 2018). The solution is not to skip breakfast. The solution is to eat smaller, more frequent morning meals with moderate carbohydrate content (to minimize the insulin-mediated vasodilation that worsens postprandial hypotension), adequate salt (to expand plasma volume), and sufficient protein and fat (to slow gastric emptying and provide sustained energy; Ganesh et al., 2020).

For MCAS patients, morning eating introduces the additional constraint of histamine management. The recipes in this chapter use exclusively low-histamine ingredients prepared fresh or from properly frozen components, consistent with the freshness management principles from section 13.2 (Comas-Basté et al., 2020). For EDS patients with gastroparesis, recipes emphasize soft textures, moderate fiber, and smaller portions that accommodate delayed gastric emptying (Thwaites et al., 2022).

15.2 Overnight Chia Pudding

Overnight chia seed pudding with coconut milk and blueberries is the single most efficient trifecta breakfast because it requires zero morning energy, delivers all four Trifecta Plate components (section 10.1), and can be batch-prepared for three to five days without histamine concerns (chia seeds and coconut milk are shelf-stable, and the pudding contains no animal protein that would accumulate histamine during refrigeration).

Chia seeds provide 10 grams of fiber per two-tablespoon serving, including both soluble and insoluble fiber types. They absorb 10 to 12 times their weight in liquid (Muñoz et al., 2012), which means a chia pudding functions as both food and fluid delivery. For POTS patients, this embedded hydration contributes meaningfully to morning fluid targets without requiring additional drinking. Chia seeds also provide approximately 4 grams of protein per serving, 5 grams of omega-3 alpha-linolenic acid (an anti-inflammatory fatty acid discussed in section 9.2; Nieman et al., 2009), and calcium, magnesium, and phosphorus.

Recipe: Overnight Chia Pudding

Combine 3 tablespoons of chia seeds, 1 cup of full-fat coconut milk (canned or carton, checking ingredient label per the three-scan method from section 13.10 for additives), 1/2 teaspoon of fine sea salt (approximately 1,150 mg sodium), 1 teaspoon of maple syrup or honey, and 1/2 teaspoon of vanilla extract in a jar or container. Stir well, refrigerate for a minimum of four hours or overnight. Top with 1/4 cup of fresh or frozen blueberries (thawed) before eating. Approximate nutrition: 380 calories, 12 g protein (with collagen peptide addition), 24 g fat, 32 g carbohydrate, 1,150 mg sodium.

Pro Tip: Collagen Boost. Stir one scoop (10 to 15 grams) of unflavored collagen peptides into the chia mixture before refrigerating. This adds protein without altering flavor, supports collagen synthesis relevant to EDS connective tissue integrity (Gensemer et al., 2021), and dissolves completely in cold liquid.

Batch method: Prepare five jars simultaneously on a prep day (section 13.9). The pudding keeps in the refrigerator for up to five days because it contains no animal protein or other histamine-accumulating ingredients. This single batch covers five weekday mornings with zero daily preparation.

15.3 Savory Morning Options

Many trifecta patients find that savory breakfasts deliver sodium more naturally than sweet breakfasts, where salt addition can feel forced. Savory morning meals also tend to contain more protein and less simple carbohydrate, which reduces the postprandial insulin spike that can worsen orthostatic symptoms in POTS (Shibao et al., 2005).

Sweet Potato and Sage Hash with Poached Eggs

Peel and dice two medium sweet potatoes into 1/2-inch cubes. Heat 2 tablespoons of olive oil in a ceramic-coated skillet over medium heat. Add the sweet potatoes, 1 teaspoon of fine sea salt, and 1/2 teaspoon of dried sage. Cook, stirring occasionally, for 12 to 15 minutes until the potatoes are tender and lightly browned. While the hash cooks, poach two eggs in simmering salted water (3 to 4 minutes for soft yolks). Serve the hash topped with poached eggs and an additional pinch of flaky salt. Serves two. Approximate per serving: 340 calories, 14 g protein, 16 g fat, 36 g carbohydrate, 1,400 mg sodium.

Sweet potatoes provide complex carbohydrates with a moderate glycemic index (GI of approximately 63 when boiled; Atkinson et al., 2008), beta-carotene (a precursor to vitamin A), and potassium (approximately 540 mg per medium potato), which supports the sodium-potassium balance discussed in section 7.4. Sage contains rosmarinic acid with anti-inflammatory properties (Bauer et al., 2012). Eggs (if individually tolerated per the reintroduction protocol from section 6.9) provide complete protein and choline.

Savory Breakfast Rice Bowl with Soft-Boiled Egg and Sautéed Greens

Reheat one individual portion of frozen cooked rice (from batch prep, section 13.9) in the microwave for 2 to 3 minutes. Meanwhile, sauté one cup of fresh baby spinach or chopped bok choy in 1 tablespoon of ghee with 1/2 teaspoon of salt and a pinch of ground ginger for 2 minutes. Prepare a soft-boiled egg (6 to 7 minutes in boiling water, then ice bath). Assemble the bowl: rice, greens, halved egg, drizzle of olive oil, and a generous pinch of flaky sea salt. Serves one. Approximate: 420 calories, 16 g protein, 18 g fat, 48 g carbohydrate, 1,300 mg sodium.

This bowl illustrates the **component assembly** approach from section 13.9. The rice was batch-cooked and frozen days earlier. The greens take two minutes of active cooking. The egg requires boiling water and a timer. Total active preparation on a low-energy morning: under 10 minutes, most of it seated at the counter on a perching stool (section 13.7).

Turkey Breakfast Patties with Herbs

Combine 1 pound of ground turkey (purchased fresh and cooked within 24 hours per section 13.2), 1 teaspoon of fine sea salt, 1/2 teaspoon of dried thyme, 1/2 teaspoon of dried rosemary (crushed), 1/4 teaspoon of ground black pepper, and 1 tablespoon of olive oil. Form into eight small patties (approximately 2 ounces each). Cook in a skillet over medium heat for 4 to 5 minutes per side until internal temperature reaches 165°F. Cool, then individually wrap and freeze within 30 minutes of cooking. Reheat from frozen in a skillet (5 to 6 minutes) or microwave (90 seconds). Makes eight patties. Approximate per two-patty serving: 220 calories, 26 g protein, 12 g fat, 0 g carbohydrate, 600 mg sodium.

These patties are the breakfast equivalent of a trifecta building block. They freeze with minimal quality loss, reheat quickly, and provide protein and sodium in a form that pairs with any carbohydrate or vegetable. Two patties alongside a reheated sweet potato or bowl of oatmeal create a complete Trifecta Plate breakfast in under five minutes from frozen components.

15.4 Clotilde's Morning Routine

Background

Clotilde, a 31-year-old elementary school teacher with POTS, hEDS, and MCAS, had been skipping breakfast for years. She described herself as "not a morning person" and explained that morning nausea (a common POTS symptom related to overnight volume depletion and gastroparesis; Thwaites et al., 2022) made the thought of eating before 10 a.m. physically unpleasant. She consumed coffee with cream as her only morning intake, arriving at school with approximately 100 calories, no sodium beyond what the cream provided, and 200 mg of caffeine that further increased her heart rate.

Presentation

Clotilde's morning symptoms were her worst of the day: heart rate spikes to 135 upon standing, persistent dizziness through her first two class periods, difficulty finding words during morning lessons (brain fog), and visible facial flushing. She had attributed these symptoms to "just how POTS is in the morning" and had not connected them to her absent breakfast. Her POTS specialist noted that her morning sodium intake was essentially zero, her morning fluid intake was limited to 8 ounces of coffee (a mild diuretic at that dose; Killer et al., 2014), and her blood glucose was at its lowest point during her highest-demand work hours.

Analysis

Clotilde's morning symptom pattern reflected the predictable hemodynamic consequences of insufficient morning sodium and fluid intake in a POTS patient. The overnight fasting period depletes intravascular volume, and the catecholamine surge upon waking raises heart rate in a system that lacks adequate volume to compensate (Vernino et al., 2021). Caffeine without food further stimulates sympathetic nervous system activity while providing no volume expansion. The nausea she experienced was itself a symptom of the volume deficit and gastroparesis, not a contraindication to eating. Small-volume, calorie-dense, high-sodium foods bypass the nausea more effectively than large-volume meals (Ganesh et al., 2020).

Intervention

Her dietitian introduced a two-phase morning routine. Phase 1, consumed within 10 minutes of waking while still in bed or seated: the electrolyte morning tonic (section 15.6, approximately 1,000 mg sodium in 8 ounces of warm water). Phase 2, consumed within 30 minutes of waking: a half-portion of overnight chia pudding (section 15.2, approximately 190 calories and 575 mg sodium). The small volumes and calorie density were chosen specifically to bypass morning nausea. Coffee was moved to after breakfast, reducing its hemodynamic impact by buffering absorption with food.

Outcome

Over three weeks, Clotilde's morning heart rate peaks decreased from 135 to 115 upon standing. Brain fog during first-period classes improved, and she reported being able to "find words faster" by 8:30 a.m. The morning nausea, paradoxically, improved rather than worsened with early eating, because the sodium and fluid in the tonic and pudding began addressing the volume deficit that was producing the nausea in the first place. She described the electrolyte tonic as "the thing I should have been doing for five years."

Teaching Points

- Morning nausea in POTS patients is frequently a symptom of overnight volume depletion rather than a contraindication to eating, and early sodium and fluid intake often reduces nausea rather than worsening it
- Small-volume, calorie-dense, high-sodium foods (chia pudding, electrolyte tonic) bypass gastroparesis-related nausea more effectively than large-volume breakfasts
- Moving caffeine consumption to after breakfast rather than before reduces sympathetic stimulation during the most hemodynamically vulnerable period of the day

15.5 Grain Based Breakfasts

Salted Maple Oatmeal with Pear and Pecans

Combine 1/2 cup of rolled oats with 1 cup of water and 1/2 teaspoon of fine sea salt in a small pot. Cook over medium heat for 5 to 7 minutes, stirring occasionally, until the oats reach desired consistency. Remove from heat and stir in 1 tablespoon of maple syrup, 1 tablespoon of ghee, half a ripe pear (diced), and 2 tablespoons of chopped pecans. Sprinkle with an additional pinch of flaky salt. Serves one. Approximate: 420 calories, 10 g protein, 20 g fat, 54 g carbohydrate, 1,200 mg sodium.

Oats provide **beta-glucan**, a soluble fiber that slows gastric emptying, moderates postprandial blood glucose spikes, and supports beneficial gut microbiota (Tosh, 2013). For POTS patients, the salt-in-oatmeal technique delivers sodium seamlessly. Salted oatmeal tastes like savory porridge rather than dessert, and the salt enhances rather than clashes with the maple and pear sweetness. Pecans contribute monounsaturated fats and a small amount of the anti-inflammatory compound gamma-tocopherol (Haddad et al., 2006). Pears are among the lowest-histamine fruits (Maintz & Novak, 2007) and provide gentle fiber appropriate for gastroparesis patients.

Rice Flour Pancakes with Fresh Fruit Compote

Whisk together 1 cup of rice flour, 1 tablespoon of tapioca starch, 1 teaspoon of baking powder (aluminum-free), 1/2 teaspoon of fine sea salt, 1 egg (beaten), 3/4 cup of coconut milk, and 1 tablespoon of melted coconut oil. Let the batter rest for 5 minutes. Cook on a lightly oiled skillet over medium heat, using approximately 3 tablespoons of batter per pancake (small pancakes are easier to flip and cook more evenly). Cook 2 to 3 minutes per side until golden.

For the compote: combine 1 cup of fresh or frozen blueberries, 2 tablespoons of water, 1 tablespoon of maple syrup, and a pinch of salt in a small saucepan. Simmer 5 to 7 minutes until berries soften and liquid thickens. Serve pancakes topped with warm compote and a drizzle of maple syrup. Makes approximately eight small pancakes (two servings). Approximate per serving: 380 calories, 8 g protein, 14 g fat, 58 g carbohydrate, 800 mg sodium.

Rice flour pancakes provide a gluten-free option that avoids wheat, which some MCAS patients identify as a personal trigger through the elimination-rechallenge protocol (section 6.9). The tapioca starch creates a lighter texture than rice flour alone. These pancakes freeze well individually (separated by parchment paper) and reheat in a toaster or skillet, making them batch-prep friendly.

15.6 Beverages and Tonics

Electrolyte Morning Tonic (Warm, Lemon-Free)

Dissolve 1/2 teaspoon of fine sea salt (approximately 1,150 mg sodium), 1/8 teaspoon of potassium-containing salt substitute (such as Morton Lite Salt, providing approximately 175 mg potassium), and 1 teaspoon of honey in 8 ounces of warm water. Add 1/4 teaspoon of ground ginger and stir. Sip over 10 to 15 minutes, ideally within the first 15 minutes after waking. Approximate: 25 calories, 1,150 mg sodium, 175 mg potassium.

This tonic deliberately excludes citrus. Lemon juice, though commonly recommended in morning tonics, is a histamine liberator that can trigger MCAS symptoms in sensitive patients (Kovacova-Hanuskova et al., 2015). The warm water temperature aids absorption and is gentler on a gastroparesis-affected stomach than cold water, which can slow gastric motility (Bateman, 1982). Ginger provides mild prokinetic effects that may improve gastric motility in gastroparesis (Giacosa et al., 2015).

Green Smoothie with Cucumber, Apple, Ginger, and Sea Salt

Blend 1 cup of peeled, seeded cucumber (approximately 2/3 of a medium cucumber), 1 medium apple (peeled, cored, and roughly chopped), 1 cup of coconut water, 1/2 inch of fresh ginger root (peeled), 1/2 teaspoon of fine sea salt, 1 scoop of collagen peptides (optional), and 4 to 5 ice cubes until smooth. Serves one. Approximate: 180 calories, 12 g protein (with collagen), 1 g fat, 34 g carbohydrate, 1,200 mg sodium.

Cucumber provides hydration (96% water content) and potassium. Apple adds natural sweetness and soluble fiber (pectin). Coconut water contributes additional potassium (approximately 600 mg per cup; Kalman et al., 2012) and natural sugars that improve sodium absorption through the sodium-glucose cotransporter described in section 7.2. This smoothie avoids all common histamine-triggering fruits (citrus, strawberries, pineapple, papaya) and fermented ingredients.

"Brain Fog Buster" Smoothie

Blend 1/2 cup of frozen blueberries, 1/2 medium frozen banana (peeled before freezing), 1 tablespoon of almond butter (or sunflower seed butter if tree nut sensitive), 1 cup of coconut milk, 1 scoop of collagen peptides, 1/2 teaspoon of fine sea salt, 1/4 teaspoon of ground turmeric, and a pinch of ground black pepper (which enhances curcumin bioavailability by approximately 2,000%; Shoba et al., 1998). Serves one. Approximate: 420 calories, 18 g protein, 24 g fat, 38 g carbohydrate, 1,200 mg sodium.

This smoothie is engineered to address brain fog through four mechanisms: protein (collagen peptides) supports neurotransmitter precursor availability, healthy fat (almond butter, coconut milk) provides sustained energy without blood sugar spikes, complex carbohydrate (blueberries, banana) fuels brain glucose metabolism, and electrolytes (salt, coconut milk potassium) support the cerebral perfusion that POTS compromises during upright posture (Raj et al., 2020). The turmeric adds the anti-inflammatory curcumin discussed in section 9.3 (Daily et al., 2016).

15.7 Erasmus Builds a System

Background

Erasmus, a 44-year-old software developer with POTS and recently diagnosed MCAS, worked from home. He had received the trifecta dietary framework from his dietitian and understood the principles intellectually. But translating those principles into daily breakfasts had stalled. He found himself standing in the kitchen each morning, fatigued and foggy, trying to decide what to make. Decision fatigue combined with physical fatigue meant he often defaulted to toast with butter (low sodium, low protein, minimal trifecta alignment) or skipped breakfast entirely.

Presentation

Erasmus's food diary (Chapter 14.0) showed a pattern: he ate well-structured trifecta meals for lunch and dinner but consumed only 150 to 250 calories at breakfast, with sodium intake averaging 200 mg before noon. His morning heart rate variability data from his wearable device showed that his lowest readings consistently occurred between 7:00 and 10:00 a.m., correlating with his lowest sodium and calorie intake window. His MCAS flares also clustered in the late morning, which his allergist hypothesized might relate to the combined stress of inadequate morning nutrition and the cortisol rise pattern of the hypothalamic-pituitary-adrenal axis (Theoharides & Cochrane, 2004).

Analysis

Erasmus's barrier was not dietary knowledge. It was the **executive function demand** of morning meal planning in the context of fatigue and brain fog. Research on executive function in POTS demonstrates that cognitive processing speed, working memory, and decision-making are all impaired during symptomatic periods, with particular deficits during orthostatic challenge (Arnold et al., 2015). A breakfast system that requires morning decision-making is a system designed to fail for POTS patients. The solution, consistent with the batch-cooking framework from section 13.9, is to eliminate all morning decisions by preparing a rotating breakfast menu in advance.

Intervention

The dietitian helped Erasmus design a five-day rotating breakfast plan using three recipes from this chapter: overnight chia pudding (Monday and Wednesday), turkey patties with reheated sweet potato (Tuesday and Thursday), and the Brain Fog Buster smoothie (Friday). All components were prepared during his Sunday batch session. The chia puddings were assembled in jars. The turkey patties and sweet potatoes were cooked, portioned, and frozen. The smoothie ingredients were pre-measured into individual freezer bags (frozen blueberries, frozen banana, almond butter packet, collagen scoop, salt, turmeric) that only required dumping into a blender with coconut milk.

Outcome

Over four weeks, Erasmus's morning caloric intake increased from 150 to 250 calories to 350 to 420 calories. Morning sodium intake rose from 200 mg to 1,100 to 1,200 mg. His morning heart rate variability improved, and late-morning MCAS flares decreased from approximately three per week to one. He described the system as "removing my brain from the equation, which is exactly what my brain needs at 7 a.m."

Teaching Points

- Executive function impairment in POTS directly undermines morning meal preparation when the breakfast system requires real-time decision-making, and pre-planned rotating menus eliminate this barrier
- Batch-prepping breakfast components (chia puddings, frozen patties, pre-measured smoothie bags) consolidates all preparation labor into a single high-energy session and distributes the results across the week
- Morning sodium intake exerts outsized influence on daily symptom burden because it addresses the overnight volume deficit during the period of greatest orthostatic vulnerability

15.8 Freezer Friendly Baking

Coconut Flour Muffins with Zucchini

Preheat oven to 350°F. Whisk together 1/3 cup of coconut flour, 1/4 teaspoon of baking soda, 1/2 teaspoon of fine sea salt, and 1/2 teaspoon of ground cinnamon. In a separate bowl, beat 4 eggs, then stir in 1/4 cup of melted coconut oil, 2 tablespoons of maple syrup, and 1 cup of finely grated zucchini (squeeze excess moisture with a clean towel). Combine wet and dry ingredients. Divide batter among 8 greased or lined muffin cups. Bake 22 to 25 minutes until a toothpick inserted in the center comes out clean. Cool completely, then individually wrap in plastic wrap and freeze in a single layer. To serve, unwrap and microwave from frozen for 45 to 60 seconds.

Makes eight muffins. Approximate per muffin: 130 calories, 4 g protein, 9 g fat, 8 g carbohydrate, 250 mg sodium.

Coconut flour behaves differently from wheat or rice flour. It absorbs approximately four times more liquid than wheat flour (Gunathilake et al., 2009), which is why this recipe requires four eggs for only 1/3 cup of flour. The result is a dense, moist muffin that holds together well after freezing and reheating. Zucchini contributes moisture, mild flavor, and small amounts of potassium and vitamin C without adding histamine or fiber dense enough to worsen gastroparesis symptoms.

These muffins function as a grab-and-go breakfast component, providing fat and moderate protein that pairs well with fruit or a morning tonic.

15.9 Recipe Adaptation Principles

Every recipe in this chapter follows five adaptation principles that readers can apply to modify their own existing recipes or create new ones.

The first principle is **sodium loading by design**. Each recipe targets 800 to 1,200 mg of sodium, contributing to the daily 6,000 to 10,000 mg target recommended for POTS management (Vernino et al., 2021). Salt appears in the ingredient list rather than as an afterthought at the table. Cooking with salt allows it to integrate into the flavor of the dish, improving palatability at therapeutic doses (Breslin & Beauchamp, 1997).

The second principle is **freshness-first protein**. Animal proteins are cooked from fresh (within 24 hours of purchase) or from frozen (flash-frozen at purchase, thawed in refrigerator on day of cooking), consistent with the histamine management framework from sections 6.2 and 13.2. Leftovers are portioned and frozen within 30 minutes (Comas-Basté et al., 2020).

The third principle is **gastroparesis-friendly textures**. Recipes emphasize soft, moist textures (puddings, scrambles, soups, smoothies) that require less mechanical digestion than raw vegetables or tough proteins. Portion sizes are moderate (300 to 450 calories per sitting rather than 600 or more), reducing the postprandial hemodynamic burden (Mehr et al., 2018).

The fourth principle is **anti-inflammatory ingredient selection**. Recipes preferentially include ingredients with documented anti-inflammatory properties: olive oil (oleocanthal; Beauchamp et al., 2005), turmeric (curcumin; Daily et al., 2016), ginger (gingerols; Giacosa et al., 2015), blueberries (anthocyanins; Kalt et al., 2020), and omega-3 sources like chia seeds (Nieman et al., 2009). These align with the anti-inflammatory strategy from Chapter 9.0.

The fifth principle is **batch-freeze-reheat architecture**. Every recipe either requires no morning cooking (chia pudding, smoothie bags), requires only reheating (turkey patties, muffins, rice), or requires less than 15 minutes of active cooking (oatmeal, hash, pancakes). This architecture matches the variable energy availability described in section 13.8.

15.10 Putting Mornings Together

The recipes in this chapter are not a menu to follow sequentially. They are a toolkit. A well-prepared trifecta patient maintains a rotating stock of three to four breakfast options at any given time, some in the refrigerator (chia puddings prepared every four to five days), some in the freezer (turkey patties, muffins, smoothie bags, pre-cooked rice portions), and some requiring only pantry staples (oatmeal, electrolyte tonic).

The match between recipe and day depends on energy level, symptom severity, and time available. On a crash day, the breakfast is whatever requires the least effort: a pre-made chia pudding and an electrolyte tonic, consumed in bed or on the couch. On a moderate day, a frozen turkey patty reheated alongside a microwaved sweet potato provides a heartier option. On a good day, fresh-cooked oatmeal with pear and pecans or a savory rice bowl offers variety and satisfaction.

The common thread across all these options is that each delivers the four trifecta priorities simultaneously: sodium (800 to 1,200 mg per breakfast), fluid (8 to 16 ounces embedded or alongside), low-histamine ingredients (all green-category or individually tested), and gastroparesis-appropriate texture and portion size. The morning tonic (section 15.6) can accompany any breakfast as an additional sodium and fluid bolus, particularly on days when orthostatic symptoms are prominent.

Chapter 16.0 extends this approach to soups, broths, and hydrating bowls, the liquid-forward preparations that serve as both meals and therapeutic sodium-fluid delivery throughout the day.

Chapter 16.0: Soups, Broths and Hydrating Bowls

A cup of well-salted broth is the closest thing to intravenous saline that a trifecta patient can administer at home. That comparison is not casual. Intravenous normal saline delivers 154 mEq of sodium per liter directly into the bloodstream to expand plasma volume. A cup of properly salted broth delivers approximately 1,000 to 1,500 mg of sodium in warm liquid form, absorbed through the intestinal sodium-glucose cotransporter (discussed in section 7.2) within 15 to 30 minutes. For POTS patients who cannot access IV fluids, and for the many days between infusion appointments for those who can, broth and soup are the oral equivalent of volume expansion therapy. Yet most commercial broths and soups are unusable for trifecta patients because they contain hidden histamine (from long-simmered bones, yeast extract, or "natural flavors"), unpredictable sodium levels (too much in some brands, too little in "low sodium" versions), and additives that trigger MCAS (Reese et al., 2017). This chapter provides 10 trifecta-compatible recipes for broths, soups, and hydrating bowls that solve these problems.

This chapter covers:

- Histamine-aware broth preparation with short cook times and immediate cooling
- Vegetable-based mineral broths as low-histamine alternatives to bone broth
- Complete meal soups that function as one-bowl Trifecta Plate servings
- Therapeutic broths designed specifically for electrolyte delivery and flare recovery
- Congee and grain-based porridge soups with customizable topping systems

16.1 Broth Science for Trifecta

Bone broth has become enormously popular in both mainstream wellness culture and chronic illness communities. The claimed benefits include improved gut lining integrity, enhanced joint health through collagen delivery, and mineral content from dissolved bone matrix (Hsu et al., 2017). Some of these claims have partial research support, while others remain unsubstantiated. What matters for trifecta patients, however, is a different question entirely: can bone broth be prepared safely for someone managing histamine sensitivity, and if so, how?

The problem is cook time. Traditional bone broth recipes call for 12 to 48 hours of simmering. Extended cooking extracts more collagen, minerals, and flavor from bones, but it also creates ideal conditions for histamine accumulation. As broth simmers in the 140 to 180°F range for hours, any bacteria present on the meat or bones (even in small quantities) can convert the amino acid histidine into histamine through the decarboxylation process described in section 6.2 (Comas-Basté et al., 2020). A 24-hour bone broth can contain substantially more histamine than a two-hour version made from the same ingredients. For MCAS patients, this difference can be the difference between a therapeutic food and a trigger.

Histamine-aware broth is bone broth prepared with a short cook time (two to four hours maximum), immediate cooling, and immediate portioning and freezing. This approach extracts meaningful amounts of collagen and minerals while keeping histamine accumulation within tolerable limits for most MCAS patients (Maintz & Novak, 2007). The trade-off is flavor intensity: a two-hour broth tastes lighter and less rich than a 24-hour broth. Salt, fresh herbs, turmeric, and ginger compensate for this flavor difference while adding therapeutic value.

16.2 Histamine Aware Bone Broth

Recipe: Short-Cook Chicken Bone Broth

Place 2 to 3 pounds of raw chicken backs, necks, or a whole carcass from a freshly roasted chicken (roasted within the past 24 hours, not a leftover carcass that has sat in the refrigerator) into a large pot. Add 8 cups of cold water, 1 tablespoon of apple cider vinegar (the small amount of vinegar is tolerated by most MCAS patients and aids mineral extraction from bones; Hsu et al., 2017), 1 teaspoon of fine sea salt, 2 peeled garlic cloves, 1 inch of fresh ginger root (peeled and sliced), and 2 to 3 fresh thyme sprigs. Bring to a gentle boil, then reduce heat to a low simmer. Skim any foam that rises to the surface during the first 15 minutes.

Simmer for a minimum of 2 hours and a maximum of 4 hours. Do not exceed 4 hours.

Immediately after turning off the heat, strain the broth through a fine-mesh strainer into a clean pot or large bowl. Discard solids. To cool rapidly, place the pot in an ice bath (a larger container filled with ice and cold water) and stir the broth occasionally. The goal is to bring the broth below 40°F within one hour. Once cool, portion into individual serving containers (8 to 12 ounce portions) and freeze immediately. Broth intended for consumption within 24 hours may be refrigerated instead.

Makes approximately 6 cups. Approximate per 1-cup serving: 40 calories, 6 g protein, 1 g fat, 0 g carbohydrate, 400 mg sodium (increase by adding more salt to taste when reheating).

Why the rapid cooling matters. Histamine accumulation accelerates in the temperature range between 40°F and 140°F, known in food safety as the **danger zone** (U.S. Department of Agriculture, 2023). Broth that sits on the counter cooling slowly passes through this range over several hours, providing extended opportunity for bacterial histamine production. The ice bath method bypasses the danger zone rapidly, minimizing histamine accumulation between cooking and freezing (Sánchez-Pérez et al., 2018).

16.3 Vegetable Mineral Broth

For patients who do not tolerate bone broth at any cook time, or who prefer a plant-based option, **vegetable mineral broth** provides an alternative that delivers sodium, potassium, magnesium, and flavor without any animal protein and without histamine concerns.

Recipe: Low-Histamine Vegetable Mineral Broth

Roughly chop 2 medium carrots, 2 celery stalks (if tolerated), 1 medium sweet potato (peeled), 1 medium zucchini, 4 garlic cloves (peeled and smashed), 1 inch of fresh ginger (sliced), and 1 cup of fresh parsley stems and leaves. Place all vegetables in a large pot with 10 cups of cold water, 1 tablespoon of fine sea salt, 1 teaspoon of ground turmeric, and 1/2 teaspoon of black pepper. Bring to a boil, reduce to a gentle simmer, and cook for 45 to 60 minutes. Strain through a fine-mesh strainer, pressing vegetables to extract liquid. Discard solids. Cool using the ice bath method, portion, and freeze.

Makes approximately 8 cups. Approximate per 1-cup serving: 15 calories, 0 g protein, 0 g fat, 3 g carbohydrate, 450 mg sodium.

This broth contains no animal protein, which means histamine accumulation during cooking is negligible compared to meat-based broths (Comas-Basté et al., 2020). The cook time of 45 to 60 minutes is sufficient to extract minerals and flavor from vegetables without the extended simmering that poses problems for meat-based preparations. The turmeric and ginger provide anti-inflammatory compounds (Daily et al., 2016; Giacosa et al., 2015), while the parsley contributes potassium, vitamin C, and mild diuretic properties that paradoxically support fluid balance by promoting renal sodium reabsorption (Kreydiyyeh & Usta, 2002).

16.4 Complete Meal Soups

The soups in this section function as full Trifecta Plate meals in bowl form: protein, carbohydrate, vegetable, and fat in a sodium-rich, hydrating liquid base. Each provides 350 to 500 calories per serving with 1,000 to 1,500 mg of sodium.

Chicken and Rice Soup with Fresh Herbs

Heat 2 tablespoons of olive oil in a large pot over medium heat. Add 1 diced medium carrot, 1 diced celery stalk (if tolerated), and 2 minced garlic cloves. Sauté 3 to 4 minutes until softened. Add 6 cups of homemade short-cook broth (section 16.2) or vegetable mineral broth (section 16.3), 1 teaspoon of fine sea salt, and 1/2 teaspoon of dried thyme. Bring to a simmer. Add 1/2 cup of uncooked white rice and cook 15 minutes until rice is tender. Add 2 cups of shredded cooked chicken (freshly cooked or thawed from frozen batch prep per section 13.9). Heat through for 3 to 4 minutes. Remove from heat and stir in 2 tablespoons of chopped fresh dill and 1 tablespoon of fresh parsley. Adjust salt to taste.

Serves four. Approximate per serving: 340 calories, 28 g protein, 10 g fat, 32 g carbohydrate, 1,200 mg sodium.

This soup can be portioned and frozen within 30 minutes of preparation for histamine-safe storage. Its high fluid content (approximately 12 ounces per serving) contributes meaningfully to daily hydration targets.

Sweet Potato and Coconut Soup

Peel and dice 3 medium sweet potatoes (approximately 1.5 pounds). Heat 1 tablespoon of coconut oil in a pot over medium heat. Add 1 diced small onion (if tolerated; omit for strict elimination phase) and 2 minced garlic cloves. Sauté 3 minutes. Add the sweet potatoes, 4 cups of vegetable mineral broth, 1 can (13.5 ounces) of full-fat coconut milk, 1 teaspoon of ground turmeric, 1/2 teaspoon of ground ginger, and 1.5 teaspoons of fine sea salt. Bring to a boil, reduce heat, and simmer 20 minutes until sweet potatoes are completely tender. Use an immersion blender (or transfer to a blender in batches) to purée until smooth. Adjust salt and add a pinch of black pepper.

Serves four. Approximate per serving: 380 calories, 5 g protein, 18 g fat, 52 g carbohydrate, 1,100 mg sodium.

The sweet potato provides beta-carotene, potassium, and complex carbohydrate with a moderate glycemic index (Atkinson et al., 2008). Coconut milk adds medium-chain triglycerides (MCTs), which are absorbed more rapidly than long-chain fatty acids and provide quick energy without requiring bile acid emulsification, making them better tolerated in patients with fat malabsorption related to EDS gastrointestinal dysfunction (Thwaites et al., 2022). The puréed texture accommodates gastroparesis by minimizing the mechanical digestion required.

Zucchini and Basil Soup

Dice 4 medium zucchini. Heat 2 tablespoons of olive oil over medium heat. Add 2 minced garlic cloves and the diced zucchini. Season with 1 teaspoon of salt. Sauté 5 to 6 minutes until zucchini softens. Add 3 cups of vegetable mineral broth and simmer 10 minutes. Remove from heat. Add 1/2 cup of loosely packed fresh basil leaves and purée until smooth with an immersion blender. Stir in 1 tablespoon of olive oil and adjust salt.

Serves three. Approximate per serving: 140 calories, 3 g protein, 10 g fat, 10 g carbohydrate, 1,000 mg sodium.

This is a light soup that works well as a starter, a snack between meals, or a flare day option when appetite is minimal but sodium and fluid are still needed. The calorie count is lower than the other complete meal soups, so pair it with a protein source (shredded chicken, a turkey patty from section 15.3, or a poached egg) for a full Trifecta Plate meal.

16.5 Ivo's Flare Day Protocol

Background

Ivo, a 38-year-old paramedic with POTS, hEDS, and MCAS, experienced MCAS flares triggered by heat exposure during summer ambulance shifts. On flare days, his symptoms included severe GI cramping, nausea, facial flushing, tachycardia, and brain fog lasting 6 to 12 hours. During active flares, he could not tolerate solid food. He had been subsisting on plain water and crackers during flare episodes, which provided minimal sodium and calories while failing to address the fluid deficit that heat exposure worsened.

Presentation

Ivo's food diary showed that flare days resulted in caloric intake dropping to 400 to 600 calories with sodium intake below 2,000 mg. On days following flares, his POTS symptoms were markedly worse than baseline, with standing heart rate increases of 40 or more beats per minute (compared to his usual 25 to 28 bpm increase). He described post-flare days as "feeling like I've been sick for a week." His pattern suggested that the nutritional deficit during flare days was compounding the hemodynamic recovery, creating a two-day event from what began as a several-hour flare.

Analysis

The combination of heat-triggered MCAS flare plus inadequate sodium and fluid replacement during the flare created a volume depletion cascade. MCAS flares themselves can cause fluid shifts (through increased vascular permeability mediated by histamine and prostaglandins; Molderings et al., 2011). When the patient simultaneously restricts fluid and sodium intake because of GI symptoms, the volume deficit deepens, worsening POTS symptoms both during and after the flare. The clinical principle from section 12.1 applies directly: flare days demand more sodium and fluid, not less, even when GI symptoms make eating difficult.

Intervention

Ivo's dietitian built a flare day liquid protocol using recipes from this chapter. Phase 1 (during active GI symptoms): sip the electrolyte broth with turmeric and ginger (section 16.7) at a rate of 2 to 4 ounces every 15 to 20 minutes, totaling 16 to 24 ounces over two hours. The small sip volume bypasses nausea by avoiding gastric distension. Phase 2 (once acute nausea subsides, typically 2 to 4 hours into the flare): consume a full cup of vegetable mineral broth with additional salt (1,200 mg sodium per cup) every one to two hours. Phase 3 (flare resolving, appetite returning): transition to a puréed soup (sweet potato and coconut soup or zucchini and basil soup) as the first solid-adjacent food. All components were pre-made and stored frozen in individual portions so that preparation during a flare required only reheating.

Outcome

Over the next four heat-triggered flares (spanning two months of summer shifts), Ivo maintained sodium intake above 5,000 mg and fluid intake above 60 ounces even on flare days. His post-flare POTS symptom worsening decreased substantially: standing heart rate increases the day after a flare dropped from 40-plus bpm to 28 to 32 bpm (near his baseline). He described the flare day protocol as "the difference between losing one day and losing three."

Teaching Points

- MCAS flare days require increased sodium and fluid intake rather than dietary restriction, because the flare itself causes volume depletion through histamine-mediated vascular permeability changes
- A phased liquid protocol (small sips of electrolyte broth progressing to full-cup broth servings to puréed soups) accommodates GI symptoms while maintaining sodium and fluid delivery throughout the flare
- Pre-portioned frozen broths and soups eliminate the preparation burden during flares, when the patient's physical capacity is at its lowest

16.6 Specialty Soups

Miso-Free "Umami" Soup

Traditional miso soup relies on fermented soybean paste, a concentrated histamine source that is incompatible with MCAS management (Maintz & Novak, 2007). This recipe achieves a similar savory, umami depth without fermentation.

Bring 4 cups of vegetable mineral broth to a simmer. Add 1 tablespoon of coconut aminos (a non-fermented, soy-free alternative to soy sauce made from coconut sap; verify the specific brand's ingredient list per section 13.10), 1 teaspoon of toasted sesame oil, 1 minced garlic clove, 1/2 teaspoon of grated fresh ginger, and 1 teaspoon of fine sea salt. Simmer 5 minutes. Add 1/2 cup of diced soft tofu (if individually tolerated; omit if soy is a confirmed trigger) and 1 cup of thinly sliced bok choy. Cook 3 minutes until bok choy wilts. Remove from heat. Garnish with thinly sliced green onion tops (green parts only, which are lower in FODMAPs than white parts) and a pinch of sesame seeds.

Serves two. Approximate per serving: 120 calories, 6 g protein, 6 g fat, 12 g carbohydrate, 1,300 mg sodium.

The umami flavor comes from the natural glutamate in the coconut aminos and sesame oil rather than from fermented sources. **Umami**, the fifth basic taste, activates specific glutamate receptors on the tongue and contributes to the satisfying "savory" quality of foods (Beauchamp, 2009). Achieving umami without fermentation is possible because free glutamate occurs naturally in many unfermented foods, including tomatoes, mushrooms, parmesan (though aged cheeses are high-histamine), and sea vegetables. For trifecta patients, coconut aminos, sesame, and well-salted broth provide the most accessible low-histamine umami sources.

Salted Cucumber and Dill Chilled Soup

Peel and seed 3 large cucumbers. Roughly chop and place in a blender with 1 cup of coconut yogurt (unsweetened, checking ingredient list for live cultures, which some MCAS patients tolerate while others do not; use coconut cream as alternative), 2 tablespoons of fresh dill (chopped), 1 small garlic clove, 1 teaspoon of fine sea salt, 1 tablespoon of olive oil, and 2 tablespoons of cold water. Blend until smooth. Adjust salt. Chill for at least one hour before serving. Garnish with a drizzle of olive oil, additional dill, and a pinch of flaky salt.

Serves three. Approximate per serving: 110 calories, 2 g protein, 8 g fat, 8 g carbohydrate, 800 mg sodium.

This cold soup is designed for hot weather, when MCAS patients face increased mast cell activation from heat (Theoharides et al., 2019) and POTS patients face worsened orthostatic intolerance from heat-induced vasodilation (Vernino et al., 2021). The cooling effect of chilled cucumber soup, combined with its sodium and fluid content, addresses both triggers simultaneously.

16.7 Therapeutic Broths

Electrolyte-Boosting Broth with Turmeric and Ginger

Combine 2 cups of vegetable mineral broth or short-cook bone broth in a small saucepan. Add 1/2 teaspoon of ground turmeric, 1/4 teaspoon of ground ginger (or 1/2 inch of fresh ginger, grated), 1/2 teaspoon of fine sea salt, and a generous pinch of black pepper. Heat gently until warm (not boiling, to preserve volatile compounds in the spices). Stir and sip slowly.

Serves one. Approximate: 25 calories, 1 g protein, 0 g fat, 4 g carbohydrate, 1,200 mg sodium.

This broth functions as a therapeutic beverage rather than a meal. Its purpose is concentrated sodium and fluid delivery with anti-inflammatory compounds. Curcumin from turmeric has demonstrated anti-inflammatory effects through inhibition of NF-kB and COX-2 pathways in multiple trials (Daily et al., 2016). Gingerols from ginger provide prokinetic effects that can ease the nausea associated with gastroparesis (Giacosa et al., 2015). Black pepper's piperine compound increases curcumin bioavailability by approximately 2,000% (Shoba et al., 1998). The combination creates a functional recovery drink that trifecta patients can sip throughout the day, particularly during flare recovery.

16.8 Congee and Grain Porridges

Congee (also called jook, rice porridge, or rice gruel) is a staple comfort food across East and Southeast Asian cuisines. It consists of rice cooked in a large volume of water or broth until the grains break down completely, creating a thick, smooth porridge. For trifecta patients, congee offers several unique advantages: its soft texture requires almost no mechanical digestion (making it ideal for severe gastroparesis days; Thwaites et al., 2022), it absorbs liquid during cooking (embedding hydration into the food itself), and its bland base accepts a wide variety of toppings that can customize it for different trifecta priorities.

Recipe: Basic Trifecta Congee

Combine 1 cup of white rice (rinsed) with 8 cups of homemade broth (either variety from sections 16.2 or 16.3) and 1 teaspoon of fine sea salt in a large pot. Bring to a boil, then reduce heat to the lowest setting that maintains a gentle simmer. Cook for 60 to 90 minutes, stirring every 15 to 20 minutes to prevent sticking, until the rice has broken down completely and the consistency is thick, smooth, and porridge-like. Add more broth or water if the congee becomes too thick before the rice has fully dissolved. Adjust salt before serving.

Serves four. Approximate per serving (base only): 190 calories, 6 g protein, 1 g fat, 40 g carbohydrate, 600 mg sodium.

Topping Variations allow customization for different days and needs:

The **High-Sodium Recovery** version adds shredded fresh-cooked chicken, a drizzle of sesame oil, sliced green onion tops, and an extra 1/2 teaspoon of salt per serving (totaling approximately 1,400 mg sodium). This version suits post-flare recovery days when sodium needs are elevated.

The **Gentle Gastroparesis** version adds a soft-poached egg (stirred into the hot congee until the whites set in ribbons), a drizzle of ghee, and fresh grated ginger. The egg adds protein without requiring chewing. The ghee provides fat for satiety. The ginger offers prokinetic benefit. This is the lowest-texture option, appropriate for the most symptomatic days.

The **Anti-Inflammatory** version adds diced roasted sweet potato, a generous pinch of ground turmeric, fresh basil leaves, and olive oil. This version incorporates the anti-inflammatory ingredients from Chapter 9.0 into a soothing, warm format.

Batch preparation: Cook a large pot of base congee, portion into individual containers, and freeze within 30 minutes. Congee reheats well in the microwave (add a splash of water or broth before microwaving, as it thickens further in the refrigerator and freezer). Frozen congee portions combined with pre-prepared toppings create a complete meal in under five minutes.

16.9 Honora's Soup System

Background

Honora, a 47-year-old school counselor with hEDS, POTS, and MCAS, had identified soups and broths as her best-tolerated food category. Liquids and puréed foods reliably bypassed the early satiety and nausea from her gastroparesis, and the warm temperature seemed to reduce GI discomfort compared to cold or room-temperature foods. She wanted to build a soup-centered eating system that could serve as her primary nutrition source on moderate to difficult days.

Presentation

Honora's food diary showed that on days she ate soups and broths, her total caloric intake averaged 1,600 calories with 7,500 mg of sodium, both within trifecta targets. On days she attempted solid meals, caloric intake dropped to 1,100 calories because early satiety prevented her from finishing meals, and sodium fell to 4,500 mg because she could not consume enough solid food volume to reach target. Her POTS symptoms were measurably better on soup-dominant days (average standing heart rate increase of 22 bpm versus 32 bpm on solid-food days), consistent with the higher sodium and fluid intake (Sheldon et al., 2015).

Analysis

Honora's experience illustrates that the Trifecta Plate framework (section 10.1) does not require traditional plate-based meals. The framework specifies the four components (protein, carbohydrate, vegetable/fruit, healthy fat) and the therapeutic targets (sodium, fluid, anti-inflammatory ingredients) but not the physical form. A bowl of chicken and rice soup with olive oil drizzled on top contains all four plate components in liquid form. A cup of sweet potato and coconut soup provides carbohydrate, fat, and vegetable in a single sip. The nutritional content is equivalent; the delivery method simply bypasses the gastroparesis barrier that limits solid food intake (Thwaites et al., 2022).

Intervention

Honora's dietitian helped her build a soup rotation using recipes from this chapter, organized by preparation complexity and nutritional density. Her weekly batch prep (aligned with section 13.9) included one large pot of short-cook bone broth portioned into 12 cups, one batch of sweet potato and coconut soup (four servings), one batch of chicken and rice soup (four servings), and one batch of base congee (four servings). This yielded approximately 24 individual soup or broth portions, enough for four to five servings daily across five days. A second shorter prep session mid-week replenished as needed.

Outcome

Over six weeks of soup-centered eating, Honora's average daily caloric intake stabilized at 1,550 calories with sodium consistently above 7,000 mg. Her weight stabilized after a three-month period of slow decline. POTS symptoms improved modestly (average standing heart rate increase decreased from 28 to 23 bpm). She described the approach as "eating the way my body actually works instead of fighting it." Her dietitian confirmed that nutritional adequacy (protein, micronutrients, fiber) was maintained through the variety of soups and the supplementation protocol from section 5.3.

Teaching Points

- The Trifecta Plate framework is defined by its nutritional components (protein, carbohydrate, vegetable, fat) and therapeutic targets (sodium, fluid, anti-inflammatory ingredients), not by the physical form of the meal, and soup-based eating can meet all framework requirements while accommodating gastroparesis
- Soup-centered eating patterns often produce higher sodium and fluid intake than solid-food patterns because the liquid base embeds hydration into every eating occasion, reducing the reliance on separate beverage consumption
- Batch preparation of multiple soup varieties provides rotation and nutritional diversity while concentrating all cooking labor into one to two sessions per week

16.10 Hearty Root Vegetable Stew

Recipe

Peel and dice into 1-inch cubes: 2 medium carrots, 1 large sweet potato, 1 medium parsnip, and 1 medium turnip. Heat 2 tablespoons of olive oil in a large pot over medium heat. Add the root vegetables and 1 teaspoon of fine sea salt. Sauté 5 minutes, stirring occasionally. Add 5 cups of homemade broth, 1/2 teaspoon of dried thyme, 1/2 teaspoon of dried rosemary (crushed), 2 minced garlic cloves, and 1 bay leaf. Bring to a boil, reduce heat, and simmer 25 to 30 minutes until all vegetables are tender. Remove bay leaf. For a thicker stew, mash approximately 1/3 of the vegetables against the side of the pot with a fork before stirring. Adjust salt. Optionally add shredded chicken for protein. Serves four.

Approximate per serving (without chicken): 200 calories, 3 g protein, 7 g fat, 32 g carbohydrate, 1,000 mg sodium. With 1/2 cup shredded chicken: 290 calories, 22 g protein.

Root vegetables are among the most reliably tolerated foods for MCAS patients because they grow underground (limiting exposure to environmental allergens and molds), have thick protective skins, and contain minimal histidine for bacterial conversion (Sánchez-Pérez et al., 2018). The variety of root vegetables in this stew provides a range of micronutrients: beta-carotene from carrots and sweet potato, vitamin C from turnips, and folate from parsnips. The partial mashing technique creates a naturally thick texture without adding flour or cream, both of which can be trigger ingredients for some trifecta patients.

16.11 Soup as Medicine Review

The recipes in this chapter serve two simultaneous purposes. They are food, providing calories, macronutrients, and micronutrients. And they are therapy, delivering sodium, fluid, anti-inflammatory compounds, and gastroparesis-appropriate textures in forms that accommodate the worst days of trifecta living.

The distinction between bone broth and vegetable mineral broth gives patients options for different tolerance levels. The short-cook method and immediate cooling protocol make bone broth accessible to MCAS patients who would react to traditional long-simmered versions. Complete meal soups (chicken and rice, sweet potato and coconut, root vegetable stew) function as full Trifecta Plate servings. Congee provides a customizable base that adapts to daily symptom variability through topping selection. Therapeutic broths (electrolyte turmeric broth) function as recovery drinks during and after flares.

Across both this chapter and Chapter 15.0, the recipes share common principles: sodium is built into the recipe rather than added as an afterthought, histamine is managed through ingredient selection and freshness protocols, textures accommodate gastroparesis, and every preparation is designed for batch cooking and freezer storage. These are not ordinary recipes adapted for chronic illness. They are engineered from the ground up around the physiological realities of POTS, EDS, and MCAS, using the evidence-based framework built across Chapters 6.0 through 14.0.

Chapter 17.0 continues the recipe section with lunch, dinner, and main dishes that apply these same trifecta principles to the larger meals of the day

.

Chapter 17.0: Main Meals and Entrées

Nephele had cooked chicken breast and rice for dinner every night for 11 weeks. Not because she loved it. Because it was the only dinner she trusted. Her MCAS had flared so unpredictably over the past year that she had retreated to the smallest possible set of foods, and by the time she reached her dietitian's office, her evening meal had collapsed to a single recipe. She ate it with the grim determination of someone taking medicine. The rice was undersalted because she feared overdoing sodium (despite her POTS specialist recommending 8,000 mg daily). The chicken was dry because she overcooked it to compensate for her anxiety about freshness and histamine. There were no vegetables because she had eliminated most of them after inconclusive reactions she never properly tracked. And there was no pleasure, which mattered more than she realized, because food aversion and eating monotony are independent predictors of further dietary restriction and malnutrition in chronic illness populations (Zickgraf & Ellis, 2018).

This chapter provides 15 protein-forward entrée recipes designed to expand the trifecta dinner table without expanding risk:

- Poultry, fish, lamb, beef, and pork options covering the full protein spectrum
- Freshness protocols specific to each protein type
- Batch-friendly preparations for cook-once-eat-three-times efficiency
- One-pan and one-pot recipes that minimize standing time and cleanup
- Sodium loading built into every recipe at therapeutic levels

17.1 Protein Selection Principles

Protein is the macronutrient that demands the most careful handling in trifecta cooking. Not because protein itself is problematic, but because protein-rich foods are the primary vehicles for histamine accumulation through bacterial decarboxylation of the amino acid histidine (Comas-Basté et al., 2020). The histamine content of a chicken thigh purchased fresh from the butcher, cooked within hours, and eaten immediately is fundamentally different from the histamine content of the same chicken thigh purchased from the back of a grocery store case, stored in the refrigerator for three days, cooked slowly, and eaten as leftovers the following evening. The protein itself hasn't changed. The bacterial activity on and within it has.

The **freshness hierarchy** for trifecta protein selection, established in sections 6.2 and 13.2, follows a consistent pattern. The safest option is flash-frozen protein purchased commercially and thawed in the refrigerator immediately before cooking. Commercial flash-freezing occurs within hours of slaughter or catch at temperatures of negative 20 to negative 40°F, halting bacterial histamine production at its lowest point (Lehane & Olley, 2000). The second-safest option is fresh protein purchased from a butcher or meat counter on the day of cooking and prepared within hours. The least safe option (and the one most commonly eaten by the general population) is fresh protein that has spent multiple days in the home refrigerator before cooking.

For **fish**, the freshness concern is amplified. Fish muscle contains higher concentrations of free histidine than poultry or red meat, and certain fish species (tuna, mackerel, sardines, anchovies) are particularly susceptible to rapid histamine formation through bacterial action (Taylor, 1986). The recipes in this chapter that include fish (salmon, cod) specify flash-frozen fillets as the preferred starting material, consistent with the recommendation from Reese et al. (2017) that frozen fish is paradoxically fresher, from a histamine perspective, than fish sold as "fresh" at most retail counters.

For **ground meats**, the surface-area-to-volume ratio creates additional risk. Grinding meat exposes far more surface area to bacterial contact than whole cuts, accelerating histamine accumulation (Sánchez-Pérez et al., 2018). Ground turkey, ground beef, and ground lamb should be purchased the day of cooking or thawed from frozen immediately before use. Cooking should occur within two hours of thawing.

17.2 Poultry Recipes

Herb-Crusted Chicken Thighs with Roasted Root Vegetables

Preheat oven to 425°F. Pat dry 6 bone-in, skin-on chicken thighs with paper towels (removing surface moisture improves browning and crispness; McGee, 2004). Combine 1 tablespoon of dried thyme, 1 tablespoon of dried rosemary (crushed), 1 teaspoon of garlic powder, 1.5 teaspoons of fine sea salt, 1/2 teaspoon of ground black pepper, and 2 tablespoons of olive oil in a small bowl. Rub this mixture over all surfaces of the chicken thighs. On a sheet pan, toss 2 cups of diced sweet potato, 2 cups of diced carrots, and 1 cup of diced parsnips with 2 tablespoons of olive oil and 1/2 teaspoon of salt. Arrange vegetables in a single layer and place chicken thighs on top, skin side up. Roast 35 to 40 minutes until chicken skin is golden and internal temperature reaches 165°F. Serves four (allow two thighs for larger appetites). Approximate per serving (1.5 thighs plus vegetables): 480 calories, 34 g protein, 26 g fat, 28 g carbohydrate, 1,400 mg sodium.

This is a single-pan meal that delivers all four Trifecta Plate components (section 10.1). The chicken fat renders during roasting and bastes the vegetables below, adding flavor without additional cooking fat. Bone-in thighs are preferable to boneless breasts for trifecta cooking because they retain moisture during roasting (reducing the need for precise timing) and provide slightly higher fat content for sustained energy.

Simple Roast Chicken with Pan Drippings Gravy

Preheat oven to 425°F. Pat dry a whole chicken (3.5 to 4 pounds, purchased fresh or thawed from frozen within 24 hours). Season the cavity with 1/2 teaspoon of salt and a few fresh thyme sprigs. Rub the exterior with 2 tablespoons of softened ghee, 1.5 teaspoons of fine sea salt, 1/2 teaspoon of garlic powder, and 1/2 teaspoon of dried sage. Place breast-side up on a rack set inside a roasting pan. Roast 60 to 75 minutes until the thickest part of the thigh reaches 165°F. Rest 10 minutes before carving.

For gravy: pour pan drippings through a strainer into a small saucepan. Skim visible fat if desired (or leave it for caloric density). Whisk in 1 tablespoon of rice flour or tapioca starch mixed with 2 tablespoons of cold water. Heat over medium, whisking constantly, until thickened (2 to 3 minutes). Add 1/2 cup of homemade broth (section 16.2 or 16.3), 1/4 teaspoon of salt, and a pinch of black pepper. Simmer 2 minutes. This gravy is dairy-free, gluten-free, and uses the collagen-rich pan drippings as its base.

Serves four to six. Approximate per serving (5 ounces meat plus gravy): 420 calories, 38 g protein, 28 g fat, 2 g carbohydrate, 1,100 mg sodium.

Pro Tip: Batch Advantage. A roast chicken yields shredded meat for three to four additional meals (chicken and rice soup from section 16.4, rice bowls from section 15.3, lettuce wraps from this chapter). Shred all leftover meat immediately after carving, portion into individual containers, and freeze within 30 minutes. The carcass can be used for short-cook bone broth (section 16.2) within 24 hours if not frozen immediately.

Slow-Cooker Pulled Chicken with Safe Seasonings

Place 2 pounds of boneless, skinless chicken thighs in a slow cooker. Add 1 cup of homemade broth, 1 tablespoon of fine sea salt, 1 teaspoon of garlic powder, 1 teaspoon of onion powder, 1/2 teaspoon of ground turmeric, 1/2 teaspoon of dried oregano, 1/2 teaspoon of ground cumin, and 1/4 teaspoon of black pepper. Cook on low for 4 to 5 hours (do not exceed 6 hours; extended cooking in the warm, moist environment of a slow cooker can promote histamine accumulation; Comas-Basté et al., 2020). Remove chicken and shred with two forks. Return shredded chicken to the cooking liquid briefly to absorb flavor and sodium. Portion immediately into individual containers and freeze any portions not being consumed within 24 hours.

Makes approximately 6 servings. Approximate per serving: 240 calories, 32 g protein, 10 g fat, 2 g carbohydrate, 1,200 mg sodium.

One-Pot Chicken and Rice with Turmeric

Heat 2 tablespoons of olive oil in a Dutch oven or large pot over medium-high heat. Season 4 boneless, skinless chicken thighs with 1 teaspoon of salt and brown on both sides (3 minutes per side). Remove chicken and set aside. In the same pot, add 1 diced medium carrot, 1 cup of diced zucchini, and 2 minced garlic cloves. Sauté 3 minutes. Add 1.5 cups of white rice (rinsed), 3 cups of homemade broth, 1 teaspoon of ground turmeric, 1 teaspoon of fine sea salt, 1/2 teaspoon of ground ginger, and 1/4 teaspoon of black pepper. Nestle the chicken thighs into the rice. Bring to a boil, reduce heat to low, cover, and cook 18 to 20 minutes until rice is tender and chicken is cooked through. Fluff rice with a fork and serve. Garnish with fresh parsley.

Serves four. Approximate per serving: 520 calories, 32 g protein, 14 g fat, 60 g carbohydrate, 1,300 mg sodium.

This recipe consolidates protein, carbohydrate, vegetable, and fat into a single pot, minimizing dishes and standing time. The turmeric provides curcumin with anti-inflammatory activity (Daily et al., 2016), while the black pepper enhances curcumin bioavailability by approximately 2,000% through piperine's inhibition of hepatic and intestinal glucuronidation (Shoba et al., 1998).

Sheet Pan Chicken with Sweet Potato and Broccoli

Preheat oven to 400°F. Toss 2 cups of cubed sweet potato with 1 tablespoon of olive oil and 1/2 teaspoon of salt. Spread on a sheet pan and roast 15 minutes. Meanwhile, season 4 boneless, skinless chicken thighs with 1 teaspoon of salt, 1/2 teaspoon of garlic powder, 1/2 teaspoon of dried thyme, and 1 tablespoon of olive oil. After the initial 15 minutes, push sweet potatoes to one side, add chicken thighs and 2 cups of broccoli florets tossed with 1 tablespoon of olive oil and 1/4 teaspoon of salt. Roast an additional 20 to 25 minutes until chicken reaches 165°F and broccoli edges are lightly charred.

Serves four. Approximate per serving: 380 calories, 28 g protein, 14 g fat, 34 g carbohydrate, 1,100 mg sodium.

Quinoa-Crusted Chicken Tenders

Preheat oven to 400°F. Cut 1.5 pounds of chicken breast into strips approximately 1 inch wide. Set up a breading station: Bowl 1 contains 1/3 cup of rice flour mixed with 1/2 teaspoon of salt. Bowl 2 contains 2 beaten eggs. Bowl 3 contains 1 cup of cooked quinoa (cooled and slightly dried) mixed with 1/2 teaspoon of garlic powder, 1/2 teaspoon of dried oregano, and 1/2 teaspoon of salt. Dredge each strip in flour, then egg, then press into the quinoa mixture. Place on a parchment-lined baking sheet. Drizzle with olive oil. Bake 18 to 22 minutes, flipping halfway, until golden and cooked through.

Serves four. Approximate per serving: 340 calories, 36 g protein, 10 g fat, 24 g carbohydrate, 900 mg sodium.

Quinoa provides a gluten-free coating with a complete amino acid profile (Vega-Gálvez et al., 2010). The baked preparation avoids the inflammatory oils used in deep frying, consistent with the anti-inflammatory strategy from Chapter 9.0.

17.3 Marius and the Rotation Plan

Background

Marius, a 52-year-old civil engineer with POTS, hEDS, and MCAS diagnosed 18 months earlier, had successfully built a small library of safe recipes over several months of careful elimination and reintroduction (section 6.9). His problem was not food intolerance. It was meal fatigue. He rotated between four dinners (chicken and rice, ground turkey with sweet potato, plain salmon with broccoli, and a beef and vegetable stir-fry) and had grown so bored that he found himself ordering takeout two to three times per week. The takeout invariably contained hidden triggers (soy sauce, vinegar-based sauces, pre-marinated proteins, unknown cooking oils) that caused MCAS flares within hours.

Presentation

Marius's food diary showed a clear pattern: weekday dinners were trifecta-compliant and symptom-free, but weekend dinners frequently deviated to takeout, followed by MCAS flares (flushing, GI cramping, tachycardia) lasting 8 to 16 hours. The flares disrupted sleep, which worsened his Monday POTS symptoms. He described the cycle as "I know what happens, but I can't eat the same four things forever." His total food repertoire had stagnated at 14 safe foods despite his dietitian confirming that he had only formally tested and failed three items during reintroduction.

Analysis

Marius's situation illustrates the distinction between **dietary restriction driven by intolerance** and **dietary stagnation driven by inertia**. His actual trigger list was small (aged cheese, fermented soy, tomatoes). Most foods remained untested rather than confirmed unsafe. The boredom he experienced was not a failure of willpower but a predictable consequence of insufficient recipe variety operating on a sufficient ingredient list (Zickgraf & Ellis, 2018). Research on dietary monotony in chronic illness populations shows that perceived food choice limitation predicts poorer dietary adherence and increased consumption of non-compliant foods (Jaeger et al., 2021). The solution is recipe expansion, not ingredient expansion. He already had the ingredients. He needed new preparations.

Intervention

His dietitian introduced a 10-day dinner rotation using recipes from this chapter, all built from Marius's 14 confirmed safe ingredients. The rotation included herb-crusted chicken thighs (section 17.2), pan-seared salmon (section 17.4), turkey meatballs (section 17.5), one-pot chicken and rice (section 17.2), beef stir-fry (section 17.4), sheet pan chicken (section 17.2), lamb chops (section 17.4), ground turkey lettuce wraps (section 17.5), baked cod (section 17.4), and pork tenderloin (section 17.4). Each recipe used only his confirmed safe foods but in different flavor combinations, textures, and cooking methods. Batch cooking on Sundays pre-prepared components for four of the 10 meals.

Outcome

Over six weeks, Marius's takeout frequency dropped from two to three times per week to once every two weeks (on occasions when he intentionally chose restaurants where he could communicate specific preparation requirements). His MCAS flare frequency decreased proportionally. He described the 10-day rotation as "I'm eating the same foods but it doesn't feel like it." His weight stabilized and his overall caloric intake improved because he was eating full portions of meals he found satisfying rather than half-portions of meals he found tedious.

Teaching Points

- Dietary stagnation in trifecta patients often results from insufficient recipe variety rather than insufficient ingredient variety, and expanding preparations using confirmed safe foods addresses boredom without introducing risk
- Meal fatigue predicts dietary non-adherence (ordering takeout with hidden triggers), creating a cycle where the monotony intended to prevent flares actually causes them indirectly

- A structured rotation plan (7 to 14 day cycle) using batch-prepared components creates the perception of variety while maintaining trifecta compliance and consolidating preparation labor

17.4 Seafood and Red Meat

Simple Pan-Seared Salmon

Thaw flash-frozen salmon fillets (6 ounces each) in the refrigerator overnight. Pat completely dry with paper towels. Season both sides with 1/2 teaspoon of fine sea salt per fillet, 1/4 teaspoon of garlic powder, and a pinch of ground black pepper. Heat 1 tablespoon of ghee in a skillet over medium-high heat until the ghee shimmers. Place fillets skin-side up and cook 3 to 4 minutes without moving until a golden crust forms. Flip and cook skin-side down for 3 minutes. The center should remain slightly translucent for medium doneness. Serve immediately.

Serves two. Approximate per serving: 380 calories, 34 g protein, 26 g fat, 0 g carbohydrate, 600 mg sodium.

Freshness note for MCAS: Flash-frozen salmon is strongly preferred over fish-counter "fresh" salmon for MCAS patients. Wild-caught salmon sold as fresh at retail has typically been out of the water for 5 to 14 days by the time it reaches the consumer (Lehane & Olley, 2000). During this time, bacterial conversion of histidine to histamine proceeds continuously, even under proper refrigeration. Flash-frozen salmon, by contrast, was frozen within hours of harvest, effectively pausing histamine accumulation at its starting point. The quality of the final product after thawing is typically superior to "fresh" fish from a histamine perspective (Reese et al., 2017).

Salmon provides omega-3 fatty acids (EPA and DHA) with documented anti-inflammatory effects (Calder, 2015). A single 6-ounce serving provides approximately 2,000 to 3,000 mg of combined EPA and DHA, exceeding the daily amount shown to reduce inflammatory markers in clinical trials (Calder, 2015).

Baked Cod with Herb Butter and Steamed Asparagus

Preheat oven to 400°F. Place 4 cod fillets (5 to 6 ounces each, thawed from frozen) on a parchment-lined baking sheet. Combine 3 tablespoons of softened ghee with 1 tablespoon of finely chopped fresh dill, 1 tablespoon of finely chopped fresh parsley, 1 teaspoon of fine sea salt, and 1/4 teaspoon of garlic powder. Spread the herb butter evenly over the top of each fillet. Bake 12 to 15 minutes until the fish flakes easily with a fork. Meanwhile, steam 1 pound of trimmed asparagus for 4 to

5 minutes until tender-crisp. Toss with 1 tablespoon of olive oil and 1/4 teaspoon of salt.

Serves four. Approximate per serving: 280 calories, 30 g protein, 16 g fat, 4 g carbohydrate, 900 mg sodium.

Cod is a lean white fish with lower histidine content than oily fish like tuna or mackerel, making it generally better tolerated by MCAS patients (Taylor, 1986). The herb butter adds flavor and fat (for satiety and fat-soluble vitamin absorption) without dairy, since ghee has had its milk solids removed during clarification.

Lamb Chops with Mint and Garlic

Pat dry 8 lamb loin chops (approximately 1.5 pounds total). Season with 1.5 teaspoons of fine sea salt, 1/2 teaspoon of garlic powder, and 1/4 teaspoon of black pepper. Heat 2 tablespoons of olive oil in a cast-iron skillet over high heat. Sear chops 3 minutes per side for medium-rare (internal temperature 130 to 135°F). During the final minute of cooking, add 2 tablespoons of finely chopped fresh mint and 2 minced garlic cloves to the pan. Toss briefly in the hot oil, then spoon the garlic-mint mixture over the chops. Rest 5 minutes before serving.

Serves four (two chops each). Approximate per serving: 340 calories, 28 g protein, 24 g fat, 1 g carbohydrate, 950 mg sodium.

Lamb is often well-tolerated by MCAS patients who react to poultry or beef, though individual variation applies. Fresh mint provides rosmarinic acid with anti-inflammatory activity (Bauer et al., 2012). Lamb is also one of the richest dietary sources of carnitine, which plays a role in mitochondrial energy production (Flanagan et al., 2010).

Beef Stir-Fry with Coconut Aminos

Slice 1 pound of fresh beef sirloin (purchased same day or thawed from frozen) against the grain into thin strips. Season with 1/2 teaspoon of salt. Heat 2 tablespoons of coconut oil in a wok or large skillet over high heat. Cook beef in a single layer (work in batches to avoid crowding) for 2 minutes per side until browned. Remove beef. In the same pan, add 1 tablespoon of coconut oil, 2 cups of broccoli florets, 1 sliced bell pepper (if tolerated), 1 cup of sliced zucchini, and 2 minced garlic cloves. Stir-fry 3 to 4 minutes. Return beef to the pan. Add 3 tablespoons of coconut aminos, 1 teaspoon of toasted sesame oil, 1/2 teaspoon of ground ginger, and 1/4 teaspoon of salt. Toss to combine and cook 1 minute. Serve over rice.

Serves four. Approximate per serving (with 3/4 cup rice): 480 calories, 30 g protein, 18 g fat, 48 g carbohydrate, 1,100 mg sodium.

This stir-fry replaces soy sauce (fermented, high-histamine) with **coconut aminos**, a non-fermented sauce made from coconut sap that provides umami flavor without the histamine load of traditional soy sauce (Beauchamp, 2009). The beef is not marinated because marinades that include acidic components (vinegar, citrus) can increase histamine release, and pre-marinating extends the time raw protein spends at refrigerator temperatures before cooking (Sánchez-Pérez et al., 2018). Instead, seasoning occurs immediately before high-heat cooking.

Pork Tenderloin with Apple and Sage

Preheat oven to 400°F. Season a 1.5-pound pork tenderloin with 1.5 teaspoons of fine sea salt, 1/2 teaspoon of ground sage, 1/2 teaspoon of garlic powder, and 1/4 teaspoon of black pepper. Heat 2 tablespoons of olive oil in an oven-safe skillet over medium-high heat. Sear the tenderloin on all sides (approximately 6 minutes total). Add 2 peeled and sliced apples (Fuji or Gala for sweetness), 1 tablespoon of fresh sage leaves, and 1/4 cup of homemade broth to the pan. Transfer to the oven and roast 15 to 20 minutes until the pork reaches an internal temperature of 145°F. Rest 5 minutes before slicing. Spoon the cooked apples and pan juices over the sliced pork.

Serves four. Approximate per serving: 310 calories, 34 g protein, 12 g fat, 18 g carbohydrate, 1,000 mg sodium.

Pork tenderloin is among the leanest cuts of red meat, and its mild flavor accepts the apple and sage combination without competing. Apples are low on the histamine scale (Maintz & Novak, 2007) and provide pectin, a soluble fiber that supports gut microbiome diversity (Koutsos et al., 2015).

17.5 Ground Meat Preparations

Turkey Meatballs in Dairy-Free Cream Sauce

Preheat oven to 400°F. Combine 1.5 pounds of ground turkey, 1/3 cup of rice flour, 1 egg, 1 teaspoon of fine sea salt, 1/2 teaspoon of dried oregano, 1/2 teaspoon of dried basil, 1/4 teaspoon of garlic powder, and 1 tablespoon of olive oil. Mix gently (overworking toughens meatballs). Form into approximately 20 meatballs. Place on a parchment-lined baking sheet and bake 18 to 20 minutes until internal temperature reaches 165°F.

For dairy-free cream sauce: heat 1 tablespoon of ghee in a saucepan over medium heat. Whisk in 1 tablespoon of rice flour and cook 1 minute. Slowly whisk in 1 cup of full-fat coconut milk and 1/2 cup of homemade broth. Add 1/2 teaspoon of salt, 1/4 teaspoon of ground nutmeg, and a pinch of black pepper. Simmer, whisking frequently, until thickened (3 to 4 minutes). Add meatballs to the sauce and serve over rice or quinoa.

Serves four. Approximate per serving (5 meatballs with sauce): 440 calories, 34 g protein, 28 g fat, 16 g carbohydrate, 1,200 mg sodium.

The cream sauce uses coconut milk instead of dairy cream. Coconut milk's medium-chain triglycerides (MCTs) are absorbed more readily than the long-chain fatty acids in dairy cream, which benefits EDS patients with gastrointestinal fat malabsorption (Thwaites et al., 2022).

Ground Turkey Lettuce Wraps

Brown 1 pound of ground turkey in a skillet over medium-high heat with 1 tablespoon of coconut oil, breaking into small pieces. Add 2 minced garlic cloves, 1 tablespoon of grated fresh ginger, 1 diced water chestnut (optional, for crunch), and 1 diced carrot. Cook 3 to 4 minutes. Add 2 tablespoons of coconut aminos, 1 teaspoon of toasted sesame oil, 1/2 teaspoon of fine sea salt, and a pinch of ground white pepper. Stir to combine. Serve in butter lettuce cups (approximately 3 to 4 per serving) topped with sliced green onion tops, chopped fresh cilantro (if tolerated), and toasted sesame seeds.

Serves three. Approximate per serving: 320 calories, 28 g protein, 18 g fat, 12 g carbohydrate, 950 mg sodium.

Stuffed Bell Peppers with Ground Turkey and Rice

Preheat oven to 375°F. Cut the tops off 4 large bell peppers and remove seeds. In a skillet, brown 1 pound of ground turkey with 1 teaspoon of salt, 1/2 teaspoon of garlic powder, and 1/2 teaspoon of dried oregano. Add 2 cups of cooked rice, 1 diced medium zucchini, and 1/2 cup of homemade broth. Mix well. Stuff the peppers with the mixture. Place upright in a baking dish. Add 1/2 cup of broth to the bottom of the dish. Cover with foil and bake 35 to 40 minutes until peppers are tender. Remove foil and bake 5 additional minutes.

Serves four. Approximate per serving: 380 calories, 28 g protein, 12 g fat, 40 g carbohydrate, 1,000 mg sodium.

17.6 Chicken and Vegetable Skewers

Chicken Skewers with Parsley Chimichurri

Cut 1.5 pounds of boneless, skinless chicken thighs into 1.5-inch pieces. Thread onto metal or soaked wooden skewers, alternating with chunks of zucchini and bell pepper (if tolerated). Season with 1 teaspoon of salt, 1/2 teaspoon of garlic powder, 1/2 teaspoon of dried oregano, and 2 tablespoons of olive oil. Grill or broil 10 to 12 minutes, turning once, until chicken reaches 165°F.

For chimichurri: finely chop 1 cup of fresh flat-leaf parsley, 2 garlic cloves, and 2 tablespoons of fresh oregano leaves. Combine with 1/3 cup of olive oil, 2 tablespoons of red wine vinegar (small amount, test individual tolerance), 1/2 teaspoon of fine sea salt, 1/4 teaspoon of crushed red pepper flakes (omit if sensitive), and 1/4 teaspoon of black pepper. Mix well. If vinegar is not tolerated, substitute 1 tablespoon of fresh lemon juice or omit the acid entirely and increase the salt slightly. Spoon chimichurri generously over grilled skewers.

Serves four. Approximate per serving: 420 calories, 34 g protein, 28 g fat, 6 g carbohydrate, 1,100 mg sodium.

Traditional chimichurri relies on citrus or vinegar for brightness. This parsley-forward version shifts the flavor emphasis to the herbal elements. Parsley contains apigenin, a flavonoid with documented mast cell stabilizing properties in preclinical studies (Lee et al., 2007), making it a particularly appropriate herb for MCAS patients (though clinical translation of these findings remains preliminary).

17.7 Practical Cooking Guidance

Across these 15 recipes, several practical principles recur. Understanding them allows readers to adapt any recipe to trifecta requirements, not just the recipes in this book.

Internal temperatures matter more than cooking times. A chicken thigh cooked to 165°F is safe regardless of how long it took to reach that temperature. An instant-read thermometer eliminates guesswork and prevents both the food safety risk of undercooking and the texture degradation of overcooking. Invest in a digital instant-read thermometer. It costs under $15 and removes one of the most common sources of cooking anxiety for patients managing food safety concerns alongside chronic illness (U.S. Department of Agriculture, 2023).

Salt at therapeutic levels tastes different than salt at conventional levels. The recipes in this chapter contain 900 to 1,400 mg of sodium per serving, which is two to three times the sodium in a typical home-cooked meal. For the general population, this would be excessive. For a POTS patient targeting 6,000 to 10,000 mg daily across four to five eating occasions, it is therapeutic (Vernino et al., 2021). The salt is not a seasoning afterthought. It is a medical intervention distributed across the day's meals.

Immediate portioning and freezing applies to all leftovers. No recipe in this chapter is designed to sit in the refrigerator for multiple days as leftovers. Any portion not consumed at the meal should be cooled, portioned, and frozen within 30 minutes. This protocol, established in sections 6.2 and 13.2, prevents the histamine accumulation that makes next-day leftovers problematic for MCAS patients (Comas-Basté et al., 2020). Reheating from frozen is always preferable to reheating from refrigerator storage that exceeds 24 hours.

17.8 Building Trifecta Dinners

The Trifecta Plate framework from section 10.1 provides the template for every dinner: protein (the recipes in this chapter), complex carbohydrate (rice, sweet potato, quinoa), vegetable (roasted, steamed, or sautéed from the options in Chapter 18.0), and healthy fat (olive oil, ghee, coconut oil, or the fats inherent in the protein). Each recipe in this chapter explicitly identifies its macronutrient composition so that readers can assess which Trifecta Plate quadrants are covered and which require a side dish to complete.

Some recipes are self-contained plates (one-pot chicken and rice, sheet pan chicken, stuffed peppers) that include all four components. Others (pan-seared salmon, lamb chops, turkey meatballs) provide protein and fat but require a carbohydrate and vegetable side to complete the plate. Chapter 18.0 provides the side dishes that fill those gaps, and Chapter 19.0 provides snacks and portable foods that bridge the spaces between meals.

Chapter 18.0: Sides, Salads and Vegetables

The entrées from Chapter 17.0 fill one quadrant of the Trifecta Plate (section 10.1). But a plate with only protein is incomplete in the same way that a foundation without walls is incomplete. The carbohydrate, vegetable, and fat quadrants need filling, and for trifecta patients, the way those quadrants get filled matters as much as the protein choice. A side of steamed broccoli becomes a sodium delivery vehicle when tossed with herb butter and flaky salt. A sweet potato becomes a potassium-sodium balancing act (section 7.4) when baked and salted at therapeutic levels. A simple salad becomes an anti-inflammatory intervention when dressed with olive oil rich in oleocanthal (Beauchamp et al., 2005) and fresh herbs containing polyphenolic compounds. Side dishes are not afterthoughts. They are the connective tissue of trifecta meals, and connective tissue, as every EDS patient knows, is where the structural integrity lives.

This chapter provides 10 side dish recipes organized by category:

- Roasted and cooked vegetables with trifecta-specific seasoning
- Fresh salads using low-histamine ingredients
- Starch sides that contribute to carbohydrate and sodium targets
- Adaptable preparations that pair with any protein from Chapter 17.0
- Low-effort options for crash days alongside higher-effort options for good days

18.1 Roasted Vegetable Foundations

Roasting concentrates flavor through the **Maillard reaction**, the chemical process in which amino acids and reducing sugars react at temperatures above 280°F to produce the browned, complex flavors associated with caramelization (McGee, 2004). For trifecta patients, roasting offers a practical advantage beyond flavor: it requires minimal hands-on time. Vegetables go into the oven on a sheet pan and emerge 25 to 40 minutes later without stirring, flipping, or monitoring. The cook can sit or lie down during the entire roasting period, making this the most energy-efficient cooking method for patients managing the fatigue of POTS and EDS.

Roasted Root Vegetable Medley with Sea Salt and Rosemary

Preheat oven to 425°F. Peel and cut into 1-inch pieces: 2 medium carrots, 1 large sweet potato, 1 medium parsnip, and 1 medium turnip. Toss with 3 tablespoons of olive oil, 1 teaspoon of fine sea salt, 1 teaspoon of dried rosemary (crushed), and

1/4 teaspoon of black pepper. Spread in a single layer on a parchment-lined sheet pan. Roast 30 to 35 minutes, tossing once halfway through, until edges are golden and vegetables are tender. Finish with a generous pinch of flaky sea salt.

Serves four. Approximate per serving: 160 calories, 2 g protein, 10 g fat, 18 g carbohydrate, 750 mg sodium.

Root vegetables are among the most reliable choices for MCAS patients. Growing underground limits their exposure to the environmental molds and pollens that can accumulate on above-ground produce, and their thick skins provide a natural barrier (Sánchez-Pérez et al., 2018). The variety of roots in this recipe provides a range of micronutrients: beta-carotene from carrots and sweet potato (converted to vitamin A, which supports mucosal immune function; Huang et al., 2018), vitamin C from turnips, and inulin from parsnips (a prebiotic fiber that nourishes beneficial gut bacteria; Shoaib et al., 2016).

Steamed Broccoli with Herbed Butter

Trim 1 pound of broccoli into uniform florets. Steam over boiling water for 4 to 5 minutes until bright green and just tender (overcooked broccoli becomes sulfurous and mushy). While broccoli steams, combine 2 tablespoons of softened ghee with 1 teaspoon of finely chopped fresh dill, 1/2 teaspoon of fine sea salt, and a pinch of garlic powder. Toss the steamed broccoli with the herb butter immediately after steaming.

Serves three. Approximate per serving: 120 calories, 4 g protein, 9 g fat, 8 g carbohydrate, 500 mg sodium.

This recipe deliberately omits lemon juice, which appears in nearly every conventional steamed broccoli recipe. Lemon is a histamine liberator that can trigger MCAS symptoms in sensitive individuals (Kovacova-Hanuskova et al., 2015). The dill provides brightness in its place, and the salt enhances all flavors, including the natural sweetness of properly steamed broccoli. Broccoli contains sulforaphane, an isothiocyanate with documented anti-inflammatory and potential mast cell modulating properties (Thimmulappa et al., 2002).

18.2 Sautéed Greens and Vegetables

Garlic-Free Sautéed Greens

Heat 2 tablespoons of olive oil in a large skillet over medium heat. Add 1 pound of trimmed, roughly chopped greens (bok choy, kale, or a combination). Season with 1/2 teaspoon of fine sea salt. Sauté 3 to 5 minutes (bok choy requires less time than kale), tossing frequently, until wilted and tender. Finish with 1 teaspoon of toasted sesame oil and an additional pinch of salt.

Serves three. Approximate per serving: 100 calories, 3 g protein, 8 g fat, 6 g carbohydrate, 500 mg sodium.

This recipe omits garlic, which some MCAS patients identify as a trigger during the elimination-rechallenge process (section 6.9). For patients who tolerate garlic, adding 2 minced cloves during the first 30 seconds of sautéing enhances flavor considerably. The recipe works either way.

Bok choy and **kale** are lower-histamine greens compared to spinach, which contains naturally occurring histamine and is a common trigger for MCAS patients (Maintz & Novak, 2007). Both provide calcium (important for patients who avoid dairy), vitamin K (relevant for connective tissue metabolism in EDS; Gensemer et al., 2021), and folate. Kale additionally provides the carotenoids lutein and zeaxanthin.

Sautéed Zucchini Noodles with Garlic Oil

Using a spiralizer or julienne peeler, create noodle-shaped strips from 4 medium zucchini. Pat the noodles dry with paper towels (removing excess moisture prevents steaming and sogginess). Heat 2 tablespoons of olive oil in a large skillet over medium-high heat. If garlic is tolerated, add 3 thinly sliced garlic cloves and cook 30 seconds until fragrant. Add the zucchini noodles and 1/2 teaspoon of fine sea salt. Toss for 2 to 3 minutes only (overcooking zucchini noodles releases water and creates a mushy texture). Remove from heat. Finish with a drizzle of olive oil and a pinch of flaky salt.

Serves four. Approximate per serving: 90 calories, 2 g protein, 7 g fat, 6 g carbohydrate, 400 mg sodium.

Zucchini noodles serve as a low-carbohydrate pasta alternative for patients who find that high-carbohydrate meals worsen postprandial POTS symptoms through insulin-mediated vasodilation (Shibao et al., 2005). They also accommodate the gastroparesis-friendly soft texture principle from section 8.3, as properly cooked zucchini noodles require minimal chewing.

18.3 Jessamine's Side Dish System

Background

Jessamine, a 26-year-old graduate student with POTS and MCAS, had mastered a set of protein preparations from her dietitian's guidance but struggled with the "rest of the plate." Her dinners consisted of well-prepared chicken or salmon accompanied by plain white rice and nothing else. She described vegetables as "something that goes bad before I can eat it" and explained that she bought fresh produce with good intentions, watched it wilt in the refrigerator over the week, and then threw it away feeling guilty. Her actual vegetable intake averaged less than one serving per day, well below the three to four servings associated with reduced inflammation markers in observational studies (Aune et al., 2017).

Presentation

Jessamine's food diary showed adequate protein and carbohydrate intake but consistently low vegetable consumption (averaging 0.8 servings daily). Her micronutrient panel revealed low vitamin A (inadequate beta-carotene intake), low vitamin K (no leafy green consumption), and borderline magnesium (Miller, 2013). Her dietitian noted that Jessamine's anti-inflammatory fat intake was also low because she used minimal cooking oil and no dressings or sauces, relying on plain salt as her only seasoning.

Analysis

Jessamine's pattern reflects the **fresh produce waste cycle** common among trifecta patients. The standard advice to "eat more vegetables" assumes a consistent daily cooking routine. But trifecta patients have variable energy and variable symptom days, meaning that produce purchased on Monday for the week may go unused if Tuesday through Thursday are flare days. The produce then deteriorates (both in freshness and in histamine content for certain vegetables), reinforcing the perception that "vegetables always go bad on me." The solution involves the same approach applied to proteins in section 13.3: buy for immediate use and freeze the rest, or buy frozen from the start.

Intervention

Her dietitian introduced a three-tier side dish system. Tier 1 (zero-effort, crash-day sides): frozen vegetables that can be steamed in the microwave (frozen broccoli, frozen green beans, frozen bok choy), finished with a pat of ghee and salt. Total preparation time: 4 minutes. Tier 2 (low-effort, moderate-day sides): roasted root vegetables that require only cutting, seasoning, and placing in the oven (no active monitoring). Tier 3 (higher-effort, good-day sides): fresh salads and sautéed preparations from this chapter. The frozen vegetables were purchased pre-cut and pre-washed, eliminating the preparation steps that consumed energy on difficult days.

Outcome

Over four weeks, Jessamine's vegetable intake increased from 0.8 servings daily to 2.4 servings. Her vitamin A and vitamin K levels improved at the eight-week lab check. She described the three-tier approach as "permission to eat frozen vegetables when I can't do anything else." Her anti-inflammatory fat intake improved because each tier included a fat component (ghee, olive oil, dressing). She reported that the roasted root vegetables became her most-used recipe because "I can chop things sitting down, throw them in the oven, and lie on the couch until the timer goes off."

Teaching Points

- The fresh produce waste cycle in trifecta patients can be interrupted by maintaining a frozen vegetable stock alongside fresh purchases, ensuring that vegetable intake continues even when fresh produce cannot be used before it deteriorates
- A tiered side dish system (zero-effort frozen, low-effort roasted, higher-effort fresh) matches the variable energy availability of POTS and EDS patients and prevents vegetable intake from dropping to zero on difficult days
- Each side dish serving should include a fat component (ghee, olive oil, dressing) to support both satiety and fat-soluble vitamin absorption from the vegetables being consumed

18.4 Starch Sides

Sweet Potato Fries with Sea Salt (Baked)

Preheat oven to 425°F. Peel 2 large sweet potatoes and cut into 1/4-inch-thick sticks. Toss with 2 tablespoons of olive oil, 1 tablespoon of tapioca starch (creates crispness on the exterior), and 1 teaspoon of fine sea salt. Arrange in a single layer on two parchment-lined sheet pans (crowding prevents crisping). Bake 20 minutes, flip, and bake an additional 10 to 15 minutes until golden and crisp at the edges. Finish with flaky sea salt immediately after removing from the oven.

Serves four. Approximate per serving: 180 calories, 2 g protein, 7 g fat, 28 g carbohydrate, 750 mg sodium.

The tapioca starch coating is a technique borrowed from commercial frozen fry production. It creates a thin crust that crisps during baking while the interior stays soft, mimicking deep-fried texture without the inflammatory oils (Calder, 2015).

Coconut Rice

Combine 1.5 cups of jasmine rice (rinsed), 1 cup of full-fat coconut milk, 1 cup of water, and 1 teaspoon of fine sea salt in a saucepan. Bring to a boil, stir once, reduce heat to the lowest setting, cover, and cook 18 minutes. Remove from heat and let stand, covered, for 5 minutes. Fluff with a fork.

Serves four. Approximate per serving: 300 calories, 5 g protein, 10 g fat, 48 g carbohydrate, 600 mg sodium.

Coconut rice transforms a basic starch into a more satisfying, calorie-dense side. The coconut milk adds MCTs for quick energy absorption (Thwaites et al., 2022) and creates a subtly sweet, creamy flavor that pairs with both Asian-inspired dishes (stir-fry, lettuce wraps) and Western preparations (roast chicken, lamb chops).

Simple Quinoa Pilaf with Fresh Herbs

Rinse 1 cup of quinoa under cold water (rinsing removes saponins that create a bitter taste). Toast the rinsed quinoa in a dry saucepan over medium heat for 2 minutes, stirring constantly, until fragrant. Add 2 cups of homemade broth, 1/2 teaspoon of fine sea salt, and a pinch of ground turmeric. Bring to a boil, reduce heat, cover, and simmer 15 minutes until liquid is absorbed. Fluff with a fork. Stir in 2 tablespoons of chopped fresh parsley, 1 tablespoon of chopped fresh dill, 1 tablespoon of olive oil, and an additional pinch of salt.

Serves four. Approximate per serving: 200 calories, 7 g protein, 5 g fat, 32 g carbohydrate, 650 mg sodium.

Quinoa is a pseudocereal that provides a complete amino acid profile, including all nine essential amino acids (Vega-Gálvez et al., 2010). It is naturally gluten-free and provides more protein per serving than rice, making it a useful carbohydrate option for patients who need to increase protein intake without increasing animal protein frequency.

Cauliflower Mash with Olive Oil and Chives

Cut 1 large head of cauliflower into florets. Steam or boil until very tender (10 to 12 minutes). Drain thoroughly (excess water creates a watery mash). Transfer to a food processor or use an immersion blender. Add 2 tablespoons of olive oil, 1/2 teaspoon of fine sea salt, 1/4 teaspoon of garlic powder, and a pinch of ground white pepper. Process until smooth. Stir in 2 tablespoons of finely chopped fresh chives.

Serves four. Approximate per serving: 90 calories, 3 g protein, 7 g fat, 6 g carbohydrate, 400 mg sodium.

Cauliflower mash serves as a lower-carbohydrate alternative to mashed potatoes for patients who find that high-glycemic carbohydrate loads worsen postprandial POTS symptoms (Shibao et al., 2005). The olive oil replaces butter for dairy-free preparation and provides oleocanthal, the phenolic compound with ibuprofen-like anti-inflammatory activity described in section 9.2 (Beauchamp et al., 2005).

18.5 Fresh Salads

Simple Cucumber, Apple, and Fresh Herb Salad

Peel and thinly slice 2 medium cucumbers. Core and thinly slice 1 large apple (Fuji or Gala). Combine in a bowl with 1/4 cup of fresh mint leaves (torn), 2 tablespoons of fresh dill (chopped), and 2 tablespoons of fresh parsley (chopped). For the dressing: whisk together 3 tablespoons of olive oil, 1 tablespoon of apple cider vinegar (if tolerated; otherwise omit), 1/2 teaspoon of fine sea salt, 1/2 teaspoon of honey, and a pinch of black pepper. Toss the salad with the dressing just before serving.

Serves four. Approximate per serving: 130 calories, 1 g protein, 10 g fat, 12 g carbohydrate, 400 mg sodium.

This salad uses exclusively low-histamine produce (Maintz & Novak, 2007). Cucumber is 96% water, contributing to hydration targets. Apple provides pectin fiber. The herb combination delivers polyphenolic compounds with anti-inflammatory properties (Bauer et al., 2012). The simplicity of this salad makes it achievable even on moderate symptom days.

Roasted Beet and Arugula Salad

Preheat oven to 400°F. Wrap 4 medium beets individually in foil. Roast 45 to 60 minutes until tender when pierced with a knife. Cool, peel (the skins slide off easily after roasting), and cut into wedges. Arrange over 4 cups of fresh arugula. Drizzle with 2 tablespoons of olive oil and 1/2 teaspoon of flaky sea salt.

Serves four. Approximate per serving: 100 calories, 2 g protein, 7 g fat, 10 g carbohydrate, 400 mg sodium.

Histamine note: Beets are classified as low-histamine by most references (Maintz & Novak, 2007), but some MCAS patients report individual sensitivity. This recipe sits in the "tested yellow" category from section 6.9: introduce through the standard reintroduction protocol (single food, small portion, 48-hour observation) before incorporating regularly. Arugula may cause issues for patients sensitive to salicylates, so individual tolerance testing applies here as well.

18.6 Pairing Sides with Proteins

Side dishes are selected based on what the protein recipe provides and what the Trifecta Plate still needs. A protein recipe that already includes carbohydrate (stuffed bell peppers, one-pot chicken and rice) needs only a vegetable side. A protein recipe that includes vegetables (sheet pan chicken with broccoli) needs only a starch. A standalone protein (pan-seared salmon, lamb chops) needs both a starch and a vegetable to complete the plate.

This modular approach is the practical expression of the Trifecta Plate framework. It prevents the common trifecta patient error of eating protein-heavy, vegetable-light dinners (which misses the anti-inflammatory benefit of plant polyphenols and the micronutrient density of vegetables), and it prevents the opposite error of eating large carbohydrate portions without adequate protein (which produces insulin-mediated vasodilation and worsens postprandial POTS symptoms; Mehr et al., 2018).

Sample pairings for common Chapter 17.0 proteins: pan-seared salmon (section 17.4) pairs with coconut rice (section 18.4) and sautéed greens (section 18.2). Lamb chops (section 17.4) pair with cauliflower mash (section 18.4) and roasted root vegetables (section 18.1). Turkey meatballs (section 17.5) pair with quinoa pilaf (section 18.4) and steamed broccoli (section 18.1). The combinations are not prescriptive. They are examples of the modular system applied.

Chapter 19.0 addresses what happens between meals: the snacks, energy bites, and portable foods that maintain sodium, calories, and blood sugar stability through the gaps in the day.

Chapter 19.0: Snacks and Portable Foods

Darian was sitting in a hospital waiting room when his POTS symptoms began escalating. He had arrived for his wife's prenatal appointment at 2:00 p.m. having eaten lunch at noon. By 3:15, his heart rate was climbing, his vision was narrowing at the periphery, and the familiar pre-syncope dizziness was tightening around his awareness. He had been sitting the entire time, so the orthostatic trigger was not positional. It was glycemic. His blood glucose, unsupported by food for over three hours, had dropped below the threshold his body needed to maintain adequate cerebral perfusion (Raj et al., 2020). He had no food with him. The waiting room vending machine offered candy bars, chips in inflammatory seed oils, and trail mix containing dried fruit (high histamine) and chocolate (a histamine liberator; Kovacova-Hanuskova et al., 2015). None of it was safe. He white-knuckled through the remaining 45 minutes, then drove home shaky and nauseated.

This is the scenario that the emergency snack box was designed to prevent. This chapter provides 10 snack recipes and one snack system (the emergency box blueprint) that keep trifecta patients fueled between meals:

- Shelf-stable snacks for bags, desks, and cars
- Freezer-friendly energy bites and bars
- High-sodium portable options for on-the-go electrolyte maintenance
- Quick-assembly snacks requiring no cooking
- Homemade versions of common snacks, reformulated for the trifecta

19.1 Snacking Strategy Explained

For the general population, snacking advice is mixed. Some nutritional frameworks recommend three meals with no snacking to minimize insulin spikes. Others advocate for smaller, more frequent eating. For POTS patients, the evidence tilts toward frequent eating. The hemodynamic consequences of extended fasting periods (blood sugar drops, volume contraction from insensible losses without compensatory intake) combine with the postprandial demands of large meals (blood flow diverted to the gut, orthostatic worsening after heavy carbohydrate loads) to create a situation where smaller, more frequent eating occasions reduce symptom burden compared to three large meals (Ganesh et al., 2020).

The practical target is eating every two to three hours during waking hours, consistent with the meal timing framework from section 11.2. For a person awake from 7:00 a.m. to 10:00 p.m., this means three meals and two to three snacks daily.

Each snack should provide 150 to 300 calories, 400 to 800 mg of sodium, and at least two of the four Trifecta Plate components (protein, carbohydrate, fat, or produce). The snack does not need to be a complete plate. It needs to bridge the gap between meals without creating its own hemodynamic challenge.

Blood sugar stability is the primary metabolic goal of trifecta snacking. Rapid blood sugar drops trigger sympathetic nervous system activation (epinephrine release, increased heart rate, sweating, anxiety) that mimics and amplifies POTS symptoms (Shibao et al., 2005). Snacks that combine protein or fat with carbohydrate slow glucose absorption and flatten the glycemic curve, preventing both the spike and the subsequent crash. A snack of apple slices alone produces a faster glucose rise and fall than apple slices paired with almond butter, because the fat and protein in the almond butter slow gastric emptying and intestinal absorption (Brand-Miller et al., 2009).

19.2 No Bake Energy Snacks

Salted Nut Butter Energy Balls

Combine 1 cup of rolled oats, 1/2 cup of almond butter (or sunflower seed butter for tree nut sensitivity), 1/3 cup of honey, 2 tablespoons of collagen peptides, 1 teaspoon of fine sea salt, 1/2 teaspoon of vanilla extract, and 2 tablespoons of unsweetened shredded coconut in a bowl. Mix well. If the mixture is too sticky, refrigerate 15 minutes. Roll into approximately 16 balls (about 1 tablespoon each). Place on a parchment-lined tray and freeze for 30 minutes. Transfer to a container and store in the freezer. They soften to a pleasant chewy texture within 5 minutes at room temperature.

Makes 16 balls. Approximate per ball: 90 calories, 3 g protein, 5 g fat, 10 g carbohydrate, 150 mg sodium.

These energy balls deliver the three-macronutrient combination (protein from collagen and nut butter, fat from nut butter, carbohydrate from oats and honey) that stabilizes blood sugar between meals. The salt provides 150 mg of sodium per ball, meaning two balls deliver 300 mg. They are shelf-stable at room temperature for approximately 24 hours, making them suitable for an emergency snack box, and they last in the freezer for up to three months.

Coconut and Seed Crackers with Sea Salt

Preheat oven to 325°F. Combine 1/2 cup of pumpkin seeds, 1/4 cup of sunflower seeds, 2 tablespoons of sesame seeds, 1/4 cup of unsweetened shredded coconut, 1 tablespoon of olive oil, 1/2 teaspoon of fine sea salt, and 3 tablespoons of water.

Stir until a thick paste forms. Spread the mixture as thinly as possible on a parchment-lined baking sheet (thinner equals crispier). Bake 20 to 25 minutes until golden and firm. Cool completely on the pan (they crisp further as they cool). Break into irregular crackers.

Makes approximately 4 servings. Approximate per serving: 200 calories, 8 g protein, 16 g fat, 6 g carbohydrate, 300 mg sodium.

These crackers are grain-free and provide a base for toppings (almond butter, mashed avocado if tolerated, turkey roll-ups). Pumpkin seeds are one of the richest food sources of magnesium (approximately 150 mg per ounce; Guerrera et al., 2009), which is relevant for EDS and POTS patients given that magnesium deficiency is associated with increased muscle cramping, vascular tone changes, and autonomic dysregulation (Gröber et al., 2015).

19.3 Protein Forward Snacks

Turkey and Cucumber Roll-Ups

Lay out 4 slices of deli turkey (purchased fresh from the deli counter on the day of use, not pre-packaged; check that no nitrates, MSG, or "natural flavors" are listed in ingredients per section 13.10). Place a thin cucumber spear (approximately 3 inches long) at one end of each slice. Add a thin smear of avocado (if tolerated) or a drizzle of olive oil. Roll the turkey around the cucumber. Secure with a toothpick if needed. Sprinkle with a pinch of flaky sea salt.

Makes 4 roll-ups (one serving). Approximate per serving: 120 calories, 16 g protein, 4 g fat, 4 g carbohydrate, 600 mg sodium.

Freshness note for deli turkey and MCAS: Pre-packaged deli meats have been sliced and exposed to air for days to weeks before purchase, allowing extensive histamine accumulation. Freshly sliced deli turkey from the counter on the day of purchase has lower histamine levels but should still be consumed within 24 hours (Comas-Basté et al., 2020). For the most histamine-sensitive patients, home-roasted turkey breast (sliced and frozen in individual portions) is the safest option.

Roasted Chickpeas with Safe Seasonings

Drain and rinse one 15-ounce can of chickpeas. Pat very dry with paper towels (moisture prevents crisping). Toss with 1 tablespoon of olive oil, 1 teaspoon of fine sea salt, 1/2 teaspoon of ground cumin, 1/2 teaspoon of garlic powder, and 1/4 teaspoon of ground turmeric. Spread in a single layer on a parchment-lined baking sheet. Bake at 400°F for 30 to 35 minutes, shaking the pan halfway through, until golden and crunchy.

Makes 4 servings. Approximate per serving: 160 calories, 7 g protein, 5 g fat, 22 g carbohydrate, 650 mg sodium.

Tolerance note: Legumes are tolerated by many trifecta patients but can cause GI distress in patients with significant gastroparesis or small intestinal bacterial overgrowth (SIBO), which co-occurs with EDS at elevated rates (Thwaites et al., 2022). Introduce through the reintroduction protocol (section 6.9) before making these a regular rotation item. For patients who tolerate chickpeas, they provide an excellent plant-based protein and fiber source with a low histamine profile (Sánchez-Pérez et al., 2018).

19.4 Salome's Emergency Kit

Background

Salome, a 33-year-old real estate agent with POTS and MCAS, spent much of her workday driving between property showings, sitting in other people's offices, and walking through houses. Her schedule was unpredictable. Showings ran long, clients wanted to see additional properties, and the distance between appointments left little time for meals. She had experienced four pre-syncope episodes in the past three months, all occurring between 2:00 and 4:00 p.m. during extended periods without food. Her cardiologist had increased her midodrine dose, but the pharmacological intervention could not fully compensate for the caloric and sodium deficit caused by missed snacks and delayed meals.

Presentation

Salome's food diary revealed a consistent gap between noon lunch and 6:00 p.m. dinner. On busy showing days (three to four per week), she ate nothing between these meals. Her blood glucose monitoring showed drops to 65 to 72 mg/dL during the afternoon gap (below the 80 mg/dL threshold at which many POTS patients begin experiencing symptomatic hypoglycemia; Raj et al., 2020). Sodium intake on these days fell to 4,000 mg, well below her 8,000 mg target, because the missing afternoon snack had been her planned sodium-loading window.

Analysis

Salome's pre-syncope episodes were not random. They were predictable consequences of the physiological gap between lunch and dinner. Blood glucose decline combined with inadequate afternoon sodium created a dual deficit: reduced substrate for cerebral metabolism and reduced intravascular volume for maintaining blood pressure during the upright posture of walking through houses (Vernino et al., 2021). Her case illustrates why the snacking framework from section 11.2 is not optional for POTS patients. The two-to-three-hour eating interval is a hemodynamic prescription, not a lifestyle preference.

Intervention

Her dietitian built an **emergency snack box** system using three containers maintained in rotation: one in her car, one in her work bag, and one in her desk. Each box contained: 4 salted nut butter energy balls (section 19.2), 1 bag of coconut-seed crackers (section 19.2), 1 bag of roasted chickpeas (section 19.3), 2 packets of individual nut butter (commercially packaged, shelf-stable, approximately 200 calories each), 2 salt packets (restaurant-style, approximately 400 mg sodium each) for adding to any food or water, and 1 electrolyte powder packet (pre-measured per the tonic recipe from section 15.6, mixed into a water bottle). The boxes were restocked weekly during her Sunday batch-prep session.

Outcome

Over eight weeks, Salome's afternoon eating gaps were eliminated. She consumed a snack between 2:00 and 3:00 p.m. daily regardless of schedule. Her afternoon blood glucose readings stabilized above 80 mg/dL. Pre-syncope episodes dropped from four in the prior three months to one in the eight-week monitoring period (that single episode occurred on a day she had forgotten to restock her car box). Afternoon sodium intake increased by approximately 1,000 mg. She described the emergency box as "insurance I actually use every day."

Teaching Points

- Pre-syncope episodes in POTS patients often correlate with identifiable nutritional gaps rather than unpredictable autonomic instability, and food diary analysis can reveal these patterns
- An emergency snack box system maintained in multiple locations (car, bag, desk) prevents the scenario where a patient recognizes the need for food but has no safe options available
- Shelf-stable, trifecta-compliant snacks (energy balls, seed crackers, roasted chickpeas, individual nut butter packets) form the core of portable nutrition and should be batch-prepared during weekly cooking sessions

19.5 Quick Assembly Snacks

Apple Slices with Salted Almond Butter

Core and slice 1 medium apple into 8 wedges. Spread 2 tablespoons of almond butter (or sunflower seed butter) across the slices. Sprinkle with a generous pinch of flaky sea salt. Consume immediately (pre-sliced apples brown quickly; a squeeze of fresh apple cider can slow oxidation if needed, but this is purely cosmetic).

Serves one. Approximate: 280 calories, 7 g protein, 16 g fat, 28 g carbohydrate, 300 mg sodium (with added salt; increase to 500 mg by adding more salt to the almond butter).

This snack requires no cooking, no reheating, and no advance preparation. It provides the three-macronutrient combination (protein and fat from almond butter, carbohydrate from apple) within 60 seconds of preparation time. For POTS patients experiencing the first signs of blood sugar decline (lightheadedness, increased heart rate, difficulty concentrating), this is among the fastest trifecta-compliant interventions.

Rice Cakes with Toppings

Plain rice cakes (salted variety, approximately 35 calories and 80 mg sodium each) serve as a portable, shelf-stable base for multiple trifecta-compliant topping combinations.

The **protein and fat topping** combines 1 tablespoon of almond butter with a drizzle of honey and a pinch of flaky salt. Approximate per topped cake: 130 calories, 3 g protein, 8 g fat, 14 g carbohydrate, 200 mg sodium.

The **savory protein topping** layers 1 slice of fresh deli turkey with a thin cucumber round and a drizzle of olive oil. Approximate per topped cake: 70 calories, 6 g protein, 3 g fat, 6 g carbohydrate, 300 mg sodium.

The **sweet recovery topping** spreads 1 tablespoon of coconut butter (also called coconut manna, made from puréed whole coconut) with a few fresh blueberries and a pinch of salt. Approximate per topped cake: 120 calories, 1 g protein, 8 g fat, 12 g carbohydrate, 150 mg sodium.

Rice cakes are among the most reliably tolerated snack bases for MCAS patients because they contain minimal ingredients (rice, salt) and have an extremely low histamine profile. They store indefinitely in a sealed bag, making them a core emergency box component.

19.6 Homemade Portable Treats

Sweet Potato Chips (Oven or Air Fryer)

Peel 2 medium sweet potatoes. Slice as thinly as possible using a mandoline or sharp knife (uniform thickness ensures even cooking). Toss with 1 tablespoon of olive oil and 1/2 teaspoon of fine sea salt. For oven: arrange in a single layer on parchment-lined baking sheets. Bake at 250°F for 1.5 to 2 hours, flipping halfway, until crisp and dry. For air fryer: cook at 300°F for 12 to 15 minutes, shaking every 5 minutes. Cool completely (they crisp further as they cool). Store in an airtight container at room temperature for up to five days.

Makes approximately 4 servings. Approximate per serving: 100 calories, 1 g protein, 3 g fat, 18 g carbohydrate, 350 mg sodium.

Homemade chips avoid the inflammatory seed oils (soybean, canola, sunflower) used in most commercial chip production. These oils are high in omega-6 fatty acids, which in excess promote the pro-inflammatory eicosanoid pathways discussed in section 9.1 (Calder, 2015). Olive oil or coconut oil provides a neutral or anti-inflammatory fat base instead.

Electrolyte Gummy Recipe

Heat 1 cup of pure fruit juice (apple, blueberry, or grape, checking ingredient list for added citric acid or "natural flavors") in a saucepan over medium heat until warm but not boiling. Remove from heat. Sprinkle 3 tablespoons of unflavored grass-fed gelatin over the warm juice and whisk until completely dissolved (no lumps). Stir in 1 teaspoon of fine sea salt (approximately 2,300 mg sodium for the whole batch) and 1/4 teaspoon of potassium-containing salt substitute (approximately 350 mg potassium). Pour into silicone molds or a parchment-lined 8x8 baking dish. Refrigerate 2 to 3 hours until firm. If using a baking dish, cut into approximately 20 squares.

Makes approximately 20 gummies. Approximate per gummy: 15 calories, 1 g protein, 0 g fat, 2 g carbohydrate, 115 mg sodium.

These gummies provide sodium, potassium, and a small amount of protein (from gelatin, which is derived from collagen) in a portable, shelf-stable-for-24-hours format (refrigerate for longer storage, freeze for weeks). Four gummies deliver approximately 460 mg of sodium. Gelatin provides glycine and proline, amino acids involved in collagen synthesis that may support connective tissue in EDS patients (Gensemer et al., 2021), though the clinical impact of dietary gelatin supplementation on connective tissue integrity is not established.

Frozen Fruit Pops with Coconut Milk

Blend 1 cup of frozen blueberries, 1 cup of full-fat coconut milk, 1 tablespoon of honey, 1/4 teaspoon of fine sea salt, and 1/2 teaspoon of vanilla extract until smooth. Pour into popsicle molds (makes approximately 4 to 6 pops depending on mold size). Freeze 4 to 6 hours until solid. To unmold, run warm water briefly over the outside of the mold.

Makes 4 to 6 pops. Approximate per pop (based on 5): 90 calories, 1 g protein, 5 g fat, 12 g carbohydrate, 120 mg sodium.

These pops serve a dual purpose: they are a snack, and they are a cooling intervention. For POTS patients whose symptoms worsen in heat (Vernino et al., 2021), consuming a frozen treat lowers core body temperature while delivering calories, sodium, and fluid. The coconut milk provides MCTs for quick energy absorption (Thwaites et al., 2022) and creates a creamy texture without dairy.

19.7 Gawain Plans His Week

Background

Gawain, a 40-year-old high school history teacher with POTS and EDS, had successfully adopted the meal planning framework from Chapters 11.0 and 12.0 but described his snacking as "chaos." Between classes, he had 5-minute passing periods and a 22-minute lunch. He ate three solid meals daily but had no structured snack routine. By his fifth-period class (1:30 p.m.), his symptoms reliably worsened: heart rate elevated, concentration fragmented, and his standing tolerance at the whiteboard decreased. He had begun sitting during instruction, which helped but did not eliminate the afternoon decline.

Presentation

Gawain's food diary confirmed the pattern Salome experienced (section 19.4): a consistent caloric and sodium gap between 12:00 and 5:30 p.m. His morning sodium intake from breakfast and a mid-morning broth was adequate (approximately 3,000 mg by noon), but his afternoon intake dropped to 500 mg between lunch and dinner. His total daily sodium averaged 6,500 mg, technically within the minimum target but poorly distributed, with 75% consumed before 1:00 p.m. and only 25% consumed during the remaining eight waking hours. Research on sodium loading in POTS indicates that distribution across the day matters as much as total daily intake (Sheldon et al., 2015), because the plasma volume expansion from a sodium bolus dissipates within hours through normal renal function.

Analysis

Gawain's afternoon symptom pattern reflected sodium distribution imbalance rather than total sodium insufficiency. The morning loading provided hemodynamic support through the first half of the day, but without afternoon sodium replenishment, the volume benefit eroded by early afternoon. The five-minute passing periods created a structural barrier: he could not prepare food, could not heat food, and could not eat a sit-down snack. His afternoon nutrition solution needed to be grab-and-eat with zero preparation, consumable in under three minutes, and trifecta-compliant.

Intervention

His dietitian designed an afternoon snack rotation stored in his desk drawer: Monday and Wednesday: 2 salted nut butter energy balls plus 1 electrolyte gummy packet (4 gummies). Tuesday and Thursday: 1 individual nut butter packet on 2 salted rice cakes. Friday: turkey and cucumber roll-ups (prepared that morning and refrigerated in the staff lounge). Each combination provided 200 to 300 calories and 500 to 700 mg of sodium. He consumed the snack during the passing period between his third and fourth classes (approximately 11:00 a.m.) and again during the passing period before fifth period (approximately 1:25 p.m.).

Outcome

Over five weeks, Gawain's afternoon sodium intake rose from 500 mg to approximately 1,400 mg. His fifth-period symptom pattern improved: standing heart rate during instruction decreased from 115 to 98 bpm, and he reported being able to stand for 10 to 15 minutes continuously at the whiteboard (compared to 3 to 5 minutes previously). His daily sodium distribution shifted from 75/25 (morning/afternoon) to approximately 55/45, better matching the all-day hemodynamic support his POTS required.

Teaching Points

- Sodium distribution across the day matters as much as total daily sodium intake in POTS management, because the plasma volume expansion from morning sodium loading dissipates through normal renal function within hours
- Structural barriers to snacking (short breaks, no preparation facilities, limited time) require snack solutions that are truly grab-and-eat, requiring zero preparation and consumable in under three minutes
- A desk drawer or bag-based snack rotation, restocked weekly during batch prep sessions, converts afternoon sodium gaps from a daily decision-making challenge into an automated system

19.8 Emergency Snack Box Blueprint

The emergency snack box is not a recipe. It is an infrastructure system. Every trifecta patient should maintain at least two boxes: one portable (bag or backpack) and one stationary (car, desk, or locker). The box contents rotate based on shelf life but follow a consistent template.

The **portable box** contains: 4 to 6 salted nut butter energy balls (shelf-stable 24 hours, freeze for longer), 1 bag of coconut-seed crackers (shelf-stable weeks), 1 to 2 individual nut butter packets (shelf-stable months), 2 to 4 salt packets (shelf-stable indefinitely), and 1 electrolyte powder packet or pre-measured salt and potassium mixture in a small container. Total approximate nutritional content of the full box: 800 to 1,000 calories, 2,500 to 3,500 mg sodium, sufficient to sustain a trifecta patient through 4 to 6 hours of unexpected delay.

The **car box** should avoid heat-sensitive items during warm months (nut butters can separate, energy balls can soften). Summer car box contents shift toward: rice cakes (sealed bag), roasted chickpeas (sealed container), salt packets, and electrolyte packets (mixed into water from a bottle kept in the car). In cooler months, the car box can mirror the portable box.

The **restocking schedule** aligns with the weekly batch prep session (section 13.9). Each Sunday (or designated prep day), check all boxes, remove expired or stale items, and replace with freshly prepared or restocked contents. This takes approximately 5 minutes and prevents the failure scenario of reaching for an emergency box and finding it empty.

19.9 Snacking and Sodium Review

The snacks in this chapter are calibrated to the same trifecta principles that govern every recipe in this book: sodium at therapeutic levels (400 to 800 mg per snack), low-histamine ingredients prepared fresh or shelf-stable, anti-inflammatory fats where possible, and textures appropriate for variable GI function. They are not treats or indulgences. They are physiological maintenance doses, distributed across the afternoon and evening to sustain the plasma volume, blood sugar stability, and energy supply that meals alone cannot maintain over a 15-hour waking day.

The progression from Chapter 15.0 (breakfast) through Chapter 16.0 (soups and broths), Chapter 17.0 (main meals), Chapter 18.0 (sides), and this chapter covers every eating occasion in a typical trifecta day. The next chapter addresses special situations: dining out, travel, holidays, and other scenarios where the controlled home kitchen is no longer available and the trifecta framework must adapt to less predictable environments.

Chapter 20.0: Hydrating Drinks and Tonics

Faustina kept a water bottle on her desk, her nightstand, and her kitchen counter. She drank 80 to 100 ounces daily. And she was still dehydrated. Her cardiologist confirmed it at her six-month follow-up: despite her diligent water intake, her plasma volume remained below the threshold needed to adequately fill her vascular space, and her POTS symptoms (tachycardia on standing, pre-syncope, cognitive fog) persisted at levels inconsistent with someone who was supposedly drinking enough. The problem was not volume. It was composition. Plain water, consumed without adequate electrolytes, passes through the gastrointestinal tract and into the kidneys without being retained in the vascular compartment (Ganesh et al., 2020). The kidneys, sensing dilute plasma, excrete the excess. The result is frequent urination and persistent intravascular depletion. She was, in a metabolic sense, pouring water through a sieve.

This chapter provides 12 drink recipes that solve the composition problem:

- Electrolyte drink bases with sodium, potassium, and optional glucose for enhanced absorption
- Anti-inflammatory tonics combining hydration with therapeutic compounds
- Warm and cold options for seasonal and symptom variation
- A cost comparison showing the economics of homemade versus commercial electrolyte products
- Recovery drinks designed for post-exercise and post-flare replenishment

20.1 Hydration Physiology Reviewed

Chapter 5.0 established the foundational science of hydration in POTS. The core principle bears brief repetition here because it governs every recipe in this chapter: water follows sodium. The movement of water across intestinal epithelial cells and into the bloodstream depends on the presence of sodium (and to a lesser extent, glucose) in the intestinal lumen, driven by the **sodium-glucose co-transporter (SGLT1)** on the apical membrane of enterocytes (Rao & Bhatt, 2021). This is the same mechanism exploited by oral rehydration solutions (ORS) developed by the World Health Organization for treating cholera-related dehydration, a discovery that has been called one of the most important medical advances of the twentieth century (Binder et al., 2014).

For POTS patients, the practical implication is that every drink should contain sodium. The target concentration for maximal intestinal absorption is approximately 40 to 80 mEq/L of sodium, which translates to roughly 900 to 1,800 mg of sodium per liter (Shirreffs et al., 2004). Adding a small amount of glucose (approximately 2 to 5% concentration, or about 10 to 25 grams per liter) further enhances absorption by activating the SGLT1 co-transporter (Leiper, 2015). This is why the WHO-ORS formula contains both sodium and glucose in specific ratios, and it is why every drink in this chapter includes salt at a minimum, with several including a glucose source.

Potassium plays a complementary role. While sodium drives extracellular fluid volume (the plasma and interstitial fluid that determine blood pressure), potassium is the primary intracellular cation, and its balance with sodium affects cardiac rhythm, muscle function, and nerve conduction (Palmer & Clegg, 2016). POTS patients who supplement sodium aggressively without attending to potassium can develop a sodium-potassium imbalance that manifests as muscle cramping, palpitations, and fatigue. The recipes in this chapter include potassium where appropriate, either through ingredients (coconut water is naturally rich in potassium) or through small additions of potassium chloride salt substitute.

20.2 Electrolyte Drink Base

DIY Electrolyte Drink with Variations

This is the foundation recipe. All variations build from this base.

Combine in a large jar or pitcher: 4 cups (32 ounces) of water, 1/2 teaspoon of fine sea salt (approximately 1,150 mg sodium), 1/8 teaspoon of potassium chloride salt substitute (approximately 350 mg potassium), and 1 tablespoon of honey or maple syrup (approximately 15 grams of glucose/fructose for SGLT1 activation). Stir or shake until dissolved. Taste and adjust salt if needed. Refrigerate and consume within 24 hours.

Makes 4 servings (8 ounces each). Approximate per serving: 15 calories, 0 g protein, 0 g fat, 4 g carbohydrate, 290 mg sodium, 88 mg potassium.

This base recipe mirrors the sodium-glucose ratio used in WHO oral rehydration therapy (Binder et al., 2014) adapted for palatability and daily use rather than acute dehydration treatment. The sodium concentration (approximately 36 mEq/L) sits at the lower end of the absorption-enhancing range, making it well-tolerated for sipping throughout the day rather than being consumed in a single clinical bolus.

Variation 1: Berry Electrolyte. Add 1/4 cup of fresh or frozen blueberries, blended or muddled, to the base recipe. The blueberries provide anthocyanins with anti-inflammatory properties (Cassidy et al., 2015) and natural sweetness that can replace the honey for patients who prefer less added sugar.

Variation 2: Ginger Electrolyte. Add 1 tablespoon of freshly grated ginger to the base recipe. Steep in refrigerator for 2 hours, then strain. Ginger provides gingerols with prokinetic activity that can ease the nausea and gastroparesis symptoms common in trifecta patients (Nikkhah Bodagh et al., 2019).

Variation 3: Cucumber Basil Electrolyte. Add 1/2 cup of thinly sliced cucumber and 4 to 5 fresh basil leaves to the base recipe. Refrigerate 2 hours before drinking. The cucumber adds additional water volume and a cooling quality; the basil provides rosmarinic acid with anti-inflammatory activity (Bauer et al., 2012).

20.3 Infused Waters and Tonics

Salted Coconut Water Refresher

Combine 2 cups of pure coconut water (check label for no added sugars, flavors, or preservatives) with 1/4 teaspoon of fine sea salt (approximately 575 mg sodium) and a squeeze of fresh lime (omit for patients sensitive to citrus). Stir and serve cold.

Makes 2 servings. Approximate per serving: 45 calories, 0 g protein, 0 g fat, 11 g carbohydrate, 400 mg sodium, 350 mg potassium.

Coconut water is naturally rich in potassium (approximately 600 mg per cup; Yong et al., 2009), making it one of the most efficient plant-based potassium delivery vehicles. However, its sodium content is low (approximately 60 mg per cup), which is why this recipe adds salt. The combination of naturally occurring potassium with added sodium creates a balanced electrolyte profile in a single glass.

Cucumber Mint Infused Water

Thinly slice 1 medium cucumber and place in a large pitcher with 8 cups of water, 10 to 12 fresh mint leaves (lightly bruised to release oils), and 1/2 teaspoon of fine sea salt. Refrigerate at least 2 hours (overnight produces stronger flavor). Serve cold.

Makes 8 servings. Approximate per serving: 5 calories, 0 g protein, 0 g fat, 1 g carbohydrate, 150 mg sodium.

Infused water serves a specific behavioral function beyond hydration: it makes drinking water more appealing. For patients who struggle to consume adequate fluid volume because plain water tastes unappealing (a common report among POTS patients experiencing chronic nausea; Ganesh et al., 2020), flavored water increases voluntary intake. The mint provides menthol, which has mild antiemetic properties, and the cucumber adds a cooling perception that patients with heat intolerance often find soothing.

Ginger Turmeric Anti-Inflammatory Tonic

Combine in a saucepan: 2 cups of water, 1 tablespoon of freshly grated ginger, 1 teaspoon of ground turmeric (or 1 tablespoon of freshly grated turmeric root), 1/4 teaspoon of ground black pepper, 1/2 teaspoon of fine sea salt, and 1 tablespoon of honey. Simmer over low heat for 10 minutes (do not boil vigorously, as this can degrade some active compounds). Strain through a fine mesh strainer. Serve warm or cool and refrigerate for a cold version.

Makes 2 servings. Approximate per serving: 35 calories, 0 g protein, 0 g fat, 9 g carbohydrate, 600 mg sodium.

This tonic combines two of the most well-studied anti-inflammatory food compounds. **Curcumin**, the active polyphenol in turmeric, inhibits the NF-kB inflammatory signaling pathway and suppresses COX-2 expression (Daily et al., 2016). **Gingerols** from fresh ginger provide prokinetic effects on gastric motility (useful for gastroparesis) and anti-inflammatory activity through suppression of prostaglandin synthesis (Nikkhah Bodagh et al., 2019). The black pepper contains **piperine**, which increases curcumin's bioavailability by approximately 2,000% by inhibiting hepatic glucuronidation (Shoba et al., 1998). This tonic was first introduced as the electrolyte morning tonic in section 15.6; this version includes a higher turmeric-to-ginger ratio for patients specifically targeting inflammation.

20.4 Berenice's Hydration Overhaul

Background

Berenice, a 29-year-old veterinary technician with POTS and MCAS, drank commercial electrolyte drinks daily. She had tried four brands over the past year, spending approximately $120 per month on individual bottles and powder packets. Two of the four brands contained citric acid (a known mast cell trigger for some MCAS patients; Kovacova-Hanuskova et al., 2015), one contained "natural flavors" (an umbrella term that can include hundreds of undisclosed compounds; U.S. Food and Drug Administration, 2023), and one contained sucralose (an artificial sweetener that some MCAS patients report triggering GI symptoms). Despite her spending, her electrolyte intake was inconsistent because she rationed the drinks to manage cost and skipped them on days she worked from home.

Presentation

Berenice's symptom diary showed a pattern: POTS symptoms (standing heart rate increases of 35+ bpm, pre-syncope, fatigue) were measurably worse on days she consumed fewer electrolyte drinks. Her sodium intake on those days dropped from approximately 7,000 mg to 5,000 mg. She also reported intermittent MCAS flares (facial flushing, GI cramping) within 30 minutes of consuming certain commercial drinks, which she had attributed to "drinking them too fast" rather than to the ingredients they contained.

Analysis

Berenice's case illustrates two common problems with commercial electrolyte products for MCAS patients. The ingredient problem is that commercial formulations contain additives (citric acid, natural flavors, artificial sweeteners, dyes) that are potential MCAS triggers, creating a situation where the hydration solution itself causes symptom flares. The cost problem is that at $120 per month ($1,440 per year), the financial burden of commercial electrolytes leads to rationing behavior, which undermines the consistent daily intake that POTS management requires (Vernino et al., 2021). Homemade electrolyte drinks solve both problems simultaneously.

Intervention

Berenice's dietitian transitioned her to the DIY electrolyte drink base (section 20.2) with the ginger variation (her preferred flavor). The cost of ingredients per batch was approximately $0.35, compared to $2.50 to $4.00 per serving for commercial products. She prepared a daily pitcher each morning (5 minutes of preparation), producing four 8-ounce servings. The recipe contained five ingredients, all of which she could verify individually for MCAS tolerance.

Outcome

Over four weeks, Berenice's monthly electrolyte spending dropped from $120 to approximately $12 (a 90% reduction). Her sodium intake became consistent because she no longer rationed for cost. The intermittent MCAS flares she had attributed to "drinking too fast" disappeared, confirming that the commercial additives, not the consumption speed, had been the trigger. Her average daily standing heart rate increase decreased from 35 bpm to 27 bpm with consistent electrolyte intake.

Teaching Points

- Commercial electrolyte products frequently contain additives (citric acid, natural flavors, artificial sweeteners, dyes) that can trigger MCAS symptoms, and patients who experience flares after consuming these products should investigate ingredients before attributing symptoms to the electrolytes themselves
- The cost of commercial electrolyte drinks ($100+ per month) leads to rationing behavior in many patients, undermining the consistent daily intake that POTS management requires, while homemade alternatives reduce cost by approximately 90%
- A daily pitcher preparation routine (5 minutes each morning) produces consistent electrolyte intake throughout the day and allows the patient to control every ingredient for MCAS safety

20.5 Warm Hydration Options

Warm Salted Broth Tea

Heat 1 cup of homemade bone broth (section 16.2) or vegetable mineral broth (section 16.3) in a saucepan or microwave until steaming but not boiling. Add 1/4 teaspoon of fine sea salt (approximately 575 mg sodium, in addition to the sodium already present in the broth), a pinch of ground turmeric, and a pinch of ground ginger. Stir and sip slowly.

Approximate per serving: 30 to 50 calories (varies by broth type), 5 g protein (bone broth) or 1 g protein (vegetable broth), 1 g fat, 2 g carbohydrate, 900 to 1,100 mg sodium.

This "broth tea" functions as both a hydration vehicle and a sodium bolus. For patients who find cold drinks aversive (particularly in winter or during nausea episodes), warm broth provides the same electrolyte delivery as cold drinks while also offering the comfort and prokinetic benefits of warm liquid on the gastrointestinal tract. The thermic effect of warm liquid can stimulate gastric motility, which may benefit patients with gastroparesis (Rao & Bhatt, 2021).

Iced Herbal Tea Blends

Brew 4 cups of herbal tea using histamine-safe options: chamomile, rooibos, or peppermint (avoid black tea, green tea, and mate, which contain varying levels of histamine or are histamine liberators in some individuals; Maintz & Novak, 2007). Allow to cool. Add 1/4 teaspoon of fine sea salt, 1 tablespoon of honey, and ice. Serve cold.

Makes 4 servings. Approximate per serving: 15 calories, 0 g protein, 0 g fat, 4 g carbohydrate, 150 mg sodium.

Chamomile provides apigenin, a flavonoid with mast cell stabilizing properties in preclinical models (Lee et al., 2007). **Rooibos** (from the South African *Aspalathus linearis* plant) is naturally caffeine-free and contains quercetin and luteolin, flavonoids with anti-inflammatory and potential antihistamine activity (Joubert et al., 2008). **Peppermint** provides menthol, which relaxes smooth muscle in the gastrointestinal tract and may alleviate some gastroparesis symptoms (Khanna et al., 2014). All three are caffeine-free, which matters for POTS patients because caffeine can worsen tachycardia and anxiety symptoms despite its temporary benefit for alertness (Raj et al., 2020).

20.6 Recovery and Performance Drinks

Protein Electrolyte Recovery Smoothie

Blend 1 cup of full-fat coconut milk, 1/2 cup of frozen blueberries, 1 scoop (approximately 10 g) of collagen peptides, 1 tablespoon of almond butter, 1/2 teaspoon of fine sea salt, 1/4 teaspoon of ground turmeric, and 1/2 cup of ice until smooth.

Makes 1 serving. Approximate: 320 calories, 14 g protein, 22 g fat, 18 g carbohydrate, 1,200 mg sodium.

This smoothie is designed for consumption within 30 minutes of exercise or following a symptom flare. The combination of protein (collagen peptides), carbohydrate (blueberries, coconut milk sugars), fat (coconut milk MCTs, almond butter), and sodium creates a recovery drink that addresses multiple post-exertion deficits simultaneously. For POTS patients who exercise (which is recommended as a frontline non-pharmacological treatment; Fu et al., 2010), the post-exercise window is a period of particular vulnerability because exercise-induced vasodilation combined with sweat sodium losses can trigger severe orthostatic symptoms if not promptly addressed.

Adrenal Cocktail Recipe

The term "adrenal cocktail" circulates widely in the POTS community on social media, and while the name is physiologically imprecise (the drink does not directly affect adrenal function), the formulation has a rational basis in electrolyte and micronutrient repletion.

Combine in a glass: 4 ounces of pure orange juice (or apple juice for patients who do not tolerate citrus), 1/4 teaspoon of fine sea salt (approximately 575 mg sodium), 1/8 teaspoon of cream of tartar (potassium bitartrate, approximately 250 mg potassium). Stir well.

Makes 1 serving. Approximate: 55 calories, 0 g protein, 0 g fat, 13 g carbohydrate, 575 mg sodium, 250 mg potassium.

The rational basis: orange juice provides vitamin C (approximately 60 mg per 4-ounce serving), which plays a role in adrenal steroid biosynthesis and is consumed at higher rates during physiological stress (Padayatty & Levine, 2016). The salt provides sodium for plasma volume. The cream of tartar provides potassium. The combination delivers a quick electrolyte-and-micronutrient bolus that many patients report subjectively improves energy and reduces lightheadedness, though controlled clinical trials specifically studying this combination in POTS are lacking.

Homemade Sports Drink for Exercise Days

Combine: 3 cups of water, 1 cup of coconut water, 1/2 teaspoon of fine sea salt (approximately 1,150 mg sodium), 2 tablespoons of honey, and 2 tablespoons of fresh lemon juice (omit for citrus-sensitive patients; substitute 1 tablespoon of apple cider vinegar if tolerated, or omit the acid entirely). Shake or stir vigorously.

Makes 4 servings. Approximate per serving: 40 calories, 0 g protein, 0 g fat, 10 g carbohydrate, 400 mg sodium, 150 mg potassium.

This drink is designed for consumption during and after exercise. The sodium concentration (approximately 45 mEq/L) falls within the range recommended by the American College of Sports Medicine for fluid replacement during physical activity (Sawka et al., 2007). The glucose from honey provides the co-transport mechanism for enhanced intestinal sodium absorption (Leiper, 2015). The coconut water adds natural potassium to compensate for sweat losses.

20.7 Cost Comparison Analysis

The following comparison illustrates the cost difference between homemade and commercial electrolyte options for a POTS patient consuming four servings per day (the approximate intake recommended in sections 5.3 and 11.2).

Homemade DIY electrolyte base (section 20.2): Ingredients cost approximately $0.08 to $0.12 per serving. At four servings daily, monthly cost is approximately $10 to $15.

Commercial powder packets (popular brands marketed to chronic illness patients): Average cost $1.50 to $2.50 per serving. At four servings daily, monthly cost is approximately $180 to $300.

Commercial ready-to-drink bottles: Average cost $2.50 to $4.00 per serving. At four servings daily, monthly cost is approximately $300 to $480.

The annual cost difference between homemade ($120 to $180) and commercial powders ($2,160 to $3,600) ranges from $2,000 to $3,400. For patients already burdened by the direct and indirect costs of chronic illness (medical visits, medications, reduced work capacity), this difference is clinically relevant because cost-driven rationing reduces adherence to the electrolyte intake levels that POTS management requires (Vernino et al., 2021).

The homemade versions also provide an advantage that no cost calculation captures: ingredient transparency. Every component is visible, verifiable, and individually testable for MCAS tolerance. Commercial products contain proprietary blends, "natural flavors," dyes, and preservatives whose specific chemical identities may not be disclosed and whose MCAS trigger potential cannot be assessed without consuming them (U.S. Food and Drug Administration, 2023).

Pro Tip: Batch Preparation Efficiency. Prepare a week's worth of electrolyte base concentrate by multiplying the recipe by seven, storing in mason jars in the refrigerator, and pouring individual servings daily. Total weekly preparation time: approximately 10 minutes. This eliminates the daily friction of mixing a fresh batch and makes consistent intake as effortless as reaching into the refrigerator.

20.8 Osric's Exercise Recovery

Background

Osric, a 36-year-old former collegiate swimmer with POTS and EDS diagnosed two years earlier, was attempting to return to structured exercise following the modified Levine Protocol recommended by his cardiologist (Fu et al., 2010). He could complete recumbent cycling sessions (30 minutes at moderate intensity) without excessive symptom provocation during exercise. But within 15 to 30 minutes of finishing each session, he experienced severe orthostatic symptoms: standing heart rate spikes to 140+ bpm (from a pre-exercise baseline of 105), nausea, visual graying, and profound fatigue that lasted 3 to 4 hours. He had begun skipping exercise sessions because "the aftermath isn't worth it."

Presentation

Osric's exercise logs showed a consistent post-exercise crash pattern. His pre-exercise sodium loading was adequate (he consumed 1,000 mg of sodium in the hour before cycling), but he drank only plain water during and after exercise. His sweat rate, estimated at approximately 500 to 700 mL per 30-minute session (consistent with moderate-intensity cycling; Baker, 2017), produced estimated sweat sodium losses of 400 to 800 mg per session (sweat sodium concentration averages 40 to 80 mEq/L; Baker, 2017). He was replacing volume (water) but not electrolytes, creating a post-exercise dilutional state: lower plasma sodium concentration, lower plasma osmolality, and reduced intravascular volume.

Analysis

Osric's post-exercise crashes illustrate the exercise-rehydration paradox in POTS: drinking plain water during and after exercise can worsen orthostatic symptoms rather than improving them, because water without sodium dilutes the plasma and triggers renal excretion of the excess volume (Shirreffs et al., 2004). The pre-exercise sodium loading provided temporary protection, but the sweat-induced sodium losses during exercise depleted those reserves. His body needed sodium-containing fluid during and immediately after exercise to replace both the volume and the electrolyte content of his sweat losses.

Intervention

His dietitian designed a three-phase exercise hydration protocol: Phase 1 (pre-exercise): his existing sodium loading was confirmed as adequate (1,000 mg sodium in the hour before exercise). Phase 2 (during exercise): he consumed 8 to 12 ounces of the homemade sports drink (section 20.6) during the 30-minute cycling session, delivering approximately 400 to 600 mg of sodium during exercise. Phase 3 (post-exercise): within 10 minutes of completing the session, he consumed the protein-electrolyte recovery smoothie (section 20.6), delivering 1,200 mg of sodium plus protein and carbohydrate for muscle recovery.

Outcome

The post-exercise crash pattern resolved within three sessions. Osric's post-exercise standing heart rate decreased from 140+ bpm to 118 bpm (still elevated above his baseline of 105, but no longer triggering pre-syncope). Post-exercise fatigue duration shortened from 3 to 4 hours to approximately 45 minutes. He resumed regular exercise three times per week and described the change as "I'm not afraid of the bike anymore." Over 12 weeks, consistent exercise combined with adequate hydration produced further cardiovascular improvements consistent with the Levine Protocol literature (Fu et al., 2010).

Teaching Points

- Post-exercise crashes in POTS patients often result from replacing sweat volume with plain water rather than sodium-containing fluid, creating a dilutional state that worsens orthostatic symptoms
- A three-phase exercise hydration protocol (pre-exercise sodium loading, during-exercise electrolyte drink, post-exercise recovery smoothie) addresses the full spectrum of exercise-induced fluid and electrolyte losses
- Adequate post-exercise hydration enables consistent exercise adherence, which is itself one of the most effective non-pharmacological treatments for POTS (Fu et al., 2010)

20.9 Drink Selection Guide

The drinks in this chapter serve different functions at different times. Matching the right drink to the right moment prevents the common trifecta patient error of treating all hydration as interchangeable.

Morning (first 30 minutes after waking): Warm salted broth tea or ginger-turmeric tonic. Warm liquids stimulate gastric motility, sodium replaces overnight losses, and the low volume (8 ounces) accommodates the morning nausea that many POTS patients experience (section 15.1).

Throughout the day (sipped between meals): DIY electrolyte base in any variation, cucumber-mint infused water, or iced herbal tea. These provide steady sodium intake distributed across waking hours, consistent with the sodium distribution principle from section 19.7.

Pre-exercise (60 minutes before): DIY electrolyte base (double concentration: use 1 teaspoon of salt per 32 ounces) or the adrenal cocktail.

During and after exercise: Homemade sports drink during, protein-electrolyte recovery smoothie after.

During MCAS flares: Warm salted broth tea sipped slowly (section 16.5 established the flare-day liquid protocol), transitioning to electrolyte base or salted coconut water as the flare subsides.

Evening: Iced herbal tea (chamomile for its mild anxiolytic properties through GABA receptor modulation; Srivastava et al., 2010), consumed at least 90 minutes before bed to allow urinary emptying before sleep.

Chapter 21.0: Desserts and Treats

The idea that trifecta patients should not eat dessert comes from nowhere in the clinical literature. It emerges instead from a psychological space where food anxiety, elimination fatigue, and the moralization of eating combine to produce a belief that pleasure and medical compliance are incompatible. Galatea's dietitian encountered this belief directly when Galatea, a 41-year-old POTS and MCAS patient who had maintained a flawless low-histamine protocol for eight months, broke down during a session and said, "I just want to eat something that feels like a treat and not a prescription." She had lost 12 pounds (she could not afford to lose any of them), her relationship with food had narrowed to a set of mechanical routines, and her dietitian recognized the early signs of avoidant/restrictive food intake disorder (ARFID), which co-occurs with MCAS at rates that research is only beginning to quantify (Zickgraf & Ellis, 2018). The prescription was dessert.

This chapter provides eight treat recipes that are trifecta-compliant without requiring compromise on taste:

- Gluten-free and dairy-free preparations using coconut milk, rice flour, and naturally low-histamine fruits
- Recipes that contribute to daily sodium, calorie, and micronutrient targets
- Options spanning cold, warm, frozen, and shelf-stable formats
- A chocolate-free alternative (carob mousse) for patients who react to chocolate's histamine-liberating properties

21.1 Food Pleasure and Compliance

The clinical rationale for including desserts in a therapeutic diet is not indulgence. It is adherence. Research on long-term dietary restriction consistently shows that rigid dietary rules without flexibility predict dietary abandonment, while flexible approaches that accommodate preferred foods (including treats) predict sustained adherence (Stewart et al., 2002). The elimination diet literature specifically warns against indefinite restriction without reintroduction and without accommodation for food pleasure, as this pattern promotes the development of disordered eating (Zickgraf & Ellis, 2018).

For trifecta patients, the adherence question is especially acute. The dietary framework established in this book involves simultaneous management of sodium targets (6,000 to 10,000 mg daily; Vernino et al., 2021), histamine avoidance (Chapter 6.0), gastroparesis accommodation (Chapter 8.0), and anti-inflammatory food selection (Chapter 9.0). Maintaining all four parameters indefinitely requires a diet that the patient is willing to eat indefinitely. And willingness requires some degree of enjoyment.

The desserts in this chapter are engineered with the same precision as every other recipe in this book. They use low-histamine ingredients, they contribute to caloric targets (which matter for patients who are underweight or losing weight due to dietary restriction), they include sodium where appropriate, and they avoid the common dessert triggers for MCAS patients: dairy, gluten, chocolate, citrus, and fermented ingredients. They are not exceptions to the trifecta framework. They are expressions of it.

21.2 Coconut Based Desserts

Coconut Milk Panna Cotta with Fresh Berries

In a small bowl, sprinkle 1 tablespoon of unflavored grass-fed gelatin over 2 tablespoons of cold water. Let stand 5 minutes (this step, called **blooming**, allows the gelatin granules to absorb water and swell, preventing lumps when heated; McGee, 2004). In a saucepan, heat 2 cups of full-fat coconut milk with 3 tablespoons of maple syrup, 1/4 teaspoon of fine sea salt, and 1/2 teaspoon of vanilla extract over medium heat until steaming (do not boil). Remove from heat. Add the bloomed gelatin and whisk until completely dissolved. Pour into 4 ramekins or small glasses. Refrigerate at least 4 hours or overnight until set. Serve topped with 1/4 cup of fresh blueberries per serving.

Makes 4 servings. Approximate per serving: 220 calories, 4 g protein, 16 g fat, 16 g carbohydrate, 180 mg sodium.

Panna cotta is traditionally made with heavy dairy cream. This version uses full-fat coconut milk, which provides MCTs for quick energy absorption (Thwaites et al., 2022) and creates a creamy, rich texture indistinguishable from dairy in most blind taste comparisons. The gelatin provides glycine and proline, amino acids involved in collagen synthesis (Gensemer et al., 2021). The blueberry topping provides anthocyanins with anti-inflammatory activity (Cassidy et al., 2015) and natural sweetness that allows the maple syrup to be reduced.

Frozen Blueberry Coconut Bark

Line a baking sheet with parchment paper. Pour 1 cup of full-fat coconut milk into a bowl. Stir in 1 tablespoon of honey, 1/4 teaspoon of fine sea salt, and 1/2 teaspoon of vanilla extract. Pour onto the prepared baking sheet and spread to approximately 1/4-inch thickness. Scatter 1/2 cup of fresh blueberries and 2 tablespoons of unsweetened shredded coconut over the surface. Freeze 2 to 3 hours until solid. Break into irregular pieces. Store in an airtight container in the freezer.

Makes approximately 6 servings. Approximate per serving: 80 calories, 1 g protein, 6 g fat, 7 g carbohydrate, 100 mg sodium.

This bark serves the same cooling function as the frozen fruit pops from section 19.6 but in a format that requires no molds and produces a satisfying snap when broken. For POTS patients with heat intolerance, frozen treats provide a dual benefit: they are a snack and they lower core body temperature (Vernino et al., 2021).

Rice Pudding with Coconut Milk and Cardamom

Combine 1 cup of short-grain white rice (rinsed), 3 cups of full-fat coconut milk, 1 cup of water, 3 tablespoons of maple syrup, 1/4 teaspoon of fine sea salt, and 1/2 teaspoon of ground cardamom in a saucepan. Bring to a boil, then reduce heat to the lowest setting. Cook uncovered, stirring every 5 minutes, for 30 to 35 minutes until the rice is very tender and the mixture has thickened to a pudding consistency. Remove from heat (it thickens further as it cools). Serve warm, room temperature, or cold.

Makes 6 servings. Approximate per serving: 260 calories, 4 g protein, 12 g fat, 36 g carbohydrate, 130 mg sodium.

Rice pudding is one of the most gastroparesis-friendly desserts because the long cooking process breaks the rice starch into a soft, easily digestible form that requires minimal mechanical digestion (section 8.3). **Cardamom** (*Elettaria cardamomum*) has been used in traditional medicine as a carminative (gas-reducing agent) and has shown anti-inflammatory activity in preclinical studies (Amma et al., 2010). It also provides a warm, complex flavor that elevates the pudding from bland to aromatic without adding any histamine-relevant ingredients.

21.3 Fruit Based Treats

Baked Pear with Cinnamon and Maple

Preheat oven to 375°F. Halve and core 4 ripe pears (Bartlett or Bosc work well). Place cut-side up in a baking dish. Drizzle each half with 1 teaspoon of maple syrup and 1/2 teaspoon of melted ghee. Sprinkle with ground cinnamon and a tiny pinch of sea salt. Add 1/4 cup of water to the bottom of the dish. Bake 25 to 30 minutes until the pears are very tender and the edges are slightly caramelized. Serve warm.

Makes 4 servings (two halves each). Approximate per serving: 120 calories, 1 g protein, 2 g fat, 26 g carbohydrate, 50 mg sodium.

Pears are among the lowest-histamine fruits available and are frequently listed as safe on MCAS elimination protocols (Maintz & Novak, 2007). Baking concentrates their natural sugars through water evaporation and caramelizes the surface through the Maillard reaction (McGee, 2004), producing a dessert that feels indulgent despite containing minimal added sugar. **Cinnamon** (*Cinnamomum verum*, Ceylon cinnamon preferred) has demonstrated anti-inflammatory properties through inhibition of NF-kB (Gunawardena et al., 2015). The ghee adds richness without dairy protein (the milk solids have been removed during clarification).

Apple Crumble with Oat Topping

Preheat oven to 375°F. Peel and slice 4 large apples (Fuji or Gala). Toss with 1 tablespoon of maple syrup, 1/2 teaspoon of ground cinnamon, and a pinch of salt. Place in a baking dish. For the topping: combine 1 cup of rolled oats, 3 tablespoons of coconut oil (melted), 2 tablespoons of maple syrup, 1/4 teaspoon of fine sea salt, and 1/4 teaspoon of ground cinnamon. Mix until crumbly. Spread evenly over the apples. Bake 30 to 35 minutes until the topping is golden and the apples are bubbling.

Makes 6 servings. Approximate per serving: 200 calories, 3 g protein, 8 g fat, 32 g carbohydrate, 130 mg sodium.

This crumble uses oats instead of traditional flour-butter crumb topping, making it both gluten-free (if using certified gluten-free oats) and dairy-free. The **beta-glucan** fiber in oats slows gastric emptying (Tosh, 2013), which may benefit glycemic control but should be considered by patients with severe gastroparesis who may find the added fiber challenging. Apples provide pectin, a soluble fiber that supports gut microbiome diversity (Koutsos et al., 2015). The coconut oil provides saturated fat that creates a buttery richness in the crumble topping.

21.4 Leocadia Reclaims Dessert

Background

Leocadia, a 38-year-old middle school art teacher with POTS, hEDS, and MCAS, had eliminated all desserts and treats from her diet 14 months earlier after an allergist suggested that "sugar feeds inflammation." She had interpreted this advice (which oversimplifies the relationship between dietary sugar and inflammatory pathways; Della Corte et al., 2018) as a mandate to avoid all sweet foods, including fruit. Over the following months, her caloric intake had declined steadily. She reported no pleasure in eating and described meals as "just fuel I have to put in."

Presentation

Leocadia's body weight had dropped from 135 to 118 pounds over 14 months. Her BMI of 19.2 was technically within normal range but represented a 13% loss of body weight, which is clinically concerning (Mehler & Brown, 2015). Her food diary showed total caloric intake averaging 1,200 to 1,400 calories daily, below the 1,500 to 1,800 calorie target established in section 10.3 for women with trifecta conditions. She reported fatigue, worsening POTS symptoms (her standing heart rate increase had risen from 30 to 42 bpm), and increasingly restrictive food attitudes. She scored in the clinical range on the Nine Item ARFID Screen (NIAS; Zickgraf & Ellis, 2018) for limited variety and lack of interest in eating.

Analysis

Leocadia's trajectory illustrates the restriction cascade described in section 6.7: medically motivated elimination (removing histamine triggers) became psychologically driven avoidance (removing all sugar, then all sweet foods, then most foods perceived as non-essential), which produced malnutrition (inadequate calories, progressive weight loss) and worsened the conditions the elimination was intended to treat (POTS symptoms worsen with reduced caloric intake and body mass). The distinction between necessary medical restriction and excessive psychological restriction had been lost. Her POTS symptoms worsened not because of what she ate but because of what she stopped eating. Insufficient calories reduced her cardiac output (the heart is a muscle that requires substrate), and insufficient sodium intake from the eliminated foods reduced her plasma volume.

Intervention

Her dietitian reintroduced desserts as a structured component of her meal plan. The initial addition was one serving of rice pudding with coconut milk (section 21.2) nightly after dinner, providing 260 calories that would not have been consumed otherwise. Over three weeks, the dessert rotation expanded to include baked pears (section 21.3), panna cotta (section 21.2), and apple crumble (section 21.3). Each dessert was framed not as a reward or indulgence but as a caloric prescription: her body needed 300 additional calories daily, and these recipes delivered them in a form she was willing to eat. The dietitian also addressed the "sugar feeds inflammation" misconception directly, explaining that moderate amounts of natural sugars (honey, maple syrup, fruit) within a low-histamine, anti-inflammatory dietary framework do not produce the chronic inflammatory response associated with sustained high-sugar diets (Della Corte et al., 2018).

Outcome

Over eight weeks, Leocadia's nightly caloric intake increased by approximately 250 calories. Her total daily intake rose from 1,300 to 1,550 calories. Her weight stabilized at 121 pounds and began slowly increasing. Her standing heart rate increase decreased from 42 to 34 bpm. She described the rice pudding as "the first thing I've looked forward to eating in over a year." Her NIAS scores moved out of the clinical range for lack of interest in eating. The dessert reintroduction also opened the door to reintroducing other foods she had unnecessarily eliminated, including fruit and honey in other recipes.

Teaching Points

- Excessive dietary restriction beyond medical necessity can worsen trifecta conditions by reducing caloric intake below the threshold needed to maintain cardiac output and plasma volume, and dietitians should monitor for the restriction cascade described in section 6.7
- Desserts that are trifecta-compliant (low-histamine, dairy-free, gluten-free) serve a legitimate clinical function by increasing caloric intake in underweight patients who have lost pleasure in eating
- The belief that "all sugar is inflammatory" oversimplifies the evidence; moderate natural sugars within an anti-inflammatory dietary framework do not produce the chronic inflammatory response associated with sustained high-sugar or high-fructose diets

21.5 Baked Goods

Sweet Potato Brownies

Preheat oven to 350°F. Bake 1 large sweet potato (approximately 200 g) until very tender (45 to 60 minutes at 400°F, or microwave 8 to 10 minutes). Scoop out the flesh and mash until smooth (you should have approximately 1 cup of mash). In a bowl, combine the sweet potato mash with 1/3 cup of carob powder (or cocoa powder if chocolate is tolerated), 1/4 cup of maple syrup, 2 tablespoons of coconut oil (melted), 1 egg, 1/4 cup of rice flour, 1/4 teaspoon of fine sea salt, 1/2 teaspoon of vanilla extract, and 1/2 teaspoon of baking soda. Mix until smooth. Pour into a greased 8x8 baking dish. Bake 20 to 25 minutes until a toothpick inserted in the center comes out mostly clean (these brownies are intentionally fudgy). Cool completely before cutting.

Makes 9 squares. Approximate per square: 110 calories, 2 g protein, 4 g fat, 18 g carbohydrate, 100 mg sodium.

These brownies use sweet potato as their structural base rather than flour and butter. The sweet potato provides natural sweetness, moisture, and beta-carotene (Huang et al., 2018), while the rice flour contributes just enough structure to create a brownie texture. **Carob** (*Ceratonia siliqua*) is the preferred option for MCAS patients because chocolate (theobroma cacao) contains both tyramine and phenylethylamine, biogenic amines that can act as histamine liberators in sensitive individuals (Maintz & Novak, 2007). Carob provides a similar rich, slightly sweet flavor without these compounds and contains polyphenols with documented antioxidant activity (Papagiannopoulos et al., 2004).

Simple Shortbread Cookies

Preheat oven to 325°F. Combine 1 cup of rice flour, 1/4 cup of tapioca starch, 1/3 cup of softened ghee, 3 tablespoons of maple syrup, 1/2 teaspoon of vanilla extract, and 1/4 teaspoon of fine sea salt. Mix until a soft dough forms. If the dough is too crumbly, add ghee 1 teaspoon at a time. Roll tablespoon-sized portions into balls, place on a parchment-lined baking sheet, and flatten slightly with a fork. Sprinkle tops with flaky sea salt. Bake 12 to 15 minutes until edges are just barely golden (these cookies firm up significantly as they cool; removing them while slightly soft produces the ideal crumbly-tender shortbread texture). Cool on the pan for 10 minutes before transferring.

Makes approximately 16 cookies. Approximate per cookie: 80 calories, 0 g protein, 4 g fat, 10 g carbohydrate, 80 mg sodium.

Traditional shortbread is butter, sugar, and wheat flour. This version replaces butter with ghee (dairy-protein-free), white sugar with maple syrup (less refined, lower glycemic impact), and wheat flour with rice flour and tapioca starch (gluten-free). The flaky sea salt finish serves both flavor and trifecta function: each cookie delivers a small sodium contribution, and the salt crystals on top enhance the perception of sweetness, allowing the maple syrup quantity to remain moderate (Breslin & Beauchamp, 1997).

21.6 Carob Mousse

Carob Mousse (Chocolate-Free Alternative)

In a saucepan, heat 1 can (13.5 ounces) of full-fat coconut milk with 3 tablespoons of carob powder, 2 tablespoons of maple syrup, 1/4 teaspoon of fine sea salt, and 1/2 teaspoon of vanilla extract. Whisk over medium heat until smooth and slightly thickened (3 to 4 minutes). Remove from heat. Sprinkle 1.5 teaspoons of unflavored gelatin over the warm mixture and whisk immediately until dissolved.

Pour into 4 small ramekins or glasses. Refrigerate at least 3 hours until set. The mousse will have a soft, creamy texture rather than the firm set of panna cotta.

Makes 4 servings. Approximate per serving: 180 calories, 3 g protein, 12 g fat, 16 g carbohydrate, 170 mg sodium.

For MCAS patients who cannot tolerate chocolate, carob provides the closest flavor analog. Carob is naturally caffeine-free and theobromine-free, eliminating both the stimulant effect (problematic for POTS tachycardia) and the biogenic amine content of chocolate (Maintz & Novak, 2007). Carob also contains tannins and polyphenols with antioxidant capacity, though at lower concentrations than cacao (Papagiannopoulos et al., 2004). The gelatin creates the mousse texture without dairy cream or eggs, and the coconut milk fat provides the richness that makes the mousse feel like a genuine dessert rather than a dietary compromise.

Pro Tip: Carob Adjustment. Carob is sweeter than cocoa powder, so recipes that substitute carob for cocoa should reduce added sweetener by approximately 25% to prevent an overly sweet result. In this recipe, the maple syrup is already calibrated for carob. If substituting cocoa powder back in for patients who tolerate chocolate, increase maple syrup to 3 tablespoons.

21.7 Dessert as Trifecta Component

These recipes contribute to daily nutritional targets in ways that patients may not initially recognize. A serving of rice pudding provides 260 calories toward daily caloric goals. Panna cotta provides 4 grams of protein from gelatin. The shortbread cookies contribute sodium from the flaky salt topping. Apple crumble provides soluble fiber from both the oat topping and the apple pectin. Frozen blueberry bark provides anthocyanins and serves as a cooling intervention for heat-intolerant patients.

The psychological contribution is equally measurable. The restriction cascade (section 6.7) progresses when food becomes exclusively utilitarian. Reintroducing foods that provide pleasure interrupts this progression. The desserts in this chapter are simple to prepare (most require under 15 minutes of active time), use ingredients already present in the trifecta pantry (section 13.4), and produce results that feel celebratory rather than clinical. A baked pear with cinnamon tastes like autumn. Rice pudding with cardamom tastes like comfort. And both taste like a life that includes more than managing symptoms.

The recipe chapters (15.0 through 21.0) now provide a full day of trifecta eating, from the first electrolyte tonic sipped in bed before standing to the last spoonful of rice pudding after dinner. The remaining chapters address the practical challenges of sustaining this framework in the real world: dining out, traveling, managing holidays, and maintaining the system when life becomes unpredictable.

PART FIVE: SUPPLEMENTS, MEDICATIONS & BEYOND

Chapter 22.0: Supplements and the Evidence

Theodora's kitchen counter told a story. Seventeen supplement bottles lined the back wall behind her coffee maker, arranged in the order she took them: morning stack (six capsules), midday stack (four capsules), evening stack (seven capsules). She spent $340 per month on this regimen, assembled over two years from recommendations gathered across online POTS forums, an MCAS Facebook group, a naturopath, her allergist, and a wellness influencer who claimed to have "cured" her own mast cell disease. When her new dietitian asked which supplements she had evidence were helping, Theodora paused. "I'm afraid to stop any of them," she said. "What if the one I stop is the one that's actually working?" She had never introduced them one at a time. She had no way to know.

This chapter examines the supplement evidence for trifecta conditions with the same rigor applied to every dietary recommendation in this book:

- Mast cell stabilizing supplements (quercetin, vitamin C, DAO enzymes) and what the research actually supports
- Connective tissue support for EDS (vitamin C, collagen peptides, MSM, hyaluronic acid)
- Autonomic and energy support for POTS (B vitamins, magnesium, CoQ10, L-carnitine, iron)
- Supplements that can worsen MCAS or interact with trifecta medications
- The "less is more" introduction protocol and why it matters
- Supplement quality, third-party testing, and how to avoid wasting money

22.1 Evaluating Supplement Claims

The supplement industry in the United States generates over $55 billion annually (Grand View Research, 2023) and operates under regulatory rules that differ fundamentally from those governing pharmaceuticals. Under the Dietary Supplement Health and Education Act of 1994 (DSHEA), supplements do not require pre-market approval from the FDA, and manufacturers bear no obligation to demonstrate efficacy before selling their products (U.S. Food and Drug Administration, 2022). This regulatory framework means that a supplement can be marketed with structure/function claims ("supports immune health") without any clinical trial evidence supporting that specific claim.

For trifecta patients, this creates a particular vulnerability. The chronic nature of POTS, EDS, and MCAS, combined with limited pharmaceutical options and the slow pace of clinical research, pushes many patients toward supplements as a form of self-directed treatment. Online patient communities amplify individual success stories, creating an **availability bias** where the most dramatic anecdotal reports receive the most attention while non-responders remain silent (Tversky & Kahneman, 1973). The result is a distorted perception of supplement efficacy.

This chapter does not dismiss supplements. Several have genuine mechanistic rationale and preliminary evidence supporting their use in trifecta conditions. But it applies a consistent standard: what does the published evidence actually show, what are the limitations of that evidence, and what practical considerations govern safe use? The distinction between "this might help based on mechanistic reasoning" and "this has been proven to help in controlled trials" matters enormously when patients are spending hundreds of dollars monthly and ingesting compounds that interact with their medications and their conditions.

22.2 Mast Cell Stabilizing Supplements

Quercetin

Quercetin is a flavonoid found in onions, apples, berries, and cruciferous vegetables. In laboratory studies, quercetin inhibits mast cell degranulation and reduces histamine release through stabilization of the mast cell membrane and inhibition of calcium influx into mast cells (Mlcek et al., 2016). It also inhibits the NF-kB inflammatory signaling pathway and suppresses production of pro-inflammatory cytokines including IL-6 and TNF-alpha (Li et al., 2016).

The preclinical evidence is consistent and reasonably strong. The clinical evidence in humans is limited. A small number of trials have studied quercetin supplementation for allergic conditions with mixed results. Quercetin at 500 mg twice daily showed reduction in contact dermatitis symptoms in one trial (Weng et al., 2012), and supplementation reduced markers of airway inflammation in some but not all studies (Jafarinia et al., 2020). No published randomized controlled trial has specifically studied quercetin supplementation in MCAS patients. The typical supplemental dose used in trifecta patient communities is 500 to 1,000 mg daily, often taken with vitamin C to enhance absorption (Boots et al., 2008).

The practical reality: quercetin has a plausible mechanism, encouraging preclinical data, and a generally favorable safety profile at standard doses. It is reasonable to trial. But it is not a proven mast cell stabilizer in the way that cromolyn sodium or ketotifen are proven mast cell stabilizers (supported by randomized controlled trials in human subjects). Patients should understand this distinction.

Vitamin C as Mast Cell Stabilizer

Vitamin C (ascorbic acid) plays a dual role in trifecta management. As a mast cell modulator, vitamin C has been shown to reduce serum histamine levels in humans. Johnston et al. (1996) demonstrated that supplementation with 2,000 mg of vitamin C reduced blood histamine levels by approximately 38% in subjects with elevated histamine. The proposed mechanism involves vitamin C's role in the enzymatic degradation of histamine through the enzyme diamine oxidase (DAO), as well as direct inhibition of histamine release from mast cells (Johnston et al., 1996; Hagel et al., 2013).

As a collagen synthesis cofactor (discussed further in section 22.3), vitamin C is required for the hydroxylation of proline and lysine residues during collagen formation. This dual function makes vitamin C one of the most rationally supported supplements for trifecta patients, addressing both mast cell instability and connective tissue fragility simultaneously.

The dosing range commonly used is 500 to 2,000 mg daily, divided into two or three doses. Higher doses may cause GI distress (diarrhea, cramping) in some patients, and the buffered form (calcium ascorbate or sodium ascorbate) is often better tolerated than pure ascorbic acid in MCAS patients with GI sensitivity (Carr & Maggini, 2017).

DAO Enzyme Supplements

Diamine oxidase (DAO) is the primary enzyme responsible for degrading ingested histamine in the intestinal lumen. Some patients with histamine intolerance have reduced DAO activity, either due to genetic variants in the AOC1 gene (which codes for DAO) or due to acquired inhibition from medications, alcohol, or intestinal inflammation (Comas-Basté et al., 2020). For these patients, supplemental DAO taken immediately before meals can theoretically degrade dietary histamine before it is absorbed.

The evidence is mixed. Izquierdo-Casas et al. (2019) found that DAO supplementation reduced the duration of migraine attacks in patients with low serum DAO activity. A small trial in histamine intolerance showed symptom improvement with DAO supplementation (Schnedl et al., 2019). But DAO supplements only address exogenous (dietary) histamine. They do not affect endogenous histamine released from the patient's own mast cells, which is the primary driver of MCAS symptoms (Comas-Basté et al., 2020). For patients whose symptoms are primarily MCAS-driven rather than dietary-histamine-driven, DAO supplements may provide minimal benefit.

Pro Tip: DAO Timing. DAO supplements must be taken 15 to 20 minutes before eating to be present in the intestinal lumen when food arrives. Taking DAO after a meal or between meals provides no benefit because the enzyme needs to encounter dietary histamine during digestion.

22.3 Connective Tissue Support

For patients with Ehlers-Danlos syndrome, the underlying collagen defect is genetic and cannot be corrected by supplementation. No supplement will fix a structural protein mutation. However, supporting the body's collagen synthesis machinery may help with tissue repair, wound healing, and the maintenance of connective tissue that is already more fragile than normal (Gensemer et al., 2021).

Vitamin C at 500 to 1,000 mg daily supports collagen synthesis as a required cofactor for prolyl hydroxylase and lysyl hydroxylase, the enzymes that modify proline and lysine residues during collagen maturation (Peterkofsky, 1991). Deficiency of vitamin C produces scurvy, a disease characterized by connective tissue breakdown (bleeding gums, poor wound healing, joint pain) that mirrors some EDS symptoms. While EDS patients are not deficient in vitamin C, ensuring adequate intake supports whatever collagen synthesis capacity their genetic variant allows.

Collagen peptides (hydrolyzed collagen supplements) are among the most controversial trifecta supplements. The proposed rationale is that ingested collagen peptides are absorbed as small peptide fragments (di-peptides and tri-peptides containing hydroxyproline) that may stimulate fibroblast activity and collagen production in connective tissues (Sato et al., 2017). Some evidence supports this in non-EDS populations: a meta-analysis found that collagen supplementation improved skin elasticity and hydration (de Miranda et al., 2021). A study in athletes showed reduced joint pain with collagen peptide supplementation (Clark et al., 2008). But no published trial has studied collagen peptides specifically in EDS patients, and the question of if supplemental collagen can meaningfully affect connective tissue that is genetically abnormal remains unanswered.

MSM (methylsulfonylmethane) provides bioavailable sulfur, which is involved in the formation of disulfide bonds in connective tissue proteins. Preliminary evidence suggests anti-inflammatory effects and possible benefit for joint pain (Butawan et al., 2017). **Silica** (as orthosilicic acid) participates in collagen cross-linking and bone mineralization (Jugdaohsingh, 2007). Both have limited clinical trial data in EDS specifically but plausible mechanisms.

Hyaluronic acid supplementation aims to support the extracellular matrix in which collagen fibers are embedded. Oral hyaluronic acid has shown benefit for skin hydration and knee osteoarthritis in some trials (Oe et al., 2016), but its relevance to the specific connective tissue dysfunction in EDS has not been established in clinical studies.

22.4 Autonomic and Energy Support

POTS patients frequently report fatigue, exercise intolerance, and cognitive dysfunction ("brain fog") that extend beyond what cardiovascular deconditioning alone explains. Several supplements target these symptoms through distinct mechanisms.

B Vitamins. Thiamine (B1) is required for aerobic energy metabolism, and subclinical thiamine deficiency can produce fatigue, orthostatic intolerance, and tachycardia that overlap with POTS symptoms (Bettendorff, 2013). Some POTS clinicians empirically recommend B1 supplementation (100 to 300 mg daily) based on case reports showing improvement (Eshak & Arafa, 2020). Methylcobalamin (B12) and methylfolate (5-MTHF) are relevant for patients with MTHFR variants that reduce their ability to convert standard folic acid and cyanocobalamin into active forms. B12 deficiency produces neuropathy and fatigue; its correction may improve autonomic function in deficient patients (Gröber et al., 2013).

Magnesium is the fourth most abundant mineral in the body and is involved in over 300 enzymatic reactions (de Baaij et al., 2015). Magnesium deficiency is common in the general population and may be more prevalent in POTS patients due to increased urinary excretion from high fluid intake and autonomic dysfunction (Raj et al., 2020). The form of magnesium matters: **magnesium glycinate** is well-absorbed and less likely to cause diarrhea than citrate or oxide forms. **Magnesium citrate** has a mild laxative effect that may benefit constipation-predominant patients. **Magnesium threonate** crosses the blood-brain barrier more effectively than other forms and may preferentially address cognitive symptoms (Slutsky et al., 2010). The typical supplemental dose is 200 to 400 mg of elemental magnesium daily, taken in divided doses.

CoQ10 (Coenzyme Q10) is a component of the mitochondrial electron transport chain required for ATP production. Supplementation at 100 to 300 mg daily has shown benefit for fatigue in conditions involving mitochondrial dysfunction (Tarnopolsky, 2008). **L-Carnitine** shuttles fatty acids into mitochondria for beta-oxidation and energy production. Some POTS patients show functional carnitine deficiency, and supplementation (500 to 1,000 mg daily) has been associated with reduced fatigue and improved orthostatic tolerance in small studies (Ruzieh et al., 2017).

Iron supplementation is appropriate only for confirmed iron deficiency (low ferritin, low serum iron, elevated TIBC). Unnecessary iron supplementation can worsen MCAS through iron-mediated oxidative stress that promotes mast cell activation (Kell & Pretorius, 2014). Ferritin levels below 30 ng/mL, even when above the laboratory "normal" cutoff, may contribute to fatigue and autonomic dysfunction and warrant supplementation in symptomatic POTS patients (Raj et al., 2020).

22.5 Cyril's Supplement Audit

Background

Cyril, a 44-year-old IT project manager with POTS, hEDS, and MCAS, presented with a supplement regimen of 14 products totaling $280 per month. He had accumulated these over three years, adding each based on recommendations from various online sources and practitioners. He could not identify which, if any, were providing benefit. His primary complaints remained fatigue, brain fog, joint pain, and intermittent MCAS flares despite (or possibly because of) his supplement load.

Presentation

Cyril's supplement list included quercetin (1,000 mg), vitamin C (2,000 mg), collagen peptides (10 g), CoQ10 (200 mg), magnesium glycinate (400 mg), a B-complex, fish oil (2,000 mg), turmeric extract, DAO enzyme, zinc, selenium, vitamin D, vitamin E, and a probiotic marketed for histamine intolerance. He took all of them daily. He reported GI distress (bloating, nausea) most mornings after his "morning stack" of eight capsules and tablets taken simultaneously on a mostly empty stomach.

Analysis

Cyril's regimen illustrates a pattern common among trifecta patients: supplement accumulation without systematic evaluation. By introducing multiple supplements simultaneously and never removing any, he had no baseline for comparison and no method for determining which supplements were producing benefit versus producing side effects versus producing nothing at all. His morning GI distress was almost certainly caused by the capsule volume itself (eight capsules overwhelming an already compromised gastroparesis-affected stomach) and possibly by the high-dose vitamin C on an empty stomach. Additionally, his fish oil supplement contained a significant amount of EPA and DHA, which in some MCAS patients can trigger mast cell activation through prostaglandin pathway modulation (Theoharides et al., 2012).

Intervention

His dietitian implemented a systematic supplement audit. All 14 supplements were discontinued except vitamin C (which had the strongest dual rationale for his conditions) and vitamin D (which his labs confirmed he was deficient in). After two weeks at this reduced baseline, they began reintroducing supplements one at a time, waiting 10 to 14 days between each addition to assess response. Each supplement was evaluated on three criteria: measurable or subjective symptom change, absence of new side effects, and acceptable cost relative to perceived benefit.

Outcome

Over 12 weeks, Cyril reintroduced eight supplements one at a time. Three produced noticeable benefit (magnesium glycinate reduced his muscle cramping and improved sleep; quercetin appeared to reduce the frequency of his minor MCAS flares; CoQ10 subjectively improved his afternoon energy). Two produced no detectable effect (collagen peptides, selenium). One worsened his symptoms (fish oil triggered GI cramping and what appeared to be an MCAS flare, confirmed by rechallenge two weeks later). His morning GI distress resolved entirely. His monthly supplement cost dropped from $280 to $95. And critically, he could now articulate exactly which supplements were helping, why, and what would happen if he stopped them.

Teaching Points

- Introducing multiple supplements simultaneously makes it impossible to determine which are beneficial, neutral, or harmful, and a systematic one-at-a-time introduction with a 10-to-14-day evaluation period between additions is the only reliable method for building an evidence-based personal regimen
- Supplement-induced GI distress in trifecta patients often results from capsule volume and timing (too many capsules on an empty or gastroparesis-affected stomach) rather than from the active ingredients themselves
- Some supplements commonly recommended in trifecta communities (fish oil, certain probiotics) can worsen MCAS symptoms in a subset of patients, reinforcing the need for individual trial-and-removal assessment

22.6 Supplements to Avoid

Several commonly marketed supplements can worsen mast cell activation or interact poorly with trifecta conditions:

Fish oil/omega-3 supplements are widely recommended for inflammation, but in some MCAS patients, high-dose EPA and DHA can modulate prostaglandin pathways in ways that trigger mast cell degranulation (Theoharides et al., 2012). Start low (500 mg combined EPA/DHA) and monitor carefully rather than beginning at the 2,000 to 3,000 mg doses commonly recommended.

Probiotics are frequently recommended for gut health, but certain strains produce histamine as a metabolic byproduct. *Lactobacillus casei*, *Lactobacillus bulgaricus*, and *Lactobacillus reuteri* are histamine-producing strains that can worsen symptoms in histamine-intolerant patients (Sánchez-Pérez et al., 2022). Patients with MCAS should select probiotic strains that degrade histamine (such as *Bifidobacterium infantis*, *Lactobacillus rhamnosus GG*) or avoid probiotics entirely during the elimination phase.

Iron (when not deficient) promotes oxidative stress and may activate mast cells through Fenton reaction-generated free radicals (Kell & Pretorius, 2014). Never supplement iron without confirmed deficiency.

Niacin (vitamin B3) triggers histamine release and can cause severe flushing in MCAS patients. If B-complex supplementation is desired, select a formula that uses niacinamide (nicotinamide) rather than niacin (nicotinic acid) (Maintz & Novak, 2007).

N-acetylcysteine (NAC) is an antioxidant that some patients tolerate well, but it contains a sulfur group that can trigger reactions in sulfite-sensitive MCAS patients. Trial cautiously.

22.7 Quality and Testing Standards

Not all supplement products contain what their labels claim. Independent testing by ConsumerLab, the United States Pharmacopeia (USP), and NSF International has repeatedly found that supplement products may contain less active ingredient than labeled, more active ingredient than labeled, or contaminants not listed on the label (Cohen, 2014). For MCAS patients, unlisted ingredients (fillers, flow agents, colorants) can trigger reactions even when the active ingredient is well-tolerated.

Third-party verification marks to look for include: USP Verified (the most stringent standard), NSF Certified for Sport, and ConsumerLab Approved. Products carrying these marks have been independently tested for identity, potency, purity, and dissolution (Cohen, 2014).

Additional quality indicators for MCAS patients: minimal inactive ingredients (avoid products with long lists of fillers, artificial colors, and "natural flavors"), capsule rather than tablet form (tablets require more binders and coatings), and avoidance of common excipient triggers including titanium dioxide, carrageenan, and certain cellulose derivatives (Castells, 2017).

22.8 Ianthe Builds a Protocol

Background

Ianthe, a 31-year-old physical therapist with POTS and MCAS (without EDS), wanted to begin supplementation but was wary after watching friends in her online POTS support group accumulate large, expensive, and apparently ineffective supplement regimens. She wanted a rational, evidence-based approach that she could evaluate systematically.

Presentation

Ianthe's lab work showed vitamin D at 22 ng/mL (deficient), ferritin at 28 ng/mL (low-normal but functionally low for a symptomatic POTS patient), and magnesium at the low end of normal range. Her primary symptoms were fatigue, brain fog, muscle cramping (especially at night), and two to three minor MCAS flares per week (flushing, GI cramping).

Analysis

Ianthe's case represents the ideal starting point for supplement introduction: clear lab-confirmed deficiencies combined with symptoms that align with known supplement mechanisms. Her vitamin D deficiency warranted correction regardless of POTS status, as deficiency is associated with increased mast cell activation and worsened autonomic symptoms (Thacher & Clarke, 2011). Her ferritin level, while technically "normal" by laboratory reference range, fell below the 30 ng/mL threshold at which many POTS specialists recommend supplementation (Raj et al., 2020). Her magnesium status and nighttime cramping aligned with the expected benefit of magnesium glycinate supplementation.

Intervention

Her dietitian designed a sequential introduction protocol. Week 1 to 2: vitamin D3 (2,000 IU daily with a fat-containing meal for absorption). Week 3 to 4: evaluate response, then add magnesium glycinate (200 mg at bedtime). Week 5 to 6: evaluate, then add iron bisglycinate (25 mg every other day with vitamin C, taken two hours apart from any antihistamines). Week 7 to 8: evaluate, then consider adding quercetin (500 mg daily) for MCAS flare frequency. Each addition period included a simple symptom log tracking energy (1 to 10 scale), flare frequency, sleep quality, and any new symptoms.

Outcome

After eight weeks, Ianthe's supplement regimen consisted of four supplements, each added individually with documented response. Vitamin D produced no immediate subjective change (expected, as correction takes months) but was continued based on lab deficiency. Magnesium glycinate reduced nighttime cramping within four days and improved sleep quality. Iron supplementation was subjectively associated with improved afternoon energy by week six, and a repeat ferritin at week eight showed increase to 38 ng/mL. Quercetin appeared to reduce her flare frequency from two to three per week to one to two per week. Her total monthly cost was $45, and she could describe the rationale, evidence base, and personal response for each supplement.

Teaching Points

- Lab-confirmed deficiencies should be corrected before trialing supplements for symptoms, as correcting deficiencies may resolve symptoms that would otherwise be attributed to the condition itself
- Sequential introduction with a 10-to-14-day evaluation window between additions allows clear attribution of benefit or harm to individual supplements
- A simple daily symptom log (energy level, flare frequency, sleep quality, new symptoms) transforms supplement evaluation from guesswork into data-driven decision-making

22.9 Putting Evidence into Practice

The supplement conversation for trifecta patients reduces to a set of practical principles. Correct confirmed deficiencies first (vitamin D, iron, B12, magnesium), because deficiency correction often resolves symptoms that patients and practitioners might otherwise attribute to the condition itself. After deficiencies are addressed, consider supplements with plausible mechanisms and at least some clinical evidence (quercetin for MCAS, vitamin C for dual mast cell and collagen support, magnesium for POTS-related cramping and sleep, CoQ10 for mitochondrial energy). Introduce one supplement at a time with a minimum 10-to-14-day evaluation window. Keep a simple symptom log. Evaluate cost relative to benefit. Use third-party-tested products with minimal inactive ingredients. And periodically reassess if each supplement is still necessary by conducting a structured removal trial.

The supplements discussed in this chapter are adjuncts. They support the dietary framework established in Chapters 6.0 through 21.0. They do not replace it. Quercetin supplementation cannot compensate for a diet that fails to manage histamine. Magnesium capsules cannot replace the magnesium delivered by the pumpkin seeds, leafy greens, and nuts woven through the recipes in Chapters 15.0 through 21.0. Supplements are, at best, the final 10 to 15% of the trifecta nutrition strategy. The food is the other 85 to 90%.

Chapter 23.0: Diet and Medication Interactions

Honora took her cromolyn sodium with breakfast. She had been doing this for three months, mixing the liquid into her morning oatmeal because the taste was unpleasant on its own. She mentioned this casually to her gastroenterologist during a follow-up visit. He paused. Cromolyn sodium, he explained, must be taken on an empty stomach, 15 to 30 minutes before eating, because food in the stomach dramatically reduces its absorption and its ability to coat the intestinal mucosa where it exerts its mast cell stabilizing effect (Mori et al., 2020). For three months, Honora had been taking an effective medication in a way that rendered it largely ineffective. The prescription was correct. The food timing made it fail.

This chapter examines how food and meal timing interact with the medications most commonly prescribed for POTS, EDS, and MCAS:

- How antihistamines, cromolyn, and other mast cell medications interact with food timing
- How beta-blockers, fludrocortisone, and midodrine intersect with dietary sodium, potassium, and blood sugar
- How proton pump inhibitors affect the absorption of nutrients that trifecta patients need most
- Why coordination between dietary planning and medication timing requires communication with prescribers and pharmacists

This chapter provides nutritional context for medication management. It does not provide dosing recommendations, prescribing guidance, or advice to start, stop, or modify any medication. Those decisions belong to the prescribing clinician and the patient working together.

23.1 Antihistamines and Food Timing

H1 antihistamines (cetirizine, loratadine, fexofenadine, hydroxyzine, diphenhydramine) are the frontline MCAS medications. Their absorption characteristics vary by compound. Cetirizine and loratadine can be taken with or without food, as food does not meaningfully alter their bioavailability (Simons & Simons, 2011). Fexofenadine, however, is an exception. Fruit juices (particularly grapefruit, orange, and apple) reduce fexofenadine absorption by 30 to 40% by inhibiting organic anion transporting polypeptides (OATPs) in the intestinal wall (Dresser et al., 2002). Patients taking fexofenadine should take it with water rather than juice and should avoid fruit juice consumption within two hours of the dose.

H2 blockers (famotidine, ranitidine) reduce gastric acid production. For trifecta patients, these serve dual purpose: they reduce acid-related GI symptoms and they block the H2 histamine receptors in the gut that contribute to MCAS-driven GI symptoms (Castells, 2017). Famotidine is best absorbed on an empty stomach, approximately 30 to 60 minutes before meals, which conveniently aligns with its therapeutic goal of reducing meal-triggered acid production (McRorie et al., 2014).

The dietary intersection: MCAS patients following the low-histamine diet described in Chapter 6.0 are already reducing their exogenous histamine load. Antihistamine medications address endogenous histamine (released from the patient's own mast cells). The combination of dietary histamine reduction and pharmacological histamine blockade produces additive benefit, which is why many MCAS specialists recommend both approaches simultaneously rather than choosing one over the other (Afrin et al., 2016).

23.2 Mast Cell Stabilizers and Diet

Cromolyn sodium (Gastrocrom) is a mast cell stabilizer that prevents degranulation by blocking calcium channels on the mast cell surface. In its oral form, cromolyn works locally on intestinal mast cells (it is poorly absorbed systemically), and its efficacy depends on direct contact with the intestinal mucosa (Mori et al., 2020).

The food timing rule is absolute: cromolyn must be taken 15 to 30 minutes before meals on an empty stomach. Food in the stomach dilutes the medication and coats the mucosal surface, preventing cromolyn from binding to mast cells. Patients who mix cromolyn into food or take it during meals are significantly reducing its effectiveness.

For patients who find cromolyn's taste unpleasant (it is salty and slightly bitter), mixing with a small amount (2 to 4 ounces) of plain water is acceptable. Mixing with juice, milk, or flavored beverages may be tolerated, but acidic beverages should be avoided as they may alter the compound's stability (Mori et al., 2020).

Ketotifen, another mast cell stabilizer with additional H1 antihistamine properties, does not have the same strict empty-stomach requirement as cromolyn. It can be taken with food to reduce its mild sedative effect. The sedation tends to diminish over two to four weeks of consistent use (Simons & Simons, 2011).

23.3 Cardiovascular Medications

Beta-blockers (propranolol, metoprolol) are commonly prescribed for POTS to reduce heart rate. Their interaction with food and nutrition involves several considerations. Propranolol absorption is increased when taken with food, particularly high-protein meals, which increase hepatic blood flow and reduce first-pass metabolism (Melander et al., 1977). Patients taking propranolol should be aware that taking it with versus without food can produce different blood levels and different therapeutic effects. Beta-blockers can also mask the symptoms of hypoglycemia (tremor, tachycardia, anxiety) by blocking the sympathetic response, which means patients on beta-blockers need to be especially attentive to the blood sugar stability strategies discussed in section 19.1, because they may not feel a blood sugar drop until it is more severe (Shorr et al., 1997).

Ivabradine (Corlanor) selectively reduces heart rate without the blood pressure lowering effect of beta-blockers. It should be taken with food, as food increases its bioavailability by approximately 20 to 30% (U.S. National Library of Medicine, 2023). Grapefruit juice must be avoided entirely, as it inhibits CYP3A4 metabolism of ivabradine and can produce dangerous heart rate reduction (Thollon & Bhatt, 2013).

Fludrocortisone (Florinef) is a synthetic mineralocorticoid that promotes sodium and water retention to expand plasma volume. The dietary interaction is direct: fludrocortisone amplifies the sodium retention that the dietary sodium loading described in Chapter 5.0 is designed to produce. This means that patients on fludrocortisone may achieve their sodium-retention goals with a lower dietary sodium intake than patients not on this medication. However, fludrocortisone also promotes potassium excretion, and patients on this medication are at increased risk for hypokalemia (low potassium) (Raj et al., 2020). Potassium-rich foods (coconut water, sweet potatoes, bananas if tolerated, leafy greens) become especially important for these patients, and serum potassium should be monitored regularly.

Midodrine (ProAmatine) is an alpha-1 agonist that constricts blood vessels to raise blood pressure. It should be taken during waking hours (not at bedtime, as it can cause supine hypertension) and is typically taken 15 to 30 minutes before rising or before periods of prolonged standing. Food does not significantly alter midodrine absorption, but caffeine's vasoconstrictive properties can interact additively with midodrine's effects. Patients combining midodrine with caffeine should monitor for elevated blood pressure, headache, or scalp tingling (Raj et al., 2020).

23.4 Remigius and Medication Timing

Background

Remigius, a 50-year-old architect with POTS and MCAS, was prescribed famotidine (20 mg twice daily), cromolyn sodium (200 mg four times daily before meals), propranolol (20 mg twice daily), and fludrocortisone (0.1 mg daily). He also took the morning electrolyte drink (section 20.2), ate breakfast within 30 minutes of waking (section 15.1), and supplemented with magnesium glycinate and quercetin (section 22.4). His complaint: "I feel like I'm managing a pharmacy instead of living my life. I can't figure out what to take when."

Presentation

Remigius's medication and supplement timing had devolved into a disorganized daily struggle. He was taking cromolyn with his breakfast oatmeal (reducing its effectiveness), propranolol on an empty stomach (missing the food-enhanced absorption), famotidine simultaneously with his electrolyte drink (which contained honey, technically not an empty stomach), and fludrocortisone at random times throughout the day. The magnesium and quercetin were taken "whenever I remember," sometimes with meals and sometimes without.

Analysis

Remigius's case illustrates a coordination failure that is common among trifecta patients on multiple medications. Each medication has its own food-timing requirement, and these requirements sometimes conflict with each other and with the dietary framework. Cromolyn needs an empty stomach before meals. Propranolol works better with food. Famotidine works best on an empty stomach before meals. Fludrocortisone timing is less critical but interacts with sodium and potassium intake. When a patient is also trying to follow the morning hydration protocol (section 15.1) and the snacking schedule (section 19.1), the timing complexity can become paralyzing.

Intervention

His dietitian and prescribing physician collaborated to create a single daily timeline. Upon waking: fludrocortisone (consistent daily timing matters more than food relationship). Fifteen minutes later: cromolyn sodium in water and famotidine (both on empty stomach). Fifteen minutes later: morning electrolyte drink, followed immediately by breakfast with propranolol (food enhances absorption). Magnesium at bedtime (promotes sleep). Quercetin with lunch (food enhances absorption). Pre-lunch and pre-dinner: cromolyn and famotidine doses 15 minutes before meals. The entire schedule was written on a single index card that Remigius kept on his kitchen counter.

Outcome

Within two weeks, the medication timing became automatic. Remigius reported that his MCAS symptoms improved (likely because cromolyn was now being taken correctly on an empty stomach rather than mixed into food), his propranolol seemed "more effective" (likely because food-enhanced absorption produced more consistent blood levels), and his sense of being overwhelmed by the daily regimen decreased substantially. He described the index card as "the most useful thing any healthcare provider has ever given me."

Teaching Points

- Medication timing in trifecta patients requires explicit coordination between the prescribing clinician, the pharmacist, and the dietary plan because food-timing requirements for medications can conflict with each other and with the meal and hydration framework
- Cromolyn sodium taken with food is a common and consequential error that reduces the medication's effectiveness; identifying and correcting this error often produces noticeable symptom improvement
- A single written daily timeline (medication + food + supplements) that is visible in the kitchen is one of the most practical interventions for patients managing complex multi-medication regimens

23.5 PPIs and Nutrient Absorption

Proton pump inhibitors (omeprazole, pantoprazole, esomeprazole, lansoprazole) reduce gastric acid production more potently than H2 blockers and are commonly prescribed for GERD and gastroparesis-related reflux in trifecta patients. While effective for acid-related symptoms, long-term PPI use (generally defined as more than one year of continuous use) impairs the absorption of several nutrients critical for trifecta patients.

Vitamin B12 requires gastric acid for its release from food proteins and for the activation of intrinsic factor that enables ileal absorption. Long-term PPI use reduces B12 absorption and is associated with B12 deficiency in approximately 10 to 15% of long-term users (Lam et al., 2013). For POTS patients already at risk for fatigue and neuropathy, B12 depletion can worsen these symptoms.

Magnesium absorption is impaired by long-term PPI use through mechanisms that are not fully understood but may involve altered intestinal pH affecting paracellular magnesium transport (Cheungpasitporn et al., 2015). Hypomagnesemia from PPI use can produce muscle cramping, cardiac arrhythmias, and worsened autonomic dysfunction, all of which overlap with existing trifecta symptoms.

Calcium absorption requires gastric acid for the dissolution of calcium salts. Long-term PPI use is associated with increased fracture risk, which is especially concerning for EDS patients whose connective tissue already provides less structural support for bone (Yang et al., 2006).

Iron absorption is reduced by PPI use, as gastric acid converts dietary ferric iron ($Fe3+$) to the more absorbable ferrous form ($Fe2+$) (Lam et al., 2017). For POTS patients with iron deficiency contributing to fatigue and orthostatic intolerance, PPI-induced iron malabsorption creates a treatment-undermining cycle.

Pro Tip: PPI Monitoring Protocol. Patients on long-term PPIs should have annual monitoring of B12, magnesium, calcium (including vitamin D), and iron/ferritin levels. If deficiencies develop despite adequate dietary intake, the prescribing clinician should consider PPI dose reduction, alternate-day dosing, or transition to an H2 blocker if clinically appropriate.

23.6 Low Dose Naltrexone

Low-dose naltrexone (LDN), typically prescribed at 0.5 to 4.5 mg (a fraction of the standard naltrexone dose used for addiction), is increasingly used off-label for MCAS-related inflammation and pain in trifecta patients. The proposed mechanism involves transient opioid receptor blockade that upregulates endogenous endorphin production and reduces microglial activation in the central nervous system (Younger et al., 2014).

The food timing consideration for LDN is straightforward: it should be taken at bedtime (its mechanism involves the nocturnal endorphin rebound), and while food does not significantly alter its absorption, some practitioners recommend taking it on an empty stomach or with a small amount of food to reduce the nausea that some patients experience during the initial titration period (Younger et al., 2014).

The more relevant dietary interaction is indirect. LDN can cause vivid dreams and initial sleep disruption in some patients. The sleep hygiene and circadian strategies discussed in section 24.5 become especially important during the first two to four weeks of LDN use.

23.7 Medication and Diet Summary

The medications prescribed for trifecta conditions do not operate in isolation from the food and drink consumed around them. Cromolyn needs an empty stomach. Propranolol works better with food. Fludrocortisone demands potassium attention. PPIs steal the very nutrients (B12, magnesium, iron, calcium) that trifecta patients need most. The dietary framework in this book was designed to complement pharmacological treatment, not to exist separately from it. Effective trifecta management requires the prescriber, the pharmacist, the dietitian, and the patient all working from the same timing schedule.

The next chapter examines how lifestyle factors (exercise, heat, hormonal cycles, sleep, stress, body positioning) interact with the dietary framework to amplify or undermine its effects.

Chapter 24.0: Lifestyle Factors and Nutrition

Erasmus could not understand why his POTS symptoms were worse in summer. His sodium intake was the same. His fluid intake was the same. His medications had not changed. His diet was identical to the one that had produced stable symptoms during the cooler months. Yet every June through September, his standing heart rate climbed 15 to 20 bpm higher than his winter baseline, his pre-syncope episodes doubled, and his exercise tolerance dropped to the point where he abandoned his reconditioning program entirely. His cardiologist's explanation was straightforward: heat causes peripheral vasodilation, which reduces venous return, which drops cardiac preload, which forces the heart to beat faster to maintain output (Raj et al., 2020). The same blood volume that kept him stable at 68°F was insufficient at 90°F. His diet was not failing. His environment was demanding more than his diet was providing.

This chapter examines the lifestyle factors that amplify or undermine the dietary framework established in Chapters 5.0 through 23.0:

- Exercise timing and nutritional support for reconditioning protocols
- Heat management and increased fluid and sodium requirements
- Hormonal fluctuations and their effects on histamine, POTS symptoms, and food tolerance
- Sleep, circadian rhythm, and mast cell reactivity
- Stress, cortisol, and the autonomic feedback loop
- Physical positioning strategies during and after meals

24.1 Exercise and Nutrition Timing

Exercise is one of the most effective non-pharmacological treatments for POTS. The modified Levine Protocol (also called the Dallas Protocol) and the CHOP (Children's Hospital of Philadelphia) Protocol are the two most widely studied exercise reconditioning programs for POTS, both showing improvements in stroke volume, cardiac output, and orthostatic tolerance (Fu et al., 2010; Pianosi et al., 2016). Both protocols begin with recumbent exercise (rowing, swimming, recumbent cycling) and gradually progress to upright exercise over three to six months.

The nutritional requirements for exercise in POTS patients differ from those of healthy athletes in two fundamental ways. The pre-exercise sodium load must be higher because POTS patients start with lower plasma volume (section 5.2) and lose sodium through sweat at the same rate as healthy individuals but cannot afford the loss. And the post-exercise recovery window is more critical because exercise-induced vasodilation in a patient with already impaired venous return creates a hemodynamic vulnerability that persists for 30 to 60 minutes after exercise cessation (Fu et al., 2010).

The three-phase exercise hydration protocol from Osric's case in section 20.8 applies here: 1,000 mg of sodium in the hour before exercise, electrolyte-containing fluid during exercise, and a protein-electrolyte recovery smoothie within 15 minutes of completion. The carbohydrate component of the post-exercise recovery matters specifically for POTS patients because exercise depletes muscle glycogen, and carbohydrate ingestion stimulates insulin release, which in turn promotes sodium reabsorption in the renal tubules (DeFronzo et al., 1976). In other words, eating carbohydrates after exercise helps the kidneys retain the sodium that the dietary framework has worked so hard to build up.

24.2 Heat and Fluid Demands

Environmental heat imposes additional hemodynamic demands that the trifecta dietary framework must accommodate. When ambient temperature exceeds approximately 77°F (25°C), the body diverts blood flow to the skin for evaporative cooling, reducing the effective circulating volume available for maintaining blood pressure (Crandall & González-Alonso, 2010). For POTS patients whose baseline plasma volume is already reduced, this redistribution can push the system past its compensatory threshold.

The practical dietary response is to increase sodium and fluid intake proportionally to heat exposure. For every hour of outdoor activity in temperatures above 80°F (27°C), trifecta patients should increase their electrolyte intake by approximately 500 mg of sodium and 8 to 12 ounces of fluid beyond their baseline targets (Sawka et al., 2007). The electrolyte drinks from Chapter 20.0 become especially important in warm months, and the emergency snack box (section 19.8) should be updated for heat stability (replacing items that melt or degrade, as described in section 19.8).

Sweat losses in warm environments can exceed 1 to 2 liters per hour during physical activity (Baker, 2017), with each liter of sweat containing approximately 500 to 1,500 mg of sodium. For a POTS patient who is already targeting 8,000 to 10,000 mg of sodium daily, a single hour of outdoor activity in heat can create a 500 to 1,500 mg sodium deficit that must be actively replaced. Failure to compensate produces the pattern Erasmus experienced: identical diet, worse symptoms, because the environmental demand exceeded the dietary supply.

24.3 Hormonal Effects on Trifecta

The menstrual cycle produces predictable fluctuations in hormone levels that directly affect mast cell reactivity, autonomic function, and food tolerance. Estrogen promotes mast cell degranulation by binding to estrogen receptors on mast cells and increasing histamine release (Zierau et al., 2012). This means that MCAS symptoms tend to worsen during the late luteal phase (the week before menstruation) when estrogen rises before dropping sharply, and during ovulation (mid-cycle) when estrogen peaks (Bonds & Bhatt, 2022).

For trifecta patients who menstruate, this creates a pattern where food tolerance varies across the cycle. A food that is well-tolerated during the follicular phase (days 1 through 14) may trigger reactions during the late luteal phase (days 21 through 28) because the mast cells are already primed for activation by the hormonal environment. This is not food inconsistency. It is hormonal modulation of the threshold for mast cell degranulation (Zierau et al., 2012).

POTS symptoms also fluctuate with the menstrual cycle. Progesterone, which dominates the luteal phase, promotes vasodilation and can worsen orthostatic intolerance (Fu et al., 2010). Many POTS patients report that their worst symptom days cluster in the late luteal phase, when both progesterone-mediated vasodilation and estrogen-mediated mast cell priming are active simultaneously.

The dietary response: increase sodium intake by approximately 1,000 mg daily during the late luteal phase to compensate for progesterone-mediated vasodilation, tighten histamine avoidance during the late luteal phase and ovulation (move toward the most restrictive end of the reintroduction spectrum from Chapter 7.0), and avoid testing new foods or reintroducing previously eliminated foods during the perimenstrual window. The food and symptom journal (Chapter 12.0) should track cycle phase alongside food intake to reveal patterns that are invisible when cycle data is not recorded.

24.4 Apollonia's Cycle Pattern

Background

Apollonia, a 27-year-old graphic designer with POTS, hEDS, and MCAS, reported that her symptoms "randomly got worse" approximately every four weeks. She had been following the trifecta dietary framework for four months with generally good results, but every three to four weeks she would experience two to three days of worsened POTS symptoms (standing heart rate jumping from her stable 95 bpm to 120+ bpm), increased MCAS flares (flushing, GI cramping, brain fog), and apparent food intolerances to foods she normally tolerated without issue.

Presentation

Her food journal showed that these "bad days" were consistently accompanied by the same dietary pattern: she would eat a food she had successfully consumed the previous week, experience an unexpected reaction, panic that she was "losing safe foods," restrict her diet further for several days, lose calories and sodium, and experience even worse POTS symptoms. She described a three-to-four-day "crash cycle" that resolved spontaneously, after which she gradually returned to her normal eating pattern. She had attributed this pattern to "random MCAS flares" and had begun to believe that her food tolerance was fundamentally unstable.

Analysis

When Apollonia added menstrual cycle tracking to her food journal (she used a period tracking app and simply noted the cycle day in her journal), the pattern became immediately visible. Every "random crash" occurred between cycle days 24 and 28 (the late luteal phase). Her food tolerance was not randomly unstable. It was systematically modulated by hormonal fluctuation. During the late luteal phase, elevated estrogen was priming her mast cells for degranulation (Zierau et al., 2012), lowering the threshold at which foods that were normally tolerated could trigger a reaction. Simultaneously, progesterone was promoting vasodilation, worsening her POTS baseline. The "crash cycle" was not random. It was as predictable as the calendar.

Intervention

Her dietitian introduced a cycle-adaptive dietary strategy. During cycle days 20 through 28 (late luteal through early menstruation), Apollonia shifted to the "tested green" foods only (the most reliably tolerated items from her reintroduction tracking in Chapter 7.0), increased her daily sodium by approximately 1,000 mg using the electrolyte drink base (section 20.2), and paused any planned food reintroduction trials. During cycle days 5 through 18 (follicular phase through mid-cycle), she maintained her standard diet and scheduled any new food reintroductions.

Outcome

Over three cycles (approximately 12 weeks), the "random crash" pattern resolved. By tightening her diet during the hormonal vulnerability window rather than after reactions had already occurred, Apollonia prevented the cascade of unexpected reactions, panic-driven restriction, caloric deficit, and worsened POTS symptoms. She described the cycle tracking as "the missing piece of the whole puzzle I didn't know existed." Her sense of control over her condition improved substantially, and the belief that her food tolerance was unstable was replaced by an understanding that her tolerance had a predictable hormonal rhythm.

Teaching Points

- Menstrual cycle fluctuations in estrogen and progesterone directly affect both mast cell reactivity and autonomic function, producing a predictable pattern of symptom worsening in the late luteal phase that patients often misattribute to random disease fluctuation
- Tracking menstrual cycle phase alongside food and symptom journals reveals cyclical patterns that are invisible without cycle data, and this tracking should be standard practice for all menstruating trifecta patients
- A cycle-adaptive dietary strategy (tighter histamine avoidance and increased sodium during the late luteal phase, food reintroductions scheduled during the follicular phase) prevents the cascade of unexpected reactions, panic restriction, and caloric deficit that worsens both MCAS and POTS symptoms

24.5 Sleep and Mast Cell Activity

Sleep deprivation increases mast cell reactivity. Animal studies show that sleep restriction increases mast cell numbers and degranulation in multiple tissues (Almeida et al., 2015), and human studies demonstrate that sleep deprivation elevates inflammatory markers including IL-6 and TNF-alpha, both of which prime mast cells for activation (Irwin et al., 2016). For trifecta patients, this means that a bad night of sleep does not simply produce next-day tiredness. It raises the mast cell activation baseline, lowers the threshold for food-triggered reactions, and worsens POTS symptoms through the inflammatory cascade's effect on autonomic function.

The dietary connection is bidirectional. What patients eat affects their sleep (high-histamine foods consumed in the evening can cause nocturnal itching, flushing, or GI distress that fragments sleep), and how they sleep affects their food tolerance the next day (poor sleep increases mast cell reactivity, making previously tolerated foods more likely to trigger reactions). This bidirectional relationship creates a potential vicious cycle: poor sleep causes food reactions, which cause dietary restriction, which causes caloric deficit, which worsens POTS fatigue, which disrupts sleep further.

Sleep-supporting dietary strategies include: chamomile tea in the evening (section 20.5, providing apigenin with mild anxiolytic properties through GABA receptor modulation; Srivastava et al., 2010), magnesium glycinate at bedtime (200 to 400 mg; promotes sleep through GABA receptor modulation; de Baaij et al., 2015), a light carbohydrate-containing snack 60 to 90 minutes before bed (the insulin response promotes tryptophan transport across the blood-brain barrier, increasing serotonin and melatonin synthesis; Wurtman et al., 2003), and avoidance of high-histamine foods within three hours of bedtime.

24.6 Stress and Autonomic Loops

Psychological stress activates the hypothalamic-pituitary-adrenal (HPA) axis, increasing cortisol production. Cortisol at acutely elevated levels promotes mast cell degranulation through direct glucocorticoid receptor activation on mast cells (Theoharides & Cochrane, 2004). This is counterintuitive, because therapeutic corticosteroids (like prednisone) suppress inflammation, but the acute stress response produces a cortisol pattern that can paradoxically worsen mast cell activation rather than suppress it (Theoharides & Cochrane, 2004).

Stress also activates the sympathetic nervous system, which is already dysregulated in POTS. The combination of stress-induced sympathetic activation and mast cell degranulation creates a feed-forward loop: stress causes cortisol release, which activates mast cells, which release histamine, which stimulates the sympathetic nervous system, which amplifies the stress response, which produces more cortisol. This loop explains why many trifecta patients report that periods of high stress produce their worst symptom clusters, even when their diet has not changed.

The dietary framework cannot eliminate stress. But it can reduce the loop's amplification. The anti-inflammatory dietary components (turmeric, ginger, omega-3 fatty acids from safe sources, polyphenol-rich fruits and vegetables established in Chapter 9.0) help modulate the inflammatory cascade that stress initiates. Consistent eating patterns (avoiding the missed-meal blood sugar crashes described in section 19.1) prevent the additional sympathetic activation that hypoglycemia produces. And the evening tonic and sleep-supporting nutrition described in section 24.5 support the parasympathetic restoration that buffers against the next day's stressors.

24.7 Simeon Addresses Meal Positioning

Background

Simeon, a 58-year-old retired police officer with POTS and EDS, experienced postprandial worsening of POTS symptoms after every large meal. His standing heart rate, which hovered around 105 bpm before eating, reliably spiked to 130+ bpm within 20 to 30 minutes of finishing dinner. He described a feeling of "all my blood draining into my gut," which is physiologically accurate: postprandial blood pooling in the splanchnic (abdominal) vascular bed diverts blood away from the brain and extremities, worsening orthostatic intolerance (Tani et al., 2000).

Presentation

Simeon ate dinner at his recliner, where he typically reclined at approximately 45 degrees while eating and then lay nearly flat for 30 to 60 minutes afterward while watching television. He also reported that his dinner portions were the largest of his three daily meals, as he tended to "save up" calories for the evening. His postprandial symptoms (tachycardia, lightheadedness, visual graying, fatigue) were severe enough that he had stopped going for evening walks, which had previously been his primary exercise.

Analysis

Simeon's postprandial POTS worsening resulted from three compounding factors. The large meal volume produced substantial splanchnic blood pooling (Tani et al., 2000). His reclined eating position eliminated gravity-assisted venous return from the legs, reducing cardiac preload during the exact period when his splanchnic bed was sequestering blood. And his post-meal reclined position maintained this hemodynamic disadvantage for an additional 30 to 60 minutes. The combination produced a predictable severe postprandial POTS response.

Intervention

Three changes were introduced. Meal size redistribution: dinner was reduced from approximately 40% of daily calories to 25%, with the redistributed calories moved to afternoon snacks (section 19.1) and a slightly larger lunch, following the principle from section 11.3 that smaller, more frequent meals reduce postprandial blood pooling. Body positioning: Simeon was instructed to eat seated upright at a table (not reclining) and to remain seated upright for at least 30 minutes after eating. Waist-high compression: an abdominal binder worn during and for 30 minutes after dinner to reduce splanchnic blood pooling (Bourne et al., 2021).

Outcome

Simeon's postprandial standing heart rate dropped from 130+ bpm to 112 bpm within two weeks. The combination of smaller dinner portions, upright positioning, and abdominal compression reduced the hemodynamic challenge enough to keep his symptoms below his subjective threshold for distress. He resumed his evening walks, timing them 45 minutes after dinner (after his upright rest period), and the mild exercise further improved his postprandial hemodynamic recovery. He described the changes as "embarrassingly simple for how much they helped."

Teaching Points

- Postprandial blood pooling in the splanchnic vascular bed is a major contributor to post-meal POTS symptom worsening, and its severity is directly related to meal size (larger meals cause more pooling)
- Eating position matters: seated upright eating produces better hemodynamic outcomes than reclining, and remaining upright for 30 minutes after meals allows gravity to assist venous return during the period of maximal splanchnic blood pooling
- Waist-high compression garments (abdominal binders) during and after meals directly reduce splanchnic blood pooling and can be combined with meal size reduction and upright positioning for additive benefit

24.8 Compression and Meal Strategy

Compression garments are a standard non-pharmacological treatment for POTS (Raj et al., 2020). Full-length graduated compression stockings (30 to 40 mmHg) and abdominal compression binders reduce venous pooling in the legs and splanchnic bed, respectively. During and after meals, abdominal compression is particularly relevant because it counteracts the meal-induced blood flow redistribution to the gut that worsens orthostatic symptoms.

The practical integration with the dietary framework: patients who experience significant postprandial symptoms should apply abdominal compression before eating, maintain it for 30 to 45 minutes after the meal, and combine it with the upright positioning strategy described in Simeon's case. Patients using graduated compression stockings should keep them on throughout the day, including during meals, rather than removing them for comfort while seated.

Compression also supports the exercise-nutrition connection. During the modified Levine Protocol sessions (section 24.1), abdominal compression worn during recumbent exercise improves venous return and exercise tolerance (Bourne et al., 2021). Post-exercise, compression helps mitigate the hemodynamic vulnerability of the recovery window while the patient consumes their recovery smoothie.

24.9 Integrating Lifestyle Factors

The dietary framework presented in Chapters 5.0 through 23.0 was designed to function within the reality of these lifestyle variables, not in isolation from them. The food, the medications, the supplements, the exercise, the sleep, the hormones, and the environment all interact. A meal plan that works at 68°F may fail at 90°F without sodium adjustment. A food tolerance that is stable during the follicular phase may shift during the luteal phase. An exercise session that produces benefit when followed by a recovery smoothie may produce a crash when followed by plain water. A medication that works correctly when timed around meals may fail when taken at the wrong point in the eating schedule.

The practical takeaway is that trifecta management is not a set of isolated interventions. It is a system. The dietary framework is the foundation, but its effectiveness depends on its integration with exercise timing, temperature adaptation, hormonal awareness, sleep support, stress management, body positioning, compression, and medication coordination. The patients who achieve the most stable symptom control are those who understand these connections and adjust their approach based on which variables are shifting on any given day.

Appendix A: Food Reference Lists

The food lists in this appendix consolidate the dietary guidance from Chapters 5.0 through 21.0 into organized, category-based references designed for daily use. These lists are not exhaustive. Individual tolerance varies, and the reintroduction framework from Chapter 7.0 should guide personal modifications. Foods that appear on multiple lists (for example, spinach appears on both the high-histamine and high-oxalate lists) reflect the overlapping dietary considerations that make trifecta nutrition more complex than single-condition management.

All histamine classifications follow the Swiss Interest Group Histamine Intolerance (SIGHI) list and peer-reviewed food chemistry data (Comas-Basté et al., 2020; Maintz & Novak, 2007). Sodium values reference the USDA FoodData Central database. FODMAP classifications follow Monash University FODMAP research (Varney et al., 2017). Oxalate values reference published food oxalate databases (Mitchell et al., 2019).

A.1 Low Histamine Foods

These foods are generally well-tolerated by MCAS and histamine-intolerant patients. Freshness matters: the same food can shift from low to high histamine depending on storage time, temperature, and preparation method (as discussed in section 6.3).

Proteins

- Fresh chicken (cooked and consumed same day, or frozen immediately after cooking)
- Fresh turkey (same freshness rules as chicken)
- Fresh lamb (less commonly reactive than beef or pork)
- Fresh-caught white fish (cod, halibut, sole, tilapia; must be cooked from frozen or consumed within hours of catch)
- Eggs (some patients tolerate egg whites only; yolks are occasionally reactive)
- Fresh pork (consumed same day; avoid processed, cured, or smoked pork products)

Grains and Starches

- White rice and brown rice
- Oats (certified gluten-free if gluten-sensitive)
- Quinoa

- Millet
- Rice pasta and rice noodles
- Sweet potatoes
- White potatoes
- Tapioca and arrowroot starch
- Rice flour and oat flour

Vegetables

- Zucchini and summer squash
- Butternut squash and other winter squashes
- Carrots
- Broccoli (fresh, not leftover)
- Cauliflower (fresh)
- Cucumbers
- Lettuce (all varieties)
- Asparagus
- Green beans
- Celery
- Beets (fresh only)
- Leeks
- Garlic (fresh)
- Onions (fresh; cooked onions are generally better tolerated)
- Bell peppers (green, red, yellow; tolerance varies)

Fruits

- Blueberries
- Blackberries
- Apples (peeled if GI-sensitive)
- Pears
- Peaches (fresh only)
- Cherries (fresh or frozen)
- Mango (fresh or frozen)
- Watermelon
- Grapes (fresh; avoid dried/raisins)
- Figs (fresh only; dried figs are higher histamine)

Fats and Oils

- Extra virgin olive oil
- Coconut oil
- Ghee (clarified butter; milk proteins removed during clarification)

- Avocado oil (note: whole avocados are high histamine, but the refined oil is generally tolerated)
- Flaxseed oil (use cold; do not heat)

Dairy Alternatives

- Coconut milk (full fat, canned; check for carrageenan and guar gum)
- Oat milk (unsweetened, minimal additives)
- Rice milk
- Coconut cream
- Coconut yogurt (if no added cultures that produce histamine)

Herbs, Spices, and Seasonings

- Sea salt and Himalayan pink salt
- Turmeric (fresh or dried)
- Ginger (fresh or dried)
- Basil (fresh)
- Oregano
- Thyme
- Rosemary
- Cardamom
- Cumin
- Coriander
- Parsley
- Sage
- Black pepper (small amounts; some MCAS patients are sensitive)
- Ceylon cinnamon (preferred over cassia for lower coumarin content)

Sweeteners

- Maple syrup (pure, not pancake syrup)
- Raw honey (local if possible; some MCAS patients react to specific pollen profiles)
- Coconut sugar

A.2 High Histamine Foods

These foods contain high levels of histamine, promote histamine release, or block the diamine oxidase (DAO) enzyme that degrades histamine. Avoidance or limitation is recommended during the elimination phase (Chapter 6.0), with systematic reintroduction guided by the protocol in Chapter 7.0 (Comas-Basté et al., 2020; Maintz & Novak, 2007).

High Histamine Content

- Aged cheeses (parmesan, cheddar, gouda, brie, camembert, blue cheese)
- Fermented foods (sauerkraut, kimchi, kombucha, kefir, miso, tempeh)
- Cured and processed meats (salami, pepperoni, hot dogs, bacon, deli meats, jerky)
- Smoked fish (smoked salmon, mackerel, sardines, anchovies)
- Canned fish (tuna, sardines, anchovies)
- Vinegar (especially wine vinegar, balsamic vinegar; apple cider vinegar is sometimes tolerated)
- Soy sauce and tamari
- Fish sauce
- Tomatoes and tomato products (sauce, paste, ketchup)
- Spinach (raw spinach is higher histamine than briefly cooked)
- Eggplant
- Avocado
- Leftover cooked meat (histamine increases with refrigerated storage time)
- Bone broth stored longer than 24 hours (freshly made and immediately frozen is lower histamine)

Histamine Liberators (trigger mast cell release)

- Citrus fruits (oranges, lemons, limes, grapefruit)
- Strawberries
- Pineapple
- Papaya
- Bananas (ripe; green bananas are lower)
- Chocolate and cacao
- Egg whites (in some individuals)
- Shellfish (shrimp, crab, lobster, mussels)
- Peanuts
- Walnuts
- Cashews
- Alcohol (especially red wine, beer, and champagne)
- Artificial food dyes (Red 40, Yellow 5, Yellow 6)
- Sulfites and preservatives (sodium bisulfite, potassium metabisulfite)
- MSG (monosodium glutamate)

DAO Blockers (inhibit histamine degradation)

- Alcohol (all forms)
- Black tea, green tea, mate tea
- Energy drinks

- Certain medications (discussed in Chapter 23.0)

A.3 High Sodium Trifecta Foods

These foods support the 6,000 to 10,000 mg daily sodium target for POTS management (section 5.2) while remaining compatible with the low-histamine framework. Sodium values are approximate and vary by brand and preparation (USDA FoodData Central, 2023).

Naturally Higher Sodium Foods

- Celery (1 cup raw: approximately 80 mg sodium)
- Beets (1 cup cooked: approximately 130 mg sodium)
- Carrots (1 cup raw: approximately 70 mg sodium)
- Sweet potatoes (1 medium: approximately 70 mg sodium)

Salt-Enhanced Trifecta Foods

- Salted rice cakes (per cake: approximately 50 to 100 mg, depending on brand)
- Olives, green (5 olives: approximately 200 to 400 mg; tolerance varies in MCAS)
- Salted nuts and seeds (if individually tolerated): pumpkin seeds, sunflower seeds, macadamia nuts
- Salted sweet potato chips (homemade preferred for ingredient control)
- Bone broth with added salt (1 cup: 400 to 900 mg depending on salt added; use fresh-made or frozen)
- Coconut aminos (1 tbsp: approximately 90 mg; a lower-histamine substitute for soy sauce)
- Miso (if fermented food is tolerated after reintroduction; 1 tbsp: approximately 600 mg)

Sodium-Dense Additions

- Sea salt (1/4 tsp: approximately 575 mg sodium)
- Himalayan pink salt (1/4 tsp: approximately 560 mg sodium)
- Salt tablets (500 to 1,000 mg per tablet; useful for portability)
- Electrolyte drink mix (DIY recipe from section 20.2: approximately 1,150 mg per batch)
- Salted ghee (1 tbsp ghee with 1/8 tsp salt: approximately 290 mg)

Strategic Salt Application Points

The recipes in Chapters 15.0 through 21.0 build sodium into every meal. Beyond those recipes, salt can be added to:

- Morning electrolyte drinks (section 20.2)
- Cooking water for rice, pasta, and potatoes
- Smoothies and recovery drinks (section 20.6)
- Snack items from the portable snack strategies (section 19.3)
- Evening chamomile or herbal tea (a pinch of salt in tea is common in some culinary traditions and adds 100 to 200 mg)

A.4 Low FODMAP Compatible Foods

For trifecta patients with concurrent irritable bowel syndrome (IBS), FODMAP restriction may be necessary alongside histamine management. This list identifies foods that are both low-histamine and low-FODMAP, the overlap zone where both dietary frameworks can coexist (Varney et al., 2017; Monash University, 2023).

Proteins (Low FODMAP and Low Histamine)

- Fresh chicken, turkey, lamb (same freshness rules apply)
- Eggs
- Fresh white fish (from frozen)
- Firm tofu (if soy is tolerated; tofu is low FODMAP in small servings)

Grains (Low FODMAP and Low Histamine)

- White rice
- Oats (1/2 cup serving; larger servings may be moderate FODMAP)
- Quinoa
- Rice noodles and rice pasta
- Millet
- Polenta/cornmeal

Vegetables (Low FODMAP and Low Histamine)

- Carrots
- Zucchini
- Cucumbers
- Green beans
- Bell peppers
- Lettuce (all varieties)
- Potato (white and sweet, peeled)
- Bok choy

- Eggplant (low FODMAP but higher histamine; use cautiously)
- Spinach (low FODMAP but higher histamine; use cautiously)

Fruits (Low FODMAP and Low Histamine)

- Blueberries (1/4 cup serving is low FODMAP)
- Grapes (1 cup)
- Kiwi (if tolerated; some MCAS patients react)
- Cantaloupe (3/4 cup)
- Honeydew melon

Fats (Low FODMAP and Low Histamine)

- Olive oil, coconut oil, ghee
- Pumpkin seeds (1 tbsp serving)
- Macadamia nuts (20 nuts)
- Walnuts (10 halves; but walnuts are a histamine liberator, so caution)

High FODMAP Foods to Avoid in Overlap

- Garlic (high FODMAP fructan; use garlic-infused oil as alternative)
- Onion (high FODMAP fructan; use green parts of scallion only)
- Apples (high FODMAP sorbitol; peel and limit to 1/2 apple if attempting)
- Pears (high FODMAP sorbitol in larger servings)
- Cauliflower (moderate to high FODMAP in larger servings)
- Mushrooms (high FODMAP mannitol)
- Honey (high FODMAP fructose; use maple syrup instead)

A.5 Oxalate Aware Foods

Oxalate awareness is relevant for trifecta patients who experience kidney stones, vulvodynia, or joint crystal deposition. Oxalate restriction is not necessary for all trifecta patients but should be considered when these conditions co-occur (Mitchell et al., 2019).

Higher Oxalate Foods (limit if oxalate-sensitive)

- Spinach (one of the highest oxalate foods; 750+ mg per cup cooked)
- Swiss chard
- Beet greens
- Rhubarb
- Sweet potatoes (moderate to high; 28 mg per medium potato)
- Almonds (122 mg per ounce)

- Cashews (49 mg per ounce)
- Dark chocolate/cacao (high oxalate and high histamine; doubly problematic)
- Peanuts and peanut butter
- Soy products
- Quinoa (moderate; 15 to 20 mg per cup cooked)
- Potatoes (moderate; varies by preparation)
- Berries (moderate in some varieties)

Lower Oxalate Alternatives

- Kale and collard greens (lower oxalate leafy greens replacing spinach)
- Romaine lettuce
- Bok choy
- Broccoli
- Cauliflower
- Zucchini
- Cucumbers
- White rice (very low oxalate)
- Oats (lower than quinoa)
- Macadamia nuts (lowest oxalate nut)
- Pumpkin seeds (lower oxalate than almonds or cashews)
- Coconut (lower oxalate)

Oxalate Management Strategies

- Pairing high-oxalate foods with calcium-rich foods (calcium binds oxalate in the GI tract, reducing absorption)
- Boiling high-oxalate vegetables (reduces oxalate content by 30 to 50% through leaching into cooking water)
- Distributing oxalate intake across meals rather than concentrating in a single meal
- Adequate hydration (Chapter 5.0) supports renal oxalate excretion

A.6 Micronutrient Rich Foods

These lists identify trifecta-compatible foods that are rich in the micronutrients most relevant to POTS, EDS, and MCAS management (as discussed in Chapter 4.0 and Chapter 22.0).

Vitamin C Sources (collagen synthesis and mast cell stabilization)

- Bell peppers, red (1 cup raw: 190 mg)

- Broccoli (1 cup cooked: 100 mg)
- Kale (1 cup cooked: 80 mg)
- Brussels sprouts (1 cup cooked: 75 mg)
- Blueberries (1 cup: 14 mg; also provides anthocyanins)
- Mango (1 cup: 60 mg)
- Pineapple (1 cup: 79 mg; but is a histamine liberator, so tolerance varies)
- Kiwi (1 medium: 64 mg; tolerance varies in MCAS)

Vitamin B12 Sources

- Fresh chicken (3 oz: 0.3 mcg)
- Fresh turkey (3 oz: 0.3 mcg)
- Fresh lamb (3 oz: 2.5 mcg)
- Eggs (1 large: 0.6 mcg)
- Fresh fish from frozen (3 oz cod: 0.9 mcg; 3 oz salmon: 4.8 mcg, but salmon is moderate histamine)
- Nutritional yeast (if tolerated; 1 tbsp fortified: 2.4 mcg; may trigger MCAS in some patients)

Vitamin D Sources (note: dietary sources are limited; supplementation often necessary)

- Egg yolks (1 large: approximately 40 IU)
- Fresh salmon (if tolerated; 3 oz: approximately 570 IU; moderate histamine)
- Cod liver oil (1 tsp: approximately 450 IU; check for additives)
- Fortified coconut or oat milk (varies by brand; typically 100 to 120 IU per cup)
- Mushrooms exposed to UV light (1 cup: approximately 400 IU; but mushrooms are moderate histamine and high FODMAP)

Iron Sources

- Fresh lamb (3 oz: 1.7 mg heme iron)
- Fresh turkey, dark meat (3 oz: 1.1 mg heme iron)
- Fresh chicken thighs (3 oz: 0.9 mg heme iron)
- Pumpkin seeds (1 oz: 2.3 mg non-heme iron)
- Quinoa (1 cup cooked: 2.8 mg non-heme iron)
- Lentils (if tolerated after reintroduction; 1 cup cooked: 6.6 mg non-heme iron; moderate histamine and FODMAP considerations)
- Pair non-heme iron sources with vitamin C to enhance absorption (section 4.3)
- Avoid taking iron with calcium, tea, or coffee, which inhibit absorption

Magnesium Sources

- Pumpkin seeds (1 oz: 168 mg)
- Dark chocolate (if tolerated; 1 oz: 65 mg; but high histamine and oxalate)
- Almonds (1 oz: 80 mg; moderate oxalate)
- Cashews (1 oz: 74 mg; moderate oxalate)
- Quinoa (1 cup cooked: 118 mg)
- Black beans (if tolerated; 1 cup cooked: 120 mg; FODMAP considerations)
- Swiss chard (1 cup cooked: 150 mg; high oxalate)
- Rice (1 cup cooked brown rice: 84 mg)
- Oats (1 cup cooked: 63 mg)
- Coconut milk (1 cup: 44 mg)

Appendix B: Quick Reference Charts

The charts and templates in this appendix are designed to be photocopied, printed, or digitally reproduced for daily use. They consolidate the clinical frameworks from the body of this book into visual tools that support decision-making without requiring the reader to search through chapter text during meal preparation, grocery shopping, or symptom tracking.

B.1 Trifecta Traffic Light Chart

This chart classifies foods into three categories based on their compatibility with the trifecta dietary framework (low-histamine, POTS-supportive sodium, anti-inflammatory, gastroparesis-accommodating). The classifications represent general patterns. Individual tolerance may differ, and the reintroduction protocol from Chapter 7.0 should guide personal modifications.

GREEN (Generally Safe, Well Tolerated)

These foods are low-histamine, anti-inflammatory, and compatible with the trifecta dietary framework for most patients. They form the foundation of the elimination phase (Chapter 6.0) and the core of the long-term maintenance diet.

- Fresh chicken, turkey, lamb (cooked and consumed or frozen same day)
- Fresh white fish (from frozen)
- Eggs (if individually tolerated)
- White rice, brown rice, oats, quinoa, millet
- Sweet potatoes, white potatoes
- Zucchini, carrots, broccoli, cauliflower, green beans, cucumbers, lettuce, celery
- Blueberries, pears, apples (peeled), cherries, mango
- Coconut milk, coconut oil, ghee, olive oil
- Fresh herbs (basil, oregano, thyme, rosemary, parsley)
- Turmeric, ginger, cardamom, cumin
- Maple syrup, raw honey
- Sea salt, Himalayan pink salt

YELLOW (Proceed with Caution, Test Individually)

These foods are tolerated by some trifecta patients but trigger reactions in others. They should be introduced one at a time during the reintroduction phase (Chapter 7.0), with at least 72 hours between each new food trial.

- Bell peppers (especially red and orange)
- Beets (fresh only)
- Asparagus
- Onions (cooked tolerated better than raw)
- Garlic (cooked tolerated better than raw)
- Bone broth (freshly made; histamine increases with storage)
- Pork (fresh only; no processed or cured)
- Salmon and fatty fish (moderate histamine; freshness critical)
- Avocado (histamine liberator, but some patients tolerate small amounts)
- Banana (green/less ripe tolerated better; ripe bananas are histamine liberators)
- Coconut yogurt with live cultures (some cultures produce histamine)
- Walnuts, almonds, cashews (varies by individual)
- Lentils and chickpeas (FODMAP considerations; moderate histamine)
- Nutritional yeast
- Apple cider vinegar (some patients tolerate small amounts)
- Black pepper (small amounts; sensitivity varies)

RED (Avoid During Elimination, Reintroduce Late if at All)

These foods are high-histamine, known histamine liberators, DAO blockers, or contain additives commonly triggering MCAS reactions. They should be strictly avoided during the elimination phase and reintroduced only after stable baseline is established and only with careful monitoring.

- Aged cheeses (all varieties)
- Fermented foods (sauerkraut, kimchi, kombucha, kefir, tempeh, miso)
- Cured and processed meats (salami, bacon, hot dogs, deli meats, jerky)
- Canned and smoked fish
- Shellfish
- Tomatoes and tomato products
- Spinach (raw; briefly cooked is lower histamine but still moderate)
- Eggplant
- Citrus fruits (oranges, lemons, limes, grapefruit)
- Strawberries, pineapple, papaya
- Chocolate and cacao
- Soy sauce, fish sauce, vinegar (wine and balsamic)
- Alcohol (all forms)
- Black tea, green tea, mate tea
- Peanuts
- Artificial food dyes, sulfites, MSG
- Leftover cooked meat (longer than 24 hours refrigerated)

B.2 Daily Tracking Template

This template can be photocopied or recreated in a notebook, spreadsheet, or digital note. It integrates the food, symptom, and medication tracking discussed in Chapter 12.0.

Date: _______________ Cycle Day (if applicable): _______________

Morning

- Time woke: _______
- Resting heart rate (lying): _______ bpm
- Standing heart rate (after 1 min): _______ bpm
- Morning medications and timing: ____
- Morning supplements: ____
- Morning electrolyte/drink: ____
- Breakfast foods: ____
- Breakfast sodium estimate: _______ mg

Midday

- Snack 1 foods and time: ____
- Lunch foods and time: ____
- Lunch sodium estimate: _______ mg
- Midday medications/supplements: ____
- Electrolyte intake since morning: _______ oz

Afternoon and Evening

- Snack 2 foods and time: ____
- Dinner foods and time: ____
- Dinner sodium estimate: _______ mg
- Evening medications/supplements: ____
- Evening drink: ____

Daily Totals (estimated)

- Total sodium: _______ mg (target: 6,000 to 10,000 mg)
- Total fluid: _______ oz (target: 80 to 100 oz with electrolytes)
- Total calories (if tracking): _______

Symptom Tracking

Rate each 0 (absent) to 5 (severe):

- Fatigue: ___ / 5
- Brain fog: ___ / 5
- Dizziness/lightheadedness: ___ / 5
- Heart palpitations: ___ / 5
- Nausea: ___ / 5
- GI symptoms (bloating/cramping/diarrhea): ___ / 5
- Flushing: ___ / 5
- Headache: ___ / 5
- Joint pain/hypermobility pain: ___ / 5
- Skin symptoms (hives/itching/rash): ___ / 5
- Anxiety: ___ / 5
- Overall POTS severity: ___ / 5
- Overall MCAS severity: ___ / 5
- Overall EDS pain: ___ / 5

Notes

- New food introduced today: ____
- Reaction to new food (if any): ____
- Exercise type and duration: ____
- Heat exposure: ____
- Stress level (1 to 5): ___
- Sleep quality last night (1 to 5): ___
- Hours slept: _______
- Any notable events or observations: ____

B.3 Weekly Meal Planning Template

This template supports the meal planning framework from Chapters 11.0 and 13.0. It includes columns for sodium tracking and batch preparation notes.

Week of: _______________

Batch Prep Day (suggested: Sunday or day off)

- Protein prepared: ____
- Grains cooked: ____
- Vegetables prepped: ____
- Electrolyte concentrate made: ____
- Snacks prepared: ____
- Broth made and portioned: ____

•	Breakfast	Snack 1	Lunch	Snack 2	Dinner	Evening Drink	Est. Na (mg)
Mon							
Tue							
Wed							
Thu							
Fri							
Sat							
Sun							

Shopping List (organized by store section)

Produce: ____

Proteins: ____

Grains/Pantry: ____

Frozen: ____

Oils/Fats: ____

Supplements/Electrolytes:

____

B.4 Symptom Severity Scale

This standardized scale (adapted from clinical tools used in POTS, MCAS, and chronic pain assessment) provides consistent language for communicating with healthcare providers and for tracking trends over time in the daily journal.

0 = Absent. No symptoms. Fully functional. Baseline feels normal.

1 = Mild. Symptoms present but do not interfere with daily activities. Aware of symptoms only when paying attention. Can complete all planned tasks without modification.

2 = Moderate. Symptoms noticeable and occasionally distracting. May need to slow down or take brief rests. Can complete most planned tasks but with increased effort. May need to avoid one or two known triggers.

3 = Moderately Severe. Symptoms interfere with daily function. Need to modify or cancel some activities. Difficulty concentrating. Physical symptoms require active management (lying down, extra electrolytes, medication). Can still perform basic self-care and some tasks.

4 = Severe. Symptoms dominate the day. Unable to perform most planned activities. Need prolonged rest periods. Physical symptoms are distressing (notable tachycardia, pre-syncope, active MCAS flare with multiple organ system involvement, severe pain). Basic self-care possible but effortful.

5 = Crisis. Symptoms at maximum intensity. Unable to function. May require emergency intervention (IV fluids, epinephrine, emergency department visit). Unable to perform self-care. This level represents the worst the condition produces.

Using the Scale

The goal of tracking is not to reach zero on every measure every day. For most trifecta patients, daily scores of 1 to 2 across most categories represent a stable, well-managed baseline. The tracking value comes from identifying trends: a gradual increase from baseline 1 to baseline 2 over two weeks may indicate a dietary trigger, medication change, hormonal shift (section 24.3), or seasonal heat increase (section 24.2). The scale also provides standardized language for healthcare visits: "My average POTS severity this month has been 2, up from 1 last month" communicates more useful information than "I've been feeling worse."

B.5 Electrolyte Comparison Chart

This chart compares the DIY electrolyte recipes from Chapter 20.0 with common commercial products. Values are approximate and represent a single serving.

Product	Sodium (mg)	Potassium (mg)	Sugar (g)	Calories	Histamine Risk	Monthly Cost (4/day)
DIY Electrolyte Base (section 20.2)	1,150 per batch (4 servings) / 288 per serving	350 per batch / 88 per serving	15 per batch / 3.75 per serving	60 per batch / 15 per serving	Very Low (5 known ingredients)	$10 to $15
LMNT (unflavored)	1,000	200	0	0	Low (minimal ingredients)	$120 to $150
Liquid IV	500	370	11	45	Moderate (natural flavors, citric acid)	$90 to $120
Drip Drop	330	185	7	35	Moderate (citric acid, natural flavors, sucralose)	$80 to $100
Nuun Sport	300	150	1	10	Moderate to High (citric acid, dyes in some flavors)	$45 to $60
Pedialyte	370	280	9	35	Moderate (artificial sweeteners, dyes in original)	$100 to $150
Gatorade	270	75	34	140	High (dyes, citric acid, high sugar)	$60 to $90
Coconut Water + 1/4 tsp salt	690 (575 from salt + 115 natural)	600 (natural)	12 (natural)	50	Low (2 ingredients)	$40 to $60

Reading This Chart

Sodium per serving is the most relevant column for POTS management. At four servings daily, the DIY recipe provides approximately 1,150 mg of sodium from drinks alone, supplementing the 5,000 to 8,000 mg consumed through food. Commercial products vary widely in sodium content, and many do not provide enough sodium per serving to meaningfully support POTS patients without consuming multiple servings (at proportionally higher cost).

Histamine risk reflects the presence of known MCAS triggers in the ingredient list: citric acid (a common mast cell trigger distinct from citrus fruit), artificial sweeteners, artificial dyes, and "natural flavors" (a proprietary umbrella term that may contain any number of undisclosed compounds). The DIY recipe scores lowest because every ingredient is known and individually testable for tolerance.

Monthly cost assumes four servings daily, the minimum recommended intake pattern for consistent POTS hydration support. The annual cost difference between DIY ($120 to $180) and mid-range commercial products ($1,000 to $1,500) is $800 to $1,300, which represents a meaningful financial burden for patients already managing high medical costs.

Appendix C: Resources and Support

This appendix lists organizations, professional directories, and educational resources relevant to the trifecta conditions. These organizations were active and accessible at the time of publication. Contact information, programs, and resources may change over time.

C.1 Dysautonomia Organizations

Dysautonomia International

Dysautonomia International is a nonprofit organization focused on research funding, physician education, and patient support for all forms of dysautonomia, including POTS. Their programs include a physician directory (searchable by location and condition), annual research grants, a medical conference for providers and researchers, and patient education materials. They maintain one of the most frequently updated lists of POTS-knowledgeable physicians in the United States and internationally.

Website: www.dysautonomiainternational.org

Standing Up to POTS

Standing Up to POTS is a nonprofit focused specifically on postural orthostatic tachycardia syndrome. Their resources include educational materials written for patients and families, a research initiative tracking POTS prevalence and demographics, exercise guideline summaries (including the Dallas Protocol and CHOP Protocol referenced in section 24.1), and a healthcare provider directory. Their website includes dietary guidance pages that align with many of the sodium and hydration principles covered in Chapter 5.0.

Website: www.standinguptopots.org

C.2 Ehlers Danlos Organizations

The Ehlers-Danlos Society

The Ehlers-Danlos Society is the primary international organization for EDS education, research, and support. Their resources include the 2017 International Classification of the Ehlers-Danlos Syndromes (the current diagnostic framework), a healthcare provider directory searchable by specialty and location, virtual and in-person support groups, educational webinars for patients and providers, and research funding programs. They also maintain clinical guidelines for EDS subtypes and frequently co-publish with researchers studying the overlap between EDS, POTS, and MCAS.

Website: www.ehlers-danlos.com

C.3 Mast Cell Organizations

The Mast Cell Disease Society (TMS)

TMS (formerly The Mastocytosis Society) is a nonprofit focused on mast cell diseases including mastocytosis and mast cell activation syndrome (MCAS). Their programs include patient and provider education, a physician referral list, support group coordination, and research advocacy. They provide educational materials explaining the distinction between mastocytosis (a clonal mast cell proliferative disorder) and MCAS (a mast cell activation disorder without clonal proliferation), a distinction that affects treatment approach and prognosis.

Website: www.tmsforacure.org

Mast Cell Action

Mast Cell Action is a UK-based charity supporting individuals with mast cell disorders. Their resources include patient guides, healthcare provider education materials, a support community, and advocacy for improved access to diagnosis and treatment in the National Health Service. For international readers, Mast Cell Action provides educational materials that complement the US-focused resources from TMS.

Website: www.mastcellaction.org

C.4 Finding Specialized Practitioners

The dietary framework in this book was designed to complement medical care, not replace it. Working with healthcare providers who understand trifecta conditions produces better outcomes than self-directed management alone. The following guidance helps readers identify and access specialized practitioners.

Finding a Registered Dietitian

A registered dietitian (RD) or registered dietitian nutritionist (RDN) with experience in MCAS, POTS, or EDS can personalize the dietary framework in this book to individual needs. To find a specialized dietitian:

- The Academy of Nutrition and Dietetics maintains a searchable provider directory (www.eatright.org) that allows filtering by specialty area
- The Ehlers-Danlos Society and Dysautonomia International provider directories sometimes include dietitians alongside physicians
- Ask your primary POTS, EDS, or MCAS specialist for dietitian referrals; many academic medical centers with dysautonomia or mast cell programs have affiliated dietitians
- Telehealth-based dietitians with trifecta experience can serve patients in areas without local specialists

Questions to ask a prospective dietitian:

- Do you have experience working with patients who have POTS, EDS, or MCAS?
- Are you familiar with low-histamine dietary protocols?
- How do you approach the high-sodium dietary requirements for POTS?
- Do you coordinate with prescribing physicians regarding medication and food timing interactions?
- Are you familiar with the intersection of elimination diets and disordered eating risk in chronic illness populations?

Finding Medical Specialists

- For POTS: cardiologists or neurologists specializing in autonomic disorders. Dysautonomia International's directory is the most widely used resource.
- For EDS: geneticists for diagnosis, physiatrists or physical medicine and rehabilitation physicians for ongoing management, physical therapists trained in hypermobility (the Ehlers-Danlos Society directory includes physical therapists).
- For MCAS: allergists/immunologists with mast cell disease experience. Some patients find that hematologists with mastocytosis experience also manage MCAS effectively. TMS maintains a referral list.

Coordinating Care Across Specialists

Trifecta patients often see multiple specialists who may not communicate with each other. The medication timing framework from Chapter 23.0 and the dietary framework from this book create coordination challenges that are best managed by one clinician (often the primary care provider or the dietitian) who maintains oversight of the complete picture. Patients can facilitate this coordination by:

- Sharing the daily timeline (like the index card from Remigius's case in section 23.4) with all providers
- Bringing the food and symptom journal (Chapter 12.0) to specialist appointments
- Requesting that specialists send records and recommendations to the coordinating provider
- Asking each specialist how their recommendations interact with the dietary and medication frameworks already in place

C.5 Additional Educational Resources

Published Clinical Guidelines

- 2017 International Classification of the Ehlers-Danlos Syndromes (Malfait et al., 2017)
- Canadian Cardiovascular Society Position Statement on POTS (Raj et al., 2020)
- Proposed Diagnostic Criteria for MCAS (Afrin et al., 2020; Valent et al., 2019)
- European Academy of Allergy and Clinical Immunology Histamine Intolerance Task Force (Comas-Basté et al., 2020)

Exercise Protocols Referenced in This Book

- The Dallas Protocol (Modified Levine Protocol) for POTS exercise reconditioning (Fu et al., 2010). The original research group at the University of Texas Southwestern Medical Center has published the exercise protocol guidelines. Dysautonomia International and Standing Up to POTS provide patient-accessible summaries.
- The CHOP Protocol (Children's Hospital of Philadelphia) for adolescent and young adult POTS reconditioning (Pianosi et al., 2016). Protocol details are available through the CHOP Autonomic Program website.

Peer-Reviewed Journals Publishing Trifecta Research

- *Autonomic Neuroscience* (dysautonomia-focused research)
- *Journal of Allergy and Clinical Immunology* (mast cell disease research)
- *American Journal of Medical Genetics* (EDS genetics and classification)
- *Clinical Nutrition* (dietary interventions including histamine intolerance)
- *Nutrients* (micronutrient and supplement research)

References

Adolphus, K., Lawton, C. L., & Dye, L. (2013). The effects of breakfast on behavior and academic performance in children and adolescents. Frontiers in Human Neuroscience, 7, 425.

Afrin, L. B. (2016). Never bet against Occam: Mast cell activation disease and the modern epidemics of chronic illness and medical complexity. Sisters Media.

Afrin, L. B., Ackerley, M. B., Bluestein, L. S., et al. (2020). Diagnosis of mast cell activation syndrome: A global "consensus-2." Diagnosis, 8(2), 137-152.

Afrin, L. B., Butterfield, J. H., Raithel, M., & Molderings, G. J. (2016). Often seen, rarely recognized: Mast cell activation disease, a guide to diagnosis and therapeutic options. Annals of Medicine, 48(3), 190-201.

Afrin, L. B., Self, S., Menk, J., & Lazarchick, J. (2016). Characterization of mast cell activation syndrome. American Journal of the Medical Sciences, 353(3), 207-215.

Almeida, M. C., Vizin, R. C., & Carrettiero, D. C. (2015). Current understanding on the neurophysiology of behavioral thermoregulation. Temperature, 2(4), 483-490.

American Heart Association. (2024). How much sodium should I eat per day?

Amma, K. P., Rani, M. P., Sasidharan, I., & Nisha, V. N. P. (2010). Chemical composition, flavonoid-phenolic contents and radical scavenging activity of four major varieties of cardamom. International Journal of Biological and Medical Research, 1(3), 20-24.

Antiel, R. M., Caudill, J. S., Burkhardt, B. E., Brands, C. K., & Fischer, P. R. (2011). Iron insufficiency and hypovitaminosis D in adolescents with chronic fatigue and orthostatic intolerance. Southern Medical Journal, 104(8), 609-611.

Arnold, A. C., Haman, K., Garland, E. M., et al. (2015). Cognitive dysfunction in postural tachycardia syndrome. Clinical Science, 128(1), 39-45.

Atkinson, F. S., Foster-Powell, K., & Brand-Miller, J. C. (2008). International tables of glycemic index and glycemic load values: 2008. Diabetes Care, 31(12), 2281-2283.

Aune, D., Giovannucci, E., Boffetta, P., et al. (2017). Fruit and vegetable intake and the risk of cardiovascular disease, total cancer and all-cause mortality: A systematic review and dose-response meta-analysis of prospective studies. International Journal of Epidemiology, 46(3), 1029-1056.

Baker, L. B. (2017). Sweating rate and sweat sodium concentration in athletes: A review of methodology and intra/interindividual variability. Sports Medicine, 47(Suppl 1), 111-128.

Bateman, D. N. (1982). Effects of meal temperature and volume on the emptying of liquid from the human stomach. Journal of Physiology, 331, 461-467.

Bauer, J., Kuehnl, S., Rollinger, J. M., et al. (2012). Carnosol and carnosic acids from Salvia officinalis inhibit microsomal prostaglandin E2 synthase-1. Journal of Pharmacology and Experimental Therapeutics, 342(1), 169-176.

Beauchamp, G. K. (2009). Sensory and receptor responses to umami: An overview of pioneering work. American Journal of Clinical Nutrition, 90(3), 723S-727S.

Beauchamp, G. K., Keast, R. S. J., Morel, D., et al. (2005). Ibuprofen-like activity in extra-virgin olive oil. Nature, 437(7055), 45-46.

Beckers, A. B., Keszthelyi, D., Vork, L., et al. (2021). The role of histamine in irritable bowel syndrome-like symptoms: A systematic review. Neurogastroenterology and Motility, 33(6), e14159.

Bettendorff, L. (2013). Thiamine. In Present knowledge in nutrition (10th ed., pp. 261-279). Wiley-Blackwell.

Binder, H. J., Brown, I., Ramakrishna, B. S., & Young, G. P. (2014). Oral rehydration therapy in the second decade of the twenty-first century. Current Gastroenterology Reports, 16(3), 376.

Björnson, M., Wijnbladh, K., Törnberg, A., et al. (2025). Prevalence and clinical impact of postural orthostatic tachycardia syndrome in highly symptomatic long COVID. Circulation: Arrhythmia and Electrophysiology, 18(10), e013629.

Blitshteyn, S. (2018). Vitamin B1 deficiency in patients with postural tachycardia syndrome (POTS). Neurological Research, 40(10), 828-831.

Blitshteyn, S., & Whitelaw, S. (2021). Postural orthostatic tachycardia syndrome (POTS) and other autonomic disorders after COVID-19 infection: A case series of 20 patients. Immunologic Research, 69(2), 211-219.

Bonds, R. S., & Bhatt, P. A. (2022). Sex differences in mast cell biology and pathology. The Journal of Allergy and Clinical Immunology: In Practice, 10(4), 944-951.

Boots, A. W., Haenen, G. R., & Bast, A. (2008). Health effects of quercetin: From antioxidant to nutraceutical. European Journal of Pharmacology, 585(2-3), 325-337.

Bourne, K. M., Sheldon, R. S., Hall, J., et al. (2021). Compression garment reduces orthostatic tachycardia and symptoms in patients with postural orthostatic tachycardia syndrome. Journal of the American College of Cardiology, 77(3), 285-296.

Bouzari, A., Holstege, D., & Barrett, D. M. (2015). Mineral, fiber, and total phenolic retention in eight fruits and vegetables: A comparison of refrigerated and frozen storage. Journal of Agricultural and Food Chemistry, 63(3), 951-956.

Brand-Miller, J. C., Stockmann, K., Atkinson, F., Petocz, P., & Denyer, G. (2009). Glycemic index, postprandial glycemia, and the shape of the curve in healthy subjects: Analysis of a database of more than 1,000 foods. American Journal of Clinical Nutrition, 89(1), 97-105.

Breslin, P. A. S., & Beauchamp, G. K. (1997). Salt enhances flavour by suppressing bitterness. Nature, 387(6633), 563.

British Dietetic Association. (2023). PoTS: How can a dietitian help to support those with postural tachycardia syndrome?

Bryarly, M., Phillips, L. T., Fu, Q., Vernino, S., & Levine, B. D. (2019). Postural orthostatic tachycardia syndrome: JACC focus seminar. Journal of the American College of Cardiology, 73(10), 1207–1228.

Butawan, M., Benjamin, R. L., & Bloomer, R. J. (2017). Methylsulfonylmethane: Applications and safety of a novel dietary supplement. Nutrients, 9(3), 290.

Calder, P. C. (2015). Marine omega-3 fatty acids and inflammatory processes: Effects, mechanisms and clinical relevance. Biochimica et Biophysica Acta, 1851(4), 469-484.

Calder, P. C. (2017). Omega-3 fatty acids and inflammatory processes: From molecules to man. Biochemical Society Transactions, 45(5), 1105-1115.

Carr, A. C., & Maggini, S. (2017). Vitamin C and immune function. Nutrients, 9(11), 1211.

Cassidy, A., Rogers, G., Peterson, J. J., et al. (2015). Higher dietary anthocyanin and flavonol intakes are associated with anti-inflammatory effects in a population of US adults. American Journal of Clinical Nutrition, 102(1), 172-181.

Castells, M. (2017). Diagnosis and management of anaphylaxis in precision medicine. Journal of Allergy and Clinical Immunology, 140(2), 321-333.

Castori, M., Morlino, S., Celletti, C., Ghibellini, G., Bruschini, M., Grammatico, P., Blundo, C., & Camerota, F. (2012). Re-writing the natural history of pain and related symptoms in the joint hypermobility syndrome/Ehlers-Danlos syndrome, hypermobility type. American Journal of Medical Genetics Part A, 158A(9), 2368-2373.

Cheung, I., & Vadas, P. (2015). A new disease cluster: Mast cell activation syndrome, postural orthostatic tachycardia syndrome, and Ehlers-Danlos syndrome. Journal of Allergy and Clinical Immunology, 135(2), AB65.

Cheungpasitporn, W., Thongprayoon, C., Kittanamongkolchai, W., et al. (2015). Proton pump inhibitors linked to hypomagnesemia: A systematic review and meta-analysis of observational studies. Renal Failure, 37(7), 1237-1241.

Chopra, P., Tinkle, B., Hamonet, C., et al. (2017). Pain management in the Ehlers-Danlos syndromes. American Journal of Medical Genetics Part C: Seminars in Medical Genetics, 175(1), 212-219.

Choudhary, A., Fikree, A., & Aziz, Q. (2021). Overlap between irritable bowel syndrome and hypermobile Ehlers-Danlos syndrome: An unexplored clinical phenotype? American Journal of Medical Genetics Part C: Seminars in Medical Genetics, 187(4), 561-569.

Clark, K. L., Sebastianelli, W., Flechsenhar, K. R., et al. (2008). 24-week study on the use of collagen hydrolysate as a dietary supplement in athletes with activity-related joint pain. Current Medical Research and Opinion, 24(5), 1485-1496.

Cleveland Clinic. (2022). Postural orthostatic tachycardia syndrome (POTS).

Cohen, P. A. (2014). Hazards of hindsight: Monitoring the safety of nutritional supplements. New England Journal of Medicine, 370(14), 1277-1280.

Comas-Basté, O., Sánchez-Pérez, S., Veciana-Nogués, M. T., Latorre-Moratalla, M. L., & Vidal-Carou, M. D. C. (2020). Histamine intolerance: The current state of the art. Biomolecules, 10(8), 1181.

Crandall, C. G., & González-Alonso, J. (2010). Cardiovascular function in the heat-stressed human. Acta Physiologica, 199(4), 407-423.

Daily, J. W., Yang, M., & Park, S. (2016). Efficacy of turmeric extracts and curcumin for alleviating the symptoms of joint arthritis: A systematic review and meta-analysis. Journal of Medicinal Food, 19(8), 717-729.

Dansinger, M. L., Gleason, J. A., Griffith, J. L., Selker, H. P., & Schaefer, E. J. (2005). Comparison of the Atkins, Ornish, Weight Watchers, and Zone diets for weight loss and heart disease risk reduction. Journal of the American Medical Association, 293(1), 43-53.

de Baaij, J. H. F., Hoenderop, J. G. J., & Bindels, R. J. M. (2015). Magnesium in man: Implications for health and disease. Physiological Reviews, 95(1), 1-46.

DeFronzo, R. A., Cooke, C. R., Andres, R., Faloona, G. R., & Davis, P. J. (1976). The effect of insulin on renal handling of sodium, potassium, calcium, and phosphate in man. Journal of Clinical Investigation, 55(4), 845-855.

Della Corte, K. W., Perrar, I., Penczynski, K. J., Schwingshackl, L., Herder, C., & Buyken, A. E. (2018). Effect of dietary sugar intake on biomarkers of subclinical inflammation: A systematic review and meta-analysis of intervention studies. Nutrients, 10(5), 606.

Dev, S., Mizugishi, K., Bhatt, A. S., et al. (2008). Regulatory effects of Bifidobacterium infantis on allergic diseases. Allergy, 63(9), 1167–1172.

DiBaise, J. K., Harris, L. A., & Goodman, B. (2019). Postural tachycardia syndrome (POTS) and the GI tract: A primer for the gastroenterologist. American Journal of Gastroenterology, 114(8), 1185-1192.

Dresser, G. K., Bailey, D. G., Leake, B. F., et al. (2002). Fruit juices inhibit organic anion transporting polypeptide-mediated drug uptake to decrease the oral availability of fexofenadine. Clinical Pharmacology & Therapeutics, 71(1), 11-20.

Dulal, D., Maraey, A., Elsharnoby, H., Chacko, P., & Grubb, B. (2025). Impact of COVID-19 pandemic on the incidence and prevalence of postural orthostatic tachycardia syndrome. European Heart Journal – Quality of Care and Clinical Outcomes, 11(5), 698–704.

Duncanson, K. R., Talley, N. J., Walker, M. M., & Burrows, T. L. (2021). Food and functional dyspepsia: A systematic review. Journal of Human Nutrition and Dietetics, 31(3), 390-407.

Eshak, E. S., & Arafa, A. E. (2020). Thiamine deficiency and cardiovascular disorders. Nutrition, Metabolism and Cardiovascular Diseases, 30(8), 1303-1310.

Fikree, A., Aziz, Q., & Grahame, R. (2013). Joint hypermobility syndrome. Rheumatic Disease Clinics of North America, 39(2), 419-430.

Fikree, A., Chelimsky, G., Collins, H., Kovacic, K., & Aziz, Q. (2017). Gastrointestinal involvement in the Ehlers-Danlos syndromes. American Journal of Medical Genetics Part C: Seminars in Medical Genetics, 175(1), 181-187.

Flanagan, J. L., Simmons, P. A., Vehige, J., Willcox, M. D., & Garrett, Q. (2010). Role of carnitine in disease. Nutrition & Metabolism, 7, 30.

Fu, Q., VanGundy, T. B., Galbreath, M. M., et al. (2010). Cardiac origins of the postural orthostatic tachycardia syndrome. Journal of the American College of Cardiology, 55(25), 2858-2868.

Ganesh, R., Bonnes, S. L., & DiBaise, J. K. (2020). Postural tachycardia syndrome: Nutrition implications. Nutrition in Clinical Practice, 35(5), 818-825.

Garland, E. M., Gamboa, A., Nwazue, V. C., et al. (2021). Effects of high dietary sodium intake in patients with postural tachycardia syndrome. Journal of the American Heart Association, 10(4), e016620.

Gazit, Y., Nahir, A. M., Grahame, R., & Jacob, G. (2003). Dysautonomia in the joint hypermobility syndrome. The American Journal of Medicine, 115(1), 33–40.

Gdynia, H. J., Muller, T., Sperfeld, A. D., et al. (2008). Severe sensorimotor neuropathy after intake of highest dosages of vitamin B6. Neuromuscular Disorders, 18(2), 156-158.

Gensemer, C., Burks, R., Kauber, M., et al. (2021). Hypermobile Ehlers-Danlos syndromes: Complex phenotypes, challenging diagnoses, and poorly understood causes. Developmental Dynamics, 250(3), 318-344.

Giacosa, A., Morazzoni, P., Bombardelli, E., Riva, A., Bianchi Porro, G., & Rondanelli, M. (2015). Can nausea and vomiting be treated with ginger extract? European Review for Medical and Pharmacological Sciences, 19(7), 1291-1296.

Gibbon, J. R., Frith, J., Raj, S. R., & Newton, J. L. (2021). The effects of caffeine in adults with neurogenic orthostatic hypotension: A systematic review. Clinical Autonomic Research, 31(4), 499-508.

Grand View Research. (2023). Dietary supplements market size, share and trends analysis report.

Grubb, B. P. (2008). Postural tachycardia syndrome. Circulation, 117(21), 2814–2817.

Gröber, U., Kisters, K., & Schmidt, J. (2013). Neuroenhancement with vitamin B12: Underestimated neurological significance. Nutrients, 5(12), 5031-5045.

Gröber, U., Schmidt, J., & Kisters, K. (2015). Magnesium in prevention and therapy. Nutrients, 7(9), 8199-8226.

Guerrera, M. P., Volpe, S. L., & Mao, J. J. (2009). Therapeutic uses of magnesium. American Family Physician, 80(2), 157-162.

Gunathilake, K. D. P. P., Yalegama, C., & Kumara, A. A. N. (2009). Use of coconut flour as a source of protein and dietary fiber in wheat bread. Asian Journal of Food and Agro-Industry, 2(3), 382-391.

Gunawardena, D., Karunaweera, N., Lee, S., et al. (2015). Anti-inflammatory activity of cinnamon (C. zeylanicum and C. cassia) extracts: Identification of E-cinnamaldehyde and o-methoxy cinnamaldehyde as the most potent bioactive compounds. Food & Function, 6(3), 910-919.

Gunning, W. T., Kvale, H., Kramer, P. M., Karabin, B. L., & Grubb, B. P. (2019). Postural orthostatic tachycardia syndrome is associated with elevated G-protein coupled receptor autoantibodies. Journal of the American Heart Association, 8(18), e013602.

Haddad, E. H., Sabate, J., & Whitten, C. G. (2006). Pecan consumption alters serum lipids of hypercholesterolemic men and women. Journal of Nutrition, 136(4), 957-961.

Hagel, A. F., Layritz, C. M., Hagel, W. H., et al. (2013). Intravenous infusion of ascorbic acid decreases serum histamine concentrations in patients with allergic and non-allergic diseases. Naunyn-Schmiedeberg's Archives of Pharmacology, 386(9), 789-793.

Hakim, A., De Wandele, I., O'Callaghan, C., Pocinki, A., & Rowe, P. (2017). Chronic fatigue in Ehlers-Danlos syndrome, hypermobile type. American Journal of Medical Genetics Part C: Seminars in Medical Genetics, 175(1), 175-180.

Hall, N. J., Rubin, G., & Charnock, A. (2009). Systematic review: Adherence to a gluten-free diet in adult patients with coeliac disease. Alimentary Pharmacology & Therapeutics, 30(4), 315-330.

Halmos, E. P., Power, V. A., Shepherd, S. J., Gibson, P. R., & Muir, J. G. (2014). A diet low in FODMAPs reduces symptoms of irritable bowel syndrome. Gastroenterology, 146(1), 67-75.

Harris, C. I. (2022). COVID-19 increases the prevalence of postural orthostatic tachycardia syndrome: What nutrition and dietetics practitioners need to know. Journal of the Academy of Nutrition and Dietetics, 122(9), 1600-1605.

Heidelbaugh, J. J. (2013). Proton pump inhibitors and risk of vitamin and mineral deficiency: Evidence and clinical implications. Therapeutic Advances in Drug Safety, 4(3), 125-133.

Hewlings, S. J., & Kalman, D. S. (2017). Curcumin: A review of its effects on human health. Foods, 6(10), 92.

Hsu, D. J., Lee, C. W., Tsai, W. C., & Chien, Y. C. (2017). Essential and toxic metals in animal bone broths. Food and Nutrition Research, 61(1), 1347478.

Huang, Z., Liu, Y., Qi, G., Brand, D., & Zheng, S. G. (2018). Role of vitamin A in the immune system. Journal of Clinical Medicine, 7(9), 258.

Irwin, M. R., Olmstead, R., & Carroll, J. E. (2016). Sleep disturbance, sleep duration, and inflammation: A systematic review and meta-analysis of cohort studies and experimental sleep deprivation. Biological Psychiatry, 80(1), 40-52.

Izquierdo-Casas, J., Comas-Basté, O., Latorre-Moratalla, M. L., et al. (2019). Diamine oxidase (DAO) supplement reduces headache in episodic migraine patients with DAO deficiency: A randomized double-blind trial. Clinical Nutrition, 38(1), 152-158.

Jaeger, S. R., Rasmussen, M. A., & Prescott, J. (2021). Relationships between food neophobia and food intake and preferences: Findings from a sample of New Zealand adults. Appetite, 116, 410-422.

Jafarinia, M., Sadat Hosseini, M., Kasiri, N., et al. (2020). Quercetin with the potential effect on allergic diseases. Allergy, Asthma & Clinical Immunology, 16, 36.

Jason, L. A., Evans, M., Brown, M., & Porter, N. (2010). What is fatigue? Pathological and nonpathological fatigue. PM&R, 2(5), 327-331.

Johnston, C. S., Martin, L. J., & Cai, X. (1996). Antihistamine effect of supplemental ascorbic acid and neutrophil chemotaxis. Journal of the American College of Nutrition, 11(2), 172-176.

Joneja, J. V. (2017). The beginner's guide to histamine intolerance. Berrydales Books.

Joubert, E., Gelderblom, W. C. A., Louw, A., & de Beer, D. (2008). South African herbal teas: Aspalathus linearis, Cyclopia spp. and Athrixia phylicoides. A review. Journal of Ethnopharmacology, 119(3), 376-412.

Jugdaohsingh, R. (2007). Silicon and bone health. Journal of Nutrition, Health & Aging, 11(2), 99-110.

Kalman, D. S., Feldman, S., Krieger, D. R., & Bloomer, R. J. (2012). Comparison of coconut water and a carbohydrate-electrolyte sport drink on measures of hydration and physical performance in exercise-trained men. Journal of the International Society of Sports Nutrition, 9(1), 1.

Kalt, W., Cassidy, A., Howard, L. R., et al. (2020). Recent research on the health benefits of blueberries and their anthocyanins. Advances in Nutrition, 11(2), 224-236.

Kell, D. B., & Pretorius, E. (2014). Serum ferritin is an important inflammatory disease marker, as it is mainly a leakage product from damaged cells. Metallomics, 6(4), 748-773.

Khanna, R., MacDonald, J. K., & Levesque, B. G. (2014). Peppermint oil for the treatment of irritable bowel syndrome: A systematic review and meta-analysis. Journal of Clinical Gastroenterology, 48(6), 505-512.

Killer, S. C., Blannin, A. K., & Jeukendrup, A. E. (2014). No evidence of dehydration with moderate daily coffee intake: A counterbalanced cross-over study in a free-living population. PLoS ONE, 9(1), e84154.

Koutsos, A., Tuohy, K. M., & Lovegrove, J. A. (2015). Apples and cardiovascular health: Is the gut microbiota a core consideration? Nutrients, 7(6), 3959-3998.

Kovacova-Hanuskova, E., Buday, T., Gavliakova, S., & Plevkova, J. (2015). Histamine, histamine intoxication and intolerance. Allergologia et Immunopathologia, 43(5), 498-506.

Kreydiyyeh, S. I., & Usta, J. (2002). Diuretic effect and mechanism of action of parsley. Journal of Ethnopharmacology, 79(3), 353-357.

Lally, P., van Jaarsveld, C. H. M., Potts, H. W. W., & Wardle, J. (2010). How are habits formed: Modelling habit formation in the real world. European Journal of Social Psychology, 40(6), 998-1009.

Lam, C. Y., Palsson, O. S., Whitehead, W. E., Sperber, A. D., Tornblom, H., Simren, M., & Aziz, Q. (2021). Rome IV functional gastrointestinal disorders and health impairment in subjects with hypermobility spectrum disorders or hypermobile Ehlers-Danlos syndrome. Clinical Gastroenterology and Hepatology, 19(2), 277-287.

Lam, J. R., Schneider, J. L., Quesenberry, C. P., & Corley, D. A. (2017). Proton pump inhibitor and histamine-2 receptor antagonist use and iron deficiency. Gastroenterology, 152(4), 821-829.

Lam, J. R., Schneider, J. L., Zhao, W., & Corley, D. A. (2013). Proton pump inhibitor and histamine 2 receptor antagonist use and vitamin B12 deficiency. JAMA, 310(22), 2435-2442.

Lee, E. J., Ji, G. E., & Sung, M. K. (2007). Quercetin and kaempferol suppress immunoglobulin E-mediated allergic inflammation in RBL-2H3 and Caco-2 cells. Inflammation Research, 59(10), 847-854.

Lehane, L., & Olley, J. (2000). Histamine fish poisoning revisited. International Journal of Food Microbiology, 58(1-2), 1-37.

Leiper, J. B. (2015). Fate of ingested fluids: Factors affecting gastric emptying and intestinal absorption of beverages in humans. Nutrition Reviews, 73(Suppl 2), 57-72.

Li, Y., Yao, J., Han, C., et al. (2016). Quercetin, inflammation and immunity. Nutrients, 8(3), 167.

Lonsdale, D. (2015). Thiamine and magnesium deficiencies: Keys to disease. Medical Hypotheses, 115, 13-17.

Maintz, L., & Novak, N. (2007). Histamine and histamine intolerance. American Journal of Clinical Nutrition, 85(5), 1185-1196.

Malfait, F., Francomano, C., Byers, P., et al. (2017). The 2017 international classification of the Ehlers-Danlos syndromes. American Journal of Medical Genetics Part C, 175(1), 8-26.

Marco, M. L., Heeney, D., Binda, S., et al. (2017). Health benefits of fermented foods: Microbiota and beyond. Current Opinion in Biotechnology, 44, 94–102.

Mast Cell Action. (2024). Diet and MCAS.

McGee, H. (2004). On food and cooking: The science and lore of the kitchen (Rev. ed.). Scribner.

McRorie, J. W., Kirby, J. A., & Miner, P. B. (2014). Histamine2-receptor antagonists: Rapid development of tachyphylaxis with repeat dosing. World Journal of Gastrointestinal Pharmacology and Therapeutics, 5(2), 57-62.

Mehdirad, A., Holmberg, M. J., & Engstrom, J. (2019). Water ingestion in postural orthostatic tachycardia syndrome: A feasible treatment option? Cureus, 11(11), e6237.

Mehler, P. S., & Brown, C. (2015). Anorexia nervosa: Medical complications. Journal of Eating Disorders, 3, 11.

Mehr, S. E., Barbul, A., & Shibao, C. A. (2018). Gastrointestinal symptoms in postural tachycardia syndrome: A systematic review. Clinical Autonomic Research, 28(4), 411–421.

Mehr, S. E., Engel, B. T., & Engel, S. E. (2018). The effects of carbohydrate loading on autonomic function in postural tachycardia syndrome. Autonomic Neuroscience, 215, 72-77.

Mehr, S. E., Engelbrecht, S., Engelbrecht, V., & Hilz, M. J. (2018). Postprandial symptoms and gastric function in postural tachycardia syndrome. Clinical Autonomic Research, 28(5), 489-499.

Melander, A., Danielson, K., Schersten, B., & Wahlin, E. (1977). Enhancement of the bioavailability of propranolol and metoprolol by food. Clinical Pharmacology & Therapeutics, 22(1), 108-112.

Melina, V., Craig, W., & Levin, S. (2016). Position of the Academy of Nutrition and Dietetics: Vegetarian diets. Journal of the Academy of Nutrition and Dietetics, 116(12), 1970-1980.

Miller, J. L. (2013). Iron deficiency anemia: A common and curable disease. Cold Spring Harbor Perspectives in Medicine, 3(7), a011866.

Mitchell, T., Kumar, P., Reddy, T., et al. (2019). Dietary oxalate and kidney stone formation. American Journal of Physiology-Renal Physiology, 316(3), F409-F413.

Mlcek, J., Jurikova, T., Skrovankova, S., & Sochor, J. (2016). Quercetin and its anti-allergic immune response. Molecules, 21(5), 623.

Molderings, G. J., Brettner, S., Homann, J., & Afrin, L. B. (2011). Mast cell activation disease: A concise practical guide for diagnostic workup and therapeutic options. Journal of Hematology & Oncology, 4, 10.

Monash University. (2023). FODMAP diet.

Mori, F., Barni, S., Liccioli, G., & Novembre, E. (2020). Oral cromolyn sodium for the treatment of gastrointestinal symptoms due to food allergy in children. Frontiers in Pediatrics, 8, 173.

Mouslmani, M. A. L., Sawano, M., Arun, A. S., et al. (2025). Characterization of postural orthostatic tachycardia syndrome in long COVID: Self-reported data from the LISTEN study. JACC: Advances, 4(8), 101873.

Muñoz, L. A., Cobos, A., Diaz, O., & Aguilera, J. M. (2012). Chia seeds: Microstructure, mucilage extraction and hydration. Journal of Food Engineering, 108(1), 216-224.

National Institutes of Health. (2021). Calcium: Fact sheet for health professionals. Office of Dietary Supplements.

Nieman, D. C., Cayea, E. J., Austin, M. D., et al. (2009). Chia seed does not promote weight loss or alter disease risk factors in overweight adults. Nutrition Research, 29(6), 414-418.

Nikkhah Bodagh, M., Maleki, I., & Hekmatdoost, A. (2019). Ginger in gastrointestinal disorders: A systematic review of clinical trials. Food Science & Nutrition, 7(1), 96-108.

Oe, M., Sakai, S., Yoshida, H., et al. (2016). Oral hyaluronan relieves wrinkles: A double-blinded, placebo-controlled study over a 12-week period. Clinical, Cosmetic and Investigational Dermatology, 10, 267-273.

Oner, T., Guven, B., Tavli, V., Mese, T., Yilmazer, M. M., & Demirpence, S. (2014). Postural orthostatic tachycardia syndrome (POTS) and vitamin B12 deficiency in adolescents. Pediatrics, 133(1), e138-e142.

Padayatty, S. J., & Levine, M. (2016). Vitamin C: The known and the unknown and Goldilocks. Oral Diseases, 22(6), 463-493.

Palmer, B. F., & Clegg, D. J. (2016). Physiology and pathophysiology of potassium homeostasis: Core curriculum 2019. American Journal of Kidney Diseases, 74(5), 682-695.

Papagiannopoulos, M., Wollseifen, H. R., Mellenthin, A., Haber, B., & Galensa, R. (2004). Identification and quantification of polyphenols in carob fruits (Ceratonia siliqua L.) and derived products by HPLC-UV-ESI/MSn. Journal of Agricultural and Food Chemistry, 52(12), 3784-3791.

Patel, T. B., Patel, L. D., & Patel, J. K. (2020). Histamine-producing and histamine-degrading bacteria: Implications for human health and disease. International Journal of Environmental Research and Public Health, 17(10), 3518.

Penny, H. A., Aziz, I., Ferber, M., et al. (2016). Is there a relationship between gluten sensitivity and postural tachycardia syndrome? European Journal of Gastroenterology & Hepatology, 28(12), 1383–1387.

Peterkofsky, B. (1991). Ascorbate requirement for hydroxylation and secretion of procollagen: Relationship to inhibition of collagen synthesis in scurvy. American Journal of Clinical Nutrition, 54(6), 1135S-1140S.

Pianosi, P. T., Schroeder, D. R., & Fischer, P. R. (2016). Cardiac responses to exercise distinguish postural tachycardia syndrome variants. Physiological Reports, 4(22), e13040.

Pimentel, M., Saad, R. J., Long, M. D., & Rao, S. S. C. (2020). ACG clinical guideline: Small intestinal bacterial overgrowth. American Journal of Gastroenterology, 115(2), 165-178.

PoTS UK. (2023). Diet and fluids.

Prochaska, J. O., & DiClemente, C. C. (1983). Stages and processes of self-change of smoking: Toward an integrative model of change. Journal of Consulting and Clinical Psychology, 51(3), 390-395.

Raithel, M., Baenkler, H. W., Naegel, A., et al. (2005). Significance of salicylate intolerance in diseases of the lower gastrointestinal tract. Journal of Physiology and Pharmacology, 56(Suppl 5), 89-102.

Raj, S. R. (2013). Postural tachycardia syndrome (POTS). Circulation, 127(23), 2336-2342.

Raj, S. R., Guzman, J. C., Harvey, P., et al. (2020). Canadian Cardiovascular Society position statement on postural orthostatic tachycardia syndrome (POTS) and related disorders of chronic orthostatic intolerance. Canadian Journal of Cardiology, 36(3), 357-372.

Rao, S. S. C. (2004). Oral rehydration therapy: New explanations for an old remedy. Annual Review of Medicine, 55, 97-113.

Rao, S. S. C., & Bhatt, T. (2021). Evaluation and management of nausea and vomiting of gastroparesis. Gastroenterology Clinics of North America, 50(1), 173-188.

Reese, I., Ballmer-Weber, B., Beyer, K., et al. (2017). German guideline for the management of adverse reactions to ingested histamine. Allergo Journal International, 26(5), 159-184.

Rowe, P. C., Barron, D. F., Calkins, H., et al. (1999). Orthostatic intolerance and chronic fatigue syndrome associated with Ehlers-Danlos syndrome. The Journal of Pediatrics, 135(4), 494–499.

Ruzieh, M., Baugh, A., Engell, C., et al. (2017). Effects of intermittent intravenous saline infusions in patients with medication-refractory postural tachycardia syndrome. Journal of Interventional Cardiac Electrophysiology, 48(3), 255-260.

Sato, K., Shigemura, Y., & Iwai, K. (2017). Food-derived collagen peptides, their biological activities and potential for use as functional food ingredients. Current Pharmaceutical Design, 23(20), 3028-3035.

Sawka, M. N., Burke, L. M., Eichner, E. R., et al. (2007). American College of Sports Medicine position stand: Exercise and fluid replacement. Medicine & Science in Sports & Exercise, 39(2), 377-390.

Schnedl, W. J., & Enko, D. (2021). Histamine intolerance originates in the gut. Nutrients, 13(4), 1262.

Schnedl, W. J., Schenk, M., Lackner, S., Enko, D., Mangge, H., & Forber, F. (2019). Diamine oxidase supplementation improves symptoms in patients with histamine intolerance. Food Science and Biotechnology, 28(3), 895-902.

Schwalfenberg, G. K., & Genuis, S. J. (2017). The importance of magnesium in clinical healthcare. Scientifica, 2017, 4179326.

Schwingshackl, L., & Hoffmann, G. (2014). Mediterranean dietary pattern, inflammation and endothelial function: A systematic review and meta-analysis of intervention trials. Nutrition, Metabolism and Cardiovascular Diseases, 24(9), 929-939.

Seneviratne, S. L., Maitland, A., & Afrin, L. (2017). Mast cell disorders in Ehlers-Danlos syndrome. American Journal of Medical Genetics Part C, 175(1), 226–236.

Shaw, B. H., Stiles, L. E., Bourne, K., et al. (2019). The face of postural tachycardia syndrome: A cross-sectional community-based survey. Heart Rhythm, 16(4), 574-580.

Sheldon, R. S., Grubb, B. P., Olshansky, B., et al. (2015). 2015 Heart Rhythm Society expert consensus statement on the diagnosis and treatment of postural tachycardia syndrome, inappropriate sinus tachycardia, and vasovagal syncope. Heart Rhythm, 12(6), e41-e63.

Shepherd, S. J., Halmos, E. P., Glance, S., & Almeshari, W. (2019). The role of a low-FODMAP diet in functional dyspepsia. Expert Review of Gastroenterology & Hepatology, 13(12), 1117-1124.

Shibao, C., Gamboa, A., Diedrich, A., et al. (2005). Acarbose, an alpha-glucosidase inhibitor, attenuates postprandial hypotension in autonomic failure. Hypertension, 46(5), 1002-1006.

Shirreffs, S. M., Armstrong, L. E., & Cheuvront, S. N. (2004). Fluid and electrolyte needs for preparation and recovery from training and competition. Journal of Sports Sciences, 22(1), 57-63.

Shoaib, M., Shehzad, A., Omar, M., et al. (2016). Inulin: Properties, health benefits and food applications. Carbohydrate Polymers, 147, 444-454.

Shoba, G., Joy, D., Joseph, T., Majeed, M., Rajendran, R., & Srinivas, P. S. S. R. (1998). Influence of piperine on the pharmacokinetics of curcumin in animals and human volunteers. Planta Medica, 64(4), 353-356.

Shorr, R. I., Ray, W. A., Daugherty, J. R., & Griffin, M. R. (1997). Antihypertensives and the risk of serious hypoglycemia in older persons using insulin or sulfonylureas. JAMA, 278(1), 40-43.

Simmonds, J. V., Herbland, A., Hakim, A., Ninis, N., Lever, W., & Aziz, Q. (2017). Exercise beliefs and behaviours of individuals with joint hypermobility syndrome/Ehlers-Danlos syndrome, hypermobility type. Disability and Rehabilitation, 41(4), 445-455.

Simons, F. E. R., & Simons, K. J. (2011). Histamine and H1-antihistamines: Celebrating a century of progress. Journal of Allergy and Clinical Immunology, 128(6), 1139-1150.

Slutsky, I., Abumaria, N., Wu, L. J., et al. (2010). Enhancement of learning and memory by elevating brain magnesium. Neuron, 65(2), 165-177.

Snapper, H., & Cheshire, W. P. (2022). Oral and intravenous hydration in the treatment of orthostatic hypotension and postural tachycardia syndrome. Autonomic Neuroscience, 238, 102951.

Srivastava, J. K., Shankar, E., & Gupta, S. (2010). Chamomile: A herbal medicine of the past with a bright future. Molecular Medicine Reports, 3(6), 895-901.

Staudacher, H. M., Lomer, M. C. E., Farquharson, F. M., et al. (2017). A diet low in FODMAPs reduces symptoms in patients with irritable bowel syndrome and a probiotic restores Bifidobacterium species: A randomized controlled trial. Gastroenterology, 153(4), 936-947.

Steiner, L., Bodensteiner, A., & Johnson, N. R. (2023). Gastrointestinal manifestations of hypermobile Ehlers-Danlos syndrome and dietary approaches related to their management. Journal of Orthopedic Research and Therapy, 8, 1313.

Stewart, T. M., Williamson, D. A., & White, M. A. (2002). Rigid vs. flexible dieting: Association with eating disorder symptoms in nonobese women. Appetite, 38(1), 39-44.

Stoffel, N. U., Cercamondi, C. I., Brittenham, G., et al. (2017). Iron absorption from oral iron supplements given on consecutive versus alternate days and as single morning doses versus twice-daily split doses in iron-depleted women: Two open-label, randomised controlled trials. Lancet Haematology, 4(11), e524-e533.

Sánchez-Pérez, S., Comas-Basté, O., Duelo, A., et al. (2022). The identification of biogenic amines in the products of lactic acid bacteria: A review. Foods, 11(16), 2539.

Sánchez-Pérez, S., Comas-Basté, O., Rabell-González, J., Veciana-Nogués, M. T., Latorre-Moratalla, M. L., & Vidal-Carou, M. C. (2018). Biogenic amines in plant-origin foods: Are they frequently underestimated in low-histamine diets? Foods, 7(12), 205.

Tai, F. W. D., Palsson, O. S., Lam, C. Y., et al. (2020). Functional gastrointestinal disorders are increased in joint hypermobility-related disorders with concomitant postural orthostatic tachycardia syndrome. Neurogastroenterology & Motility, 32(12), e13975.

Tani, H., Singer, W., McPhee, B. R., et al. (2000). Splanchnic-mesenteric capacitance bed in the postural tachycardia syndrome (POTS). Autonomic Neuroscience, 86(1-2), 107-113.

Tarnopolsky, M. A. (2008). The mitochondrial cocktail: Rationale for combined nutraceutical therapy in mitochondrial cytopathies. Advanced Drug Delivery Reviews, 60(13-14), 1561-1567.

Taylor, S. L. (1986). Histamine food poisoning: Toxicology and clinical aspects. Critical Reviews in Toxicology, 17(2), 91-128.

Thacher, T. D., & Clarke, B. L. (2011). Vitamin D insufficiency. Mayo Clinic Proceedings, 86(1), 50-60.

The Mast Cell Disease Society. (2022). Nutrition.

Theoharides, T. C., & Cochrane, D. E. (2004). Critical role of mast cells in inflammatory diseases and the effect of acute stress. Journal of Neuroimmunology, 146(1-2), 1-12.

Theoharides, T. C., Asadi, S., & Patel, A. B. (2012). Focal brain inflammation and autism. Journal of Neuroinflammation, 10, 46.

Theoharides, T. C., Tsilioni, I., & Ren, H. (2019). Recent advances in our understanding of mast cell activation or should it be mast cell mediator disorders? Expert Review of Clinical Immunology, 15(6), 639-656.

Thimmulappa, R. K., Mai, K. H., Srisuma, S., Kensler, T. W., Yamamoto, M., & Biswal, S. (2002). Identification of Nrf2-regulated genes induced by the chemopreventive agent sulforaphane by oligonucleotide microarray. Cancer Research, 62(18), 5196-5203.

Thollon, C., & Bhatt, D. L. (2013). Ivabradine: A selective and specific If channel inhibitor. Cardiovascular Therapeutics, 32(3), 101-110.

Thwaites, P. A., Gibson, P. R., & Burgell, R. E. (2022). Hypermobile Ehlers-Danlos syndrome and disorders of the gastrointestinal tract: What the gastroenterologist needs to know. Journal of Gastroenterology and Hepatology, 37(9), 1693-1709.

Tinkle, B., Castori, M., Berglund, B., et al. (2017). Hypermobile Ehlers-Danlos syndrome: Clinical description and natural history. American Journal of Medical Genetics Part C, 175(1), 48–69.

Topan, R., Pandya, S., Williams, S., et al. (2024). Comprehensive assessment of nutrition and dietary influences in hypermobile Ehlers-Danlos syndrome: A cross-sectional study. American Journal of Gastroenterology, 119(4), 727-738.

Tosh, S. M. (2013). Review of human studies investigating the post-prandial blood-glucose lowering ability of oat and barley food products. European Journal of Clinical Nutrition, 67(4), 310-317.

Tripkovic, L., Lambert, H., Hart, K., et al. (2012). Comparison of vitamin D2 and vitamin D3 supplementation in raising serum 25-hydroxyvitamin D status: A systematic review and meta-analysis. American Journal of Clinical Nutrition, 95(6), 1357-1364.

Tseng, A. S., Heidari, B., Engel, D., et al. (2021). Nutritional concerns in pediatric patients with postural orthostatic tachycardia syndrome. Journal of Pediatric Gastroenterology and Nutrition, 73(2), 201-206.

Tseng, A. S., Shen, W. K., & DiBaise, J. K. (2021). Nutritional implications of patients with dysautonomia and hypermobility syndromes. Current Nutrition Reports, 10(4), 328-338.

Tversky, A., & Kahneman, D. (1973). Availability: A heuristic for judging frequency and probability. Cognitive Psychology, 5(2), 207-232.

U.S. Department of Agriculture & U.S. Department of Health and Human Services. (2020). Dietary guidelines for Americans, 2020-2025 (9th ed.).

U.S. Department of Agriculture. (2023). Danger zone. Food Safety and Inspection Service.

U.S. Department of Agriculture. (2023). FoodData Central.

U.S. Department of Agriculture. (2023). Freezing and food safety. Food Safety and Inspection Service.

U.S. Department of Agriculture. (2023). Safe minimum internal temperatures. Food Safety and Inspection Service.

U.S. Food and Drug Administration. (2022). Dietary Supplement Health and Education Act of 1994.

U.S. Food and Drug Administration. (2023). CFR - Code of Federal Regulations Title 21: Natural flavoring substances and natural substances used in conjunction with flavors.

U.S. National Library of Medicine. (2023). DailyMed: Ivabradine.

USDA Agricultural Research Service. (2016). Fluid intake from beverages: National Health and Nutrition Examination Survey, 2015-2016.

Valdes, A. M., Walter, J., Segal, E., & Spector, T. D. (2018). Role of the gut microbiota in nutrition and health. BMJ, 361, k2179.

Valent, P., Akin, C., Bonadonna, P., et al. (2019). Proposed diagnostic algorithm for patients with suspected mast cell activation syndrome. Journal of Allergy and Clinical Immunology: In Practice, 7(4), 1125-1133.

Vally, H., & Misso, N. L. A. (2012). Adverse reactions to the sulphite additives. Gastroenterology and Hepatology from Bed to Bench, 5(1), 16-23.

Varney, J., Barrett, J., Scarlata, K., Catsos, P., Gibson, P. R., & Muir, J. G. (2017). FODMAPs: Food composition, defining cutoff values and international application. Journal of Gastroenterology and Hepatology, 32(Suppl 1), 53-61.

Vega-Gálvez, A., Miranda, M., Vergara, J., Uribe, E., Puente, L., & Martínez, E. A. (2010). Nutrition facts and functional potential of quinoa. Journal of the Science of Food and Agriculture, 90(15), 2541-2547.

Vernino, S., Bourne, K. M., Stiles, L. E., et al. (2021). Postural orthostatic tachycardia syndrome (POTS): State of the science and clinical care from a 2019 National Institutes of Health Expert Consensus Meeting. Autonomic Neuroscience, 235, 102828.

Vlieg-Boerstra, B. J., van der Heide, S., Oude Elberink, J. N. G., Kluin-Nelemans, J. C., & Dubois, A. E. J. (2005). Mastocytosis and adverse reactions to biogenic amines and histamine-releasing foods: What is the evidence? Netherlands Journal of Medicine, 63(7), 244-249.

Vojdani, A., & Vojdani, C. (2015). Immune reactivity to food coloring. Alternative Therapies in Health and Medicine, 21(Suppl 1), 52-62.

Volpe, R., Okrent, A., & Leibtag, E. (2013). The effect of supercenter-format stores on the healthfulness of consumers' grocery purchases. American Journal of Agricultural Economics, 95(3), 568-589.

Weinstock, L. B., Brook, J. B., Walters, A. S., Goris, A., Afrin, L. B., & Molderings, G. J. (2021). Mast cell activation symptoms are prevalent in Long-COVID. International Journal of Infectious Diseases, 112, 217-226.

Weng, Z., Zhang, B., Asadi, S., et al. (2012). Quercetin is more effective than cromolyn in blocking human mast cell cytokine release and inhibits contact dermatitis and photosensitivity in humans. PLoS ONE, 7(3), e33805.

World Health Organization. (2006). Oral rehydration salts: Production of the new ORS.

Wurtman, R. J., Wurtman, J. J., Regan, M. M., et al. (2003). Effects of normal meals rich in carbohydrates or proteins on plasma tryptophan and tyrosine ratios. American Journal of Clinical Nutrition, 77(1), 128-132.

Yang, Y. X., Lewis, J. D., Epstein, S., & Metz, D. C. (2006). Long-term proton pump inhibitor therapy and risk of hip fracture. JAMA, 296(24), 2947-2953.

Yong, J. W. H., Ge, L., Ng, Y. F., & Tan, S. N. (2009). The chemical composition and biological properties of coconut (Cocos nucifera L.) water. Molecules, 14(12), 5144-5164.

Younger, J., Parkitny, L., & McLain, D. (2014). The use of low-dose naltrexone (LDN) as a novel anti-inflammatory treatment for chronic pain. Clinical Rheumatology, 33(4), 451-459.

Zha, K., Brook, J., & Engstrom, J. (2022). Gluten-free diet in postural tachycardia syndrome: A pilot survey. Practical Neurology, 21(5), 62-65.

Zickgraf, H. F., & Ellis, J. M. (2018). Initial validation of the Nine Item Avoidant/Restrictive Food Intake Disorder screen (NIAS): A measure of three restrictive eating patterns. Appetite, 123, 32-42.

Zierau, O., Zenclussen, A. C., & Jensen, F. (2012). Role of female sex hormones, estradiol and progesterone, in mast cell behavior. Frontiers in Immunology, 3, 169.

Made in United States
Orlando, FL
04 November 2026

90201508R00177